Munchausen Syndrome  al Approach

ST BART

Munchausen Syndrome by Proxy Abuse:

A Practical Approach

Edited by

Mary Eminson MA MB ChB FRCPCH FRCPsych
Consultant Child and Adolescent Psychiatrist, Child and Family Services,
Royal Bolton Hospitals NHS Trust, UK

R. J. Postlethwaite MB ChB FRCP FRCPCH
Consultant Paediatric Nephrologist, Manchester Children's Hospital NHS
Trust, UK

A member of the Hodder Headline Group
LONDON • NEW YORK • NEW DELHI

First published in Great Britain in 2000 by Butterworth Heinemann.

This impression published in 2001 by
Arnold, a member of the Hodder Headline Group,
338 Euston Road, London NW1 3BH

http://www.arnoldpublishers.com

Distributed in the USA by
Oxford University Press Inc.,
198 Madison Avenue, New York, NY10016
Oxford is a registered trademark of Oxford University Press

Whilst the advice and information in this book are believed to be true and
accurate at the date of going to press, neither the authors nor the publisher
can accept any legal responsibility or liability for any errors or omissions
that may be made. In particular (but without limiting the generality of the
preceding disclaimer) every effort has been made to check drug dosages;
however, it is still possible that errors have been missed. Furthermore,
dosage schedules are constantly being revised and new side-effects
recognized. For these reasons the reader is strongly urged to consult the
drug companies' printed instructions before administering any of the drugs
recommended in this book.

British Library Cataloguing in Publication Data
A catalogue record for this book is available from the British Library

Library of Congress Cataloging-in-Publication Data
A catalog record for this book is available from the Library of Congress

ISBN 0 7506 4072 3

1 2 3 4 5 6 7 8 9 10

Printed and bound in India by Replika Press PVT Ltd

What do you think about this book? Or any other Arnold title?
Please send your comments to feedback.arnold@hodder.co.uk

Contents

I have striven not to laugh at human actions,
not to weep at them,
nor to hate them,
but to understand them.

Spinoza, 1632–1677
Tractatus Politicus, 1, iv

Acknowledgements

This book would not have been possible without the help of numerous people. Dr Peter Powell kindly provided detailed constructive comments on a number of chapters. Dr G. M. Addison made helpful suggestions about the sections on toxicology and Dr M. A. Lewis has contributed his considerable experience to some of the vignettes.

We are extremely grateful for the assistance of nursing staff from Central Manchester Healthcare NHS Trust, Manchester Children's Hospitals NHS Trust, Prescot Acute Hospitals NHS Trust, Rochdale Healthcare NHS Trust and Salford Community Healthcare NHS Trust. Contributions have also been received from nursing staff in colleges of nursing at the Faculty of Health, University of Central Lancashire; the School of Nursing, Midwifery and Health Visiting, the University of Manchester; and the University of Salford, Department of Nursing.

Mrs Jennifer Kelly the medical librarian at the Manchester Children's Hospitals NHS Trust has saved many hours by her efficient service in chasing up references and reprints.

Family and friends are always victims of a project such as this. Social activities have to be severely curtailed and we are grateful for both forbearance and great support whilst we have been engaged on this task.

The unsung heroes (more often heroines!) of any book are the secretaries. Mrs Amanda Jackson-Mallender has typed and re-typed versions of a number of chapters with good will and great accuracy and speed. Mrs Wendy Coupe has similarly produced and tidied up chapters, and undertaken other sub-editing tasks. We are very grateful for this invaluable assistance. The major load of the co-ordination of this book, however, has been assumed by Mrs Sue Marland. Previous experience has shown that anybody is foolish to embark on a project such as this without the support of a 'dedicated' co-ordinator. We are not sure if Sue really knew what she was letting herself in for, but we would not have started this book without her commitment and there is no way the task would have been completed without her indefatigable support.

The vignettes used throughout this book have been chosen to reflect real life clinical situations but are *not* case reports. They show some bias towards nephrological examples which reflects the specialism of one of the editors. We have altered important key elements to protect the privacy of families, but maintain the important psychological truths of the situations. It is possible that by manufacturing these examples we have inadvertently created similarities to other cases unknown to us.

Foreword

Know, one false step is ne'er retrieved,
And be with caution bold.
Not all that tempts your wandering eyes
And heedless hearts is lawful prize,
Nor all that glisters gold.

T. Gray, 1716–1771
Ode on the death of a favourite cat drowned in a tub of goldfishes

Medical practitioners are used to the fact that the information offered to them by their patients might be inaccurate, incomplete or irrelevant, and sometimes exaggerated, distorted or seriously understated. Their job always includes not being misled by such presentations. The importance of not being misled is relatively recent. Nowadays effective intervention might be possible in many of the sicknesses caused by disease. Diagnosis really matters but this step is still based on information. This new effectiveness of medicine in treating those sicknesses that are due to diseases has highlighted the contrast with those that are not. These latter sicknesses raise serious legal, moral and philosophical issues.

In the last century, and in the past fifty years in particular, we have had to learn that we can be systematically misled, in several different ways, about the true nature and purpose of the consultation in which we are engaged. We have had to come to terms with the fact that the implicit trust expected on either side of a medical engagement might very well be misplaced. The commonest coinage on the patient's side has been lying for gain. Seeking remission of work is probably the longest established practice in this regard. The term 'malinger' dates from 1820 when it would be relevant to attempts at removal from military duties or the work this entailed. It combines the French *malin* ('wicked') with *malingre* ('sickly'). DSM-IV still interprets it as 'intentional' and for gain. Fraudulent claims to sickness benefits arose as soon as they became available (consider A. J. Cronin's *The Citadel*, 1973). Access to drug-induced sensation has also been sought, universally and by a variety of means, throughout history as an antidote to toil. Later it was sought to relieve ennui and pain of mind. Access to such drugs is only institutionalized in medicine. Doctors are just convenient potential providers, combining ready with ostensibly guiltless availability.

Then there are the many variations on assuming a sick role where the conceit is that it is somehow 'unconscious' or at least unintended. The hysterias have always existed. We more recently realized that some complex and recurrent presentations of sickness were so flagrant, so cleverly dissembled, so well rehearsed, as to suggest that they were purposive. They were so persistent as to suggest an addictive element. Their locus in 'consciousness' seems uncertain. These gross parodies, which often threaten the life of the patient at their physician's hands, were given the alluring name Munchausen's syndrome. Perhaps it allowed open reference to the patient's sickness which would be opaque to them? The divertingly amusing fictional Baron would blush at his eponym. Perhaps, since the claim to be sick when not sick became another form of sickness, Kafka's syndrome might be preferred? Even so it has not escaped moral connotation and opprobrium any more than the other forms of sickness enactment referred to above.

The inescapable fact is that being sick in any way at all is a public performance. At issue is the potential threat it offers to others. The threats are of contagion, the effect on others of loss of role performance by the sick person, and potential loss of life. Presentation to a physician also threatens the physician's capacity to perform appropriately. It is a physician's natural preference to give credence to the information offered and act as if this characterized a possible disease. When this tactic fails, as it must in the situations outlined above, an entirely new situation arises. This new situation is outside medical bioscience and can confuse health care professionals whose orientation is primarily within the constructs of bioscientific medicine.

Children can be involved in most of these anomalous presentations of sickness. Since children are not autonomous their involvement has to be regarded as being at the behest or the instigation of others. The involvement of children is to their detriment. When doctors become aware of such a situation child protection becomes an issue. Some of the most recently described child protection issues are addressed in this book.

The Editors, in their 1992 paper 'Factitious illness: recognition and management' (which is cited several times within this book) made a great conceptual leap forward when they showed that parents' concerns for their children's health could be seen to be dimensional, ranging from severe neglect to gross over-concern. The value of accepting the notion of a dimension is that it reveals satisfactorily the great variety of modes of presentation of children when they are sick. That is entirely in line with my first statement in this foreword. What might be considered is whether the gross abuses of health issues seen under the rubric of Munchausen by proxy or factitious illness are within that dimension of concern. Might they not be alien to anything belonging to that dimension, requiring us to discover individual reasons for the actions of those who hurt their children by misrepresenting their state of health? It is for this reason that we should look outside bioscience (as, by definition, the child is not ill or diseased) and into the biography of those caught up in this fiction. The truth is discoverable only in terms of an account of the fabric of the lives of the participants. The participants, in my view, include the professionals who have been caught up (or out) in the fiction. Some doctors have spent hours of concerned care for years, and sleepless, anxious nights only to find that they were being duped. Their responses of outrage and frustration at the deception that has been practised on them can lead to revengeful feelings.

In a real sense what the doctors have to report is a crime against the person. The matter could be dealt with entirely by a process of criminal investigation. What makes us pause? First, we know that we have been engaged by parents in problem solving and have hitherto failed to solve the problem. Second, once considered from the point of view of psychopathology, it will be strikingly obvious that there is deviance and it is our inclination to try and understand the type of mind-set that might have given rise to such dishonesty. It is our tendency to see the events as another sort of sickness. Doctors do not react in this way when they come upon crimes against the person in the emergency room. In the case of factitious illness, as this book will show, the law can be used to further the therapeutic ambitions of those who deal with the results of this type of abuse of trust. The fact of the matter is that the parental psychopathology, when seen as sick, is often irremediable. Motivation is, however, diverse and the purpose to hurt *per se* rare. The behaviour is best seen as a stifled scream for help. The hurt is, however, so severe it must not be shared. The raising of children is fraught for the best of us. For most of us our Achilles heel remains undisclosed.

The book also gives an account of the various situations in which abuse of trust through perversion of health care arises. The history of medicine reminds doctors that they need not feel too self-righteous about abuse through the vehicle of health care. Faced by situations that frustrated their therapeutic ambitions they, in the past, descended to barbarity. By such a book as this, the field of medicine responds compassionately to an issue that is forced upon it but which, in several important ways, does not really belong to it. 'All that glisters...'

David C. Taylor
Emeritus Professor of Child and Adolescent Psychiatry
University of Manchester

Contributors

Eileen Baildam MB, ChB, FRCP, DCH, MRCGP, FRCPCH
Consultant Paediatrician, Manchester Children's Hospitals NHS Trust,
Manchester, UK

Christopher Bools MB, ChB, M(Med)Sc, MRCPsych, MRCPCH
Consultant in Child and Adolescent Psychiatry with special interest in paediatric liaison work, Royal United Hospital, Bath, UK

Gerry Byrne BA
Clinical Nurse Specialist, Park Hospital for Children, Oxford, UK

Lesley-Anne Cull BA
Barrister at Law and Open University Lecturer, Milton Keynes, UK

Mary Eminson MA, MB, ChB, FRCPCH, FRCPsych
Consultant Child and Adolescent Psychiatrist, Child and Family Services,
Bolton Hospitals NHS Trust, Bolton, UK

Jonathan Green MA, MB, BS, MRCPsych, DCH
Senior Lecturer in Child Psychiatry, Department of Child and Family
Psychiatry, Booth Hall Children's Hospital, Manchester Children's Hospitals
NHS Trust, Manchester, UK

David P. H. Jones MB, ChB, FRCPsych, DCH
Consultant Child and Family Psychiatrist and Honorary Senior Lecturer,
University of Oxford, Park Hospital for Children, Oxford, UK

Hilary Lloyd MB, ChB, MRCPsych
Consultant Child and Adolescent Psychiatrist, Department of Child and
Adolescent Psychiatry, Manchester Children's Hospitals NHS Trust,
Manchester, UK

Anne MacDonald RGN, RSCN, Dip N(Lon)
Independent Paediatric Nursing Consultant, Lymm, Cheshire, UK

Vera Mayer BA, MSc Child Development (Lon)
Practising Barrister

Caroline Newbould BA, CQSW
Senior Social Work Practitioner, Park Hospital for Children, Oxford, UK

Richard Newton MD, FRCPCH
Consultant Paediatric Neurologist, Department of Neurology, Manchester
Children's Hospitals NHS Trust, Manchester, UK

Dymphna Pearce BSc (Hons) Soc, Dip App Soc Studies, CQSW
Member of the Bucks and Oxon Panels of Guardians ad litem and Reporting
Officers

R. J. Postlethwaite MB, ChB, FRCP FRCPCH
Consultant Paediatric Nephrologist, Manchester Children's Hospitals NHS
Trust, Manchester, UK

Martin Samuels BSc, MD, FRCP, FRCPCH
Consultant Paediatrician, North Staffordshire Hospital, Stoke-on-Trent, UK

Hilary Smith MB, ChB, FRCP, FRCPCH
Consultant Paediatrician, Manchester Children's Hospitals NHS Trust
Manchester,UK

Ian Tofler MB, BS
Chairman to the Sports Psychiatry Committee of the American Academy of
Child and Adolescent Psychiatry, affiliated to Children's Hospital, Los Angeles,
USA

1

Munchausen syndrome by proxy abuse – an introduction

Mary Eminson

Introduction

The aim of this book is to help those who work with children, particularly those whose primary concern is children's physical health, to recognize, to understand and, if possible, to prevent Munchausen syndrome by proxy (MSBP) abuse. This headline title, first used in 1977 by Meadow, encompasses many different situations in which children are presented as 'sick'. They have in common the fact that a child's illness is not due to a disease or an openly acknowledged external cause such as an accident. Instead, the child's illness has arisen as a result of the parent's actions in producing a factitious illness: by making the child ill by suffocating, poisoning or physically harming the child to produce sickness (induced illness), or by the adult telling a story of symptoms which leads health professionals to believe the child has an illness. The professional then investigates and treats the child's supposed condition (invented illness). In the second case, the professional harms the child on the parent's behalf. Both of these scenarios may constitute Munchausen syndrome by proxy abuse for the purposes of this volume, as both result in unnecessary and preventable harm to children, enacted through the health care system.

This initial chapter outlines the area with which we are concerned, followed by a brief history of the awareness of this form of abuse, a description of the terminology used here and the provision of a framework both for the book and for use clinically. The final section of this introductory chapter is devoted specifically to the role of primary care professionals at all stages of MSBP abuse assessment and management. In the book as a whole our aim has been to integrate an understanding and awareness of MSBP abuse into the ordinary practice of doctors, nurses and other health and social work professionals. To do so we have drawn upon the experience of paediatricians, child psychiatrists, nursing, legal and social work professionals, practitioners who continue to work with many types of illness and family, and who have a special interest in the area of MSBP abuse.

The ingredients of MSBP abuse

To start at the most basic level, three ingredients are required for Munchausen syndrome by proxy abuse. These may be summarized as:

1 A health care system in which doctors, nurses and other health care personnel have almost unlimited capacity in terms of resources and technology to undertake investigations and interventions with children.
2 A dependent child is available for a parent (or person *in loco parentis*) and is under her or his control, influence or behest.
3 A parent, or person *in loco parentis*, presents the child to the health care system with invented symptoms or fabricated signs.

For practical purposes, this triad provides the boundary within which MSBP abuse takes place and defines this book's focus. In the next chapter, the background factors involved in each component of the triad and their interactions are explored, but before turning to this the background to our current understanding is examined.

The history of recognition of Munchausen syndrome by proxy abuse

In the mind of the British public the term 'Munchausen syndrome by proxy' is irrevocably linked to Beverley Allitt, the paediatric nurse convicted in 1993 of murdering children under her care. An immature young woman with a personality disorder and a history of major somatization herself (i.e. severe handicapping somatic complaints without evidence of organic disease: probably Munchausen syndrome), she appears to have been attracted to the role of nursing (and harming) children as a way of resolving her own substantial interpersonal difficulties. It is surmised that this was partly for the attention the role gave her as the centre of rescue attempts after she had endangered the children, partly for the gratitude of the victims' families to whom she became close, and also for the sheer power over life and death her actions involved. She was often said to be suffering from MSBP despite not being the children's mother or guardian. The confusion, which arises essentially from the mistaken view that a particular behaviour can constitute a 'disease' with the diagnostic label of a medical condition, has set back clear thinking but has also brought a lot of public attention to a topic which was previously largely the province of health professionals.

Historically, two major strands lead to the current position where MSBP abuse is sufficiently severe yet common enough a problem to merit its first international research conference sponsored by the USA's National Institutes of Mental Health (held in Stockholm in 1998). The first strand historically is the 'psychiatric' one, of which a major landmark was Asher's paper in the *Lancet* (Asher, 1951) using the term 'Munchausen syndrome' to describe a persistent pattern seen in adults, of presentation to health services with factitious somatic complaints. The patients in this original paper were extremely persistent in their demands, often persuasive and readily exploited the goodwill of nurses and doctors. They used their own bodies as collateral in their search for operations and care (and injectable painkillers sometimes), and are readily identified as having disturbed personalities. By using the eponymous title, Asher brought such patients to a new prominence, although by using a jokey title for the 'syndrome' – the name of a hazy, foreign, fantastic tale-telling character, drawn to deceit – Asher obscured the 'dreadful import of the situation' (Taylor, 1992). The risks the patients took with themselves and the flagrant abuse of trust and the resources of the health service are somewhat glossed over.

The second strand was the identification by paediatricians of perverse parental behaviour in medical settings and the recognition of the implications for child protection. Early papers on factitious presentations of children to doctors are clearly making links intellectually with the contemporary terminology of physical abuse, beginning in the 1960s with a literature on non-accidental poisoning. Pickering (1964) described three cases of salicylate poisoning in which the parents denied administration and in 1968 he described this as 'a manifestation of the battered child syndrome'. Dine (1976) published a single case report entitled 'Tranquillizer poisoning: an example of child abuse'. Rogers *et al.* (1976) produced a systematic review of six cases of non-accidental poisoning, calling this form of abuse 'an extended syndrome of child abuse'. In the 1970s a wider recognition of the different forms of paediatric presentations began, and by 1977 in a seminal paper 'Munchausen syndrome by proxy: the hinterland of child abuse', Meadow brought together the psychiatric and paediatric terminology and introduced the term 'Munchausen syndrome by proxy' into the clinical vernacular.

Burman and Stevens (1977), two weeks after Meadow's paper, reported a family in whom the mother had exhibited features of Munchausen syndrome herself. One of the children was treated for diabetes and the other had 'bizarre neurological symptoms', eventually found to be due to promethazine poisoning. Both diseases disappeared after separation from the mother. It was suggested that 'Polle syndrome' might be an appropriate term. Polle was the son of Baron Munchausen and his second wife Berhardine Brun, and died at the age of one year. The initial debate about 'Polle syndrome' or 'Munchausen syndrome by proxy', and the fact that some of the mothers in Meadow's initial report showed abnormal illness behaviour on their own account, strengthened the link with Munchausen syndrome. This, in turn, encouraged the use of medical and pseudo-medical terminology rather than integration within the social sciences in the canon of child abuse: again this tends to distance the more uncomfortable aspects of the abuse of children and of professionals.

Thus, by 1977 the various strands were woven together: the paediatric (and child protection) components, linked through non-accidental poisoning and recognition of physical and emotional abuse, and the psychiatric contribution, with recognition of the adult's abnormal illness behaviour and somatization disorders, whether for themselves or for their children. The linking element between adult somatizing patients and adults presenting children was both deception of professionals and 'pretend' somatic symptoms. This was faced more honestly in the title of a paper by Sigal, Gelkopf and Meadow in 1989: 'Munchausen by proxy syndrome: the triad of abuse, self-abuse, and deception'. Taylor (1992) has further clarified the relationships between 'ordinary illness behaviour', 'hysterias' and 'abuse from active, calculated, hands-on tampering'. He describes 'another group of sicknesses, straddling the two categories' of clearly induced illness and strongly maintained handicapping 'hysteria': he called this group 'outlandish factitious illness'. In that article many of the themes of this book are touched upon: the difficulty of acknowledging the harm caused and the disruption of the development of children, the failure of child protection systems, the involvement of doctors and the failure of parenting, which is central. This book attempts to explore more of these areas.

Since the 1970s the literature on MSBP abuse has followed a familiar pattern, beginning with case reports of different types of presentation in medical settings. Until recently these reports have continued, steadily and relentlessly, to increase in number, cataloguing the ways in which children's bodies are damaged. Perhaps something can be learned from this infinite variation in manifestations of cruelty, even if only the unlimited parental ability to dupe doctors. However, 'the plural of anecdote is not data', and this catalogue of the *results* of such duplicity has manifestly failed to increase understanding and awareness of the *processes* which have allowed its growth.

More recently this sequence has been followed by more systematic case series (Bools, Neale and Meadow, 1992; Gray and Bentovim, 1996; Southall *et al.*, 1997) which started to appear in the 1990s. This decade has seen the development of much greater theorizing about this abuse, largely expressed in books which are devoted specifically to this subject (Schreier and Libow, 1993; Day and Parnall, 1998; Levin and Sheridan, 1995; Horwath and Lawson, 1995) of which more are planned. There has been increasing recognition of the problem within the international medical literature and, finally, there has been popularization, with TV programmes and books written for an audience outside the scientific community. This progression is described in detail by Brown and Feldman (1999) who have reviewed the international literature from both a historical and developmental perspective. Contributions made by professionals from both a child health and a mental health perspective are a feature of the literature in this area, (e.g. Bools, Neale and Meadow, 1992; Donald and Jureidini, 1996; Eminson and Postlethwaite, 1992; Fisher and Mitchell, 1995). As in many areas of child abuse, research driven by theoretical hypotheses remains virtually non-existent. The hope of the recent NIMH conference is that the time for this has now arrived and with this must come a new level of clarity about terms and concepts.

Terminology

The language of this area is very confused. In this book we have attempted to be both clear and consistent. Throughout the book we refer to Munchausen syndrome by proxy abuse or MSBP abuse as a shorthand term synonymous with harm to children resulting from factitious illness, which includes that induced or fabricated directly by parents or invented by means of false stories or specimens. We acknowledge that 'factitious illness by proxy' (Bools, 1996) is a more accurate term to describe the same area, but have retained the MSBP title because of its overwhelming popularity and hence superiority as a way of communicating with other professionals.

We use the term Munchausen syndrome by proxy *abuse* to signify that children are harmed as a result of the fabrications. We take it as axiomatic that the pattern of inventing or inducing illness, in the broadest sense, is abusive to the children who are its victims, although judgement concerning the severity of the harm can, on occasions, be difficult. There is a wide spectrum of harm and it is not axiomatic that the 'significant harm' necessary for Children Act (1989) procedures is either invariably reached or easy to judge. The most cursory glance at this issue makes it obvious that we are describing a range of behaviours which vary in terms of how common they are and how harmful they are to the child. Identification of the harm caused by fabrications and good scientific evidence about the psychological impact of many of the behaviours on children's physical and emotional well-being are areas ripe for research, difficult though this may be.

We describe those who are responsible for this abuse, by their direct or indirect actions, as *perpetrators*, consistent with the child protection terminology. We do not find it helpful to describe the perpetrators as suffering from Munchausen syndrome by proxy or factitious disorder by proxy, or accurate to consider the behaviour of the perpetrators as a form of disease, warranting a unique diagnostic label under a psychiatric categorization, any more than the behaviour of those who carry out 'ordinary' child abuse would. These issues are discussed in more detail in the next chapter, but in summary, our experience suggests that detailed studies of adults who demonstrate these behaviour patterns, involving children as the subjects and victims of their abnormal illness behaviour, demonstrate a variety of different sorts of psychological pathology, just like parents who carry out more 'ordinary' child abuse.

In relation to the children who are the victims, we again reserve the term 'diagnosis' for medical conditions with characteristics that may be specified and are replicable. We have not employed the term 'diagnosis' to encompass the discovery of a fabrication as the cause of a child's symptoms, but subscribe to the view that paediatricians should 'diagnose the specific fabricated or induced medical illness(es) or condition(s) they encounter' (Fisher and Mitchell, 1995). In less technical terms, the children may be described as being victims of 'Munchausen syndrome by proxy abuse'. Perhaps because the behaviours are so shocking and counter-intuitive to our views of parenting, and because those discovering the behaviours are generally working with diseases (i.e. disorders whose intrinsic causes can be specified, sometimes at a molecular level), it has been hard to dislodge the 'medicalizing' language despite cogent criticisms (Morley, 1995; Fisher and Mitchell, 1995). As editors we have tried to ensure consistency in the use of language throughout this book.

A staged approach to assessment and management

The process of understanding and evaluating MSBP abuse is a complex one. We believe a staged approach to the situation assists professionals in determining which task they should concentrate upon at any one time and in deciding what information needs to be gathered to answer specific questions. The chapters of this book are organized to reflect the tasks of these stages.

Stage 1: The dawning of private concerns in the mind to identification of paediatric factitious illness by proxy

Before Stage 1 can be reached, professionals working with children in the health care system need an awareness of all the ingredients of the triad in which MSBP abuse may occur. In other words, they need to be intellectually and psychologically prepared with an awareness of the way parents (or those *in loco parentis*) may behave towards their children and use their children to meet their own needs. Professionals then require an understanding of the way consultations in medical settings may interact with these relationships. This in turn requires knowledge of the processes that take place between doctors and parents, especially in Westernized, high technology medical systems. In addition to an awareness of the social and psychological context of their own role, health care professionals working with parents and children may benefit from understanding something about the psychological difficulties and 'pathways' that lead parents, mothers especially, to behave abusively to their children. We might say that these areas (covered in Chapter 2) are a necessary prerequisite for being a thoughtful health care worker with children in Britain today.

Armed with such understanding, the doctor or nurse meets a parent and child whose presentation defies explanation, usually because of the discrepancy between the child's health state and history, or because a diagnosis cannot be found which explains the sick child's presentation in terms of known disease. The possibility of fabrication by a parent (or person *in loco parentis*) is considered quickly by astute clinicians who are aware of the full range of parents' behaviours: Stage 1 begins here when the possibility of fabrication is considered. The early part of Chapter 3 sets the scene for approaching paediatric consultations so that the parental contribution to the process and indeed the possibility of abuse may be considered. Whilst often still exploring other possibilities in the differential diagnosis, the task of Stage 1 is to establish the extent of the paediatric fabrication. This painstaking process involves a scrupulous approach to history taking which widens as records from other settings, other professionals and interviews with other family members are included to establish whether fabrication for the child, the mother herself and for other children, is identified. This too is described in detail in Chapter 3.

Stage 1 may be very extensive, lasting many years when a situation arises which worries professionals but is judged to be not sufficiently clearly factitious, or not sufficiently harmful, to approach social services. Then the professional may need to manage a family for many years in a vigilant way, before a sufficient level of concern is reached to move towards a more formal child protection forum: Stage 2 may never be reached for many families. When the critical threshold of harm is reached in the clinician's judgement, then he or she involves social services and this marks the end of Stage 1.

Chapters 3–8 concern themselves with the different settings in which these fabrications may present and the way in which paediatric specialists can manage the different presentations. Chapter 9 deals with some complex and unusual situations causing high levels of uncertainty and with assessment of risk, hence spanning Stages 1 and 2.

Stage 2: Integrating existing knowledge and assessing risk

Stage 2 begins when the paediatric team has satisfied themselves that either a fabrication has occurred, or the level of concern about significant harm to the child or children is so great that the circumstances need to be examined in a wider arena, including the child protection system. This is the stage of assessment. The areas to be examined include all those that have a bearing on the child and family, including areas of functioning and of support. This may involve an integration of information from primary care, paediatrics, social services and education. During the course of this stage decisions will need to be made about who is best placed to gather certain information and precisely how it will help in understanding the family and the level of harm and risk. Depending upon the severity and type of fabrication suspected, the child protection actions also vary widely, between waiting for further health care seeking in an out-patient or community setting, up to covert video surveillance and constant observations of mother and child in hospital, and including temporary separations. Professionals apart from the paediatric team, whether in a hospital or community setting, will certainly need to be involved and it may be worthwhile at this stage to involve mental health professionals, either to assist directly in the assessments, to help other professionals to undertake relevant assessments or to help other professionals think about the case and its management. Chapters 9 and 11 are relevant here.

Stage 3: Judgement of harm and risk

Stage 3 brings together the work of Stages 1 and 2, leading to conclusions about the extent and severity of the injury to the child, as a result of which decisions may be made by the courts about this and the child's future. This stage involves a synthesis of medical, child protection (social services), forensic and legal skills, views and opinions. These decisions will be based upon judgements about whether in fact harm has occurred and, if so, the capacity of individuals or families to change and reduce the risk of harm in future. Such decisions rest upon the skill used in earlier stages, and often involve the use of outside experts to integrate the mass of information gathered. This area is dealt with in Chapters 11, 12 and 13.

Stage 4: Treatment and further management

This stage has several different aspects, depending upon the decisions made earlier. For those families that remain together, further monitoring and treatment goes on, with integration of the work of primary care, social services, mental

health teams and secondary paediatrics. The primary care section of this chapter
and Chapters 11 and (most centrally) 13 are concerned with this.

For families where permanent separation of parent perpetrator and child victim
is undertaken, it is necessary to consider the impact of the abuse on the child, who
may need further therapeutic work, as may the new family into which the child or
children are integrated. Chapter 13 also deals with these issues, and concentrates
upon that small group of families where harm has occurred but where the perpetrator is considered to have made sufficient acknowledgement of their actions to
merit intensive in-patient work for the family. Abusive parents from permanently
separated families may also be able to undertake therapeutic work at this stage, or
later, or sometimes not at all: this may alter decisions about subsequent children.

Table 1.1 gives an overview of this staged approach to assessment and management of factitious illness in children.

Other contributions

As in any book with different contributions around a central, very broad theme,
we are aware of structural flaws. Although the staged approach is appropriate for
straightforward classical MSBP abuse, it is less helpful for many of the 'grey'
areas where clinicians are uncertain about parental behaviour and harm. We have
deliberately included these within the range of the book and Chapter 9, 'Dealing
with uncertainty', is not easily placed within the staged structure. It is therefore
placed between Stages 2 and 3, as is Chapter 10, 'Parental and adult professional
gain from exceptional children: achievement by proxy', which is included to
provide a thought-provoking tangent to our central themes. Certain subjects, most
notably factitious sexual abuse, are dealt with in more than one section (Chapter
5, p. 140–142 and in Chapter 8, p. 167–171), which is not ideal. Inevitably there
is some redundancy in certain themes, particularly those of information gathering
and independent corroboration, but these merit over-learning and the repetition
has therefore been welcomed. There are other important themes that have not
been included. We have chosen not to explore in detail the psychodynamic understandings of adult perpetrators, or assessment and therapeutic work with them.
The details of therapeutic work with the child, and literature about the impact of
both physical and emotional trauma on children are not explored. This is not
because we deem these subjects unimportant but because we have concentrated
upon the professionals who work with children and on the early stages of the
sequences of MSBP abuse, in the hope that a combined paediatric and psychiatric
approach to these matters will help professionals to be better equipped in future.

Finally, the professionals who have been caught up in this complex and distressing saga may also need attention: for some, for example nurses on an acute
paediatric ward, this work may be needed earlier in the process, but for those
caught up in the legal arena, help may be required later. Chapter 14 considers the
impact of MSBP abuse on helping professionals and identifies methods of both
preventing the most serious effects by proactive strategies and of managing the
distress such cases may cause.

Table 1.1 A staged approach to assessment and management of factitious illness in children

---

Stage 1: Identifying or refuting the presence of factitious illness or establishing the extent of paediatric fabrication (see Chapters 3 and 9).

- Dawning of private concern in the mind.
- Collection of paediatric evidence of fabrication or induction by a parent or person *in loco parentis.*
- Preliminary consultation with colleague.
- Preliminary risk assessment.

Stage 1 ends with either:

1 A decision that there has been no fabrication or the behaviour is insufficiently harmful to approach social services: move to 'Managing situations where harm *is not* deemed to have occurred' (Chapter 9) *or*
2 A strategy meeting and a move to child protection.

CRITICAL THRESHOLD OF CONCERN ABOUT HARM AND INVOLVING SOCIAL SERVICES.

Stage 2: Integrating existing knowledge and assessing risk (Chapters 4–11).

- Referral to social services; strategy phase.
- Investigation in progress. Integration and corroboration of information from different professionals and perspectives:
  1 Existing knowledge about paediatric fabrications, child development and health.
  2 Historical information (medical and social) about family members.
  3 Dynamic understanding (of relationships and systems, past and present).
- Initial child protection conference.
- Putting concerns to parents.

Stage 3: Judgement of harm and risk (see Chapters 9, 11 and 12).

- Child protection and legal 'judgement' phase, drawing conclusions about:
  1 Severity.
  2 Harm.
  3 The perpetrator's and family's potential for changes.
- Formal risk assessment.
- Legal process.

Stage 4: Management and treatment (see Chapter 13).

Primary care and MSBP abuse

There is no chapter in this book about the role of primary care professionals, the GP especially. However, implicit throughout is a pivotal role for primary care professionals in prevention, both primary and secondary. Their contribution is also crucial at several of the other stages of MSBP abuse assessment and management.

Role of the general practitioner and primary care team

Stage 1: Identifying the possibility of factitious illness

Many GPs and other primary care professionals are aware of one or two families on their case load whose perceptions of their children's health and use of health care resources is chronically or intermittently distorted and could be damaging to the children if not firmly contained. This may include inconsistent and undesirable use of any medication which the children are taking (see Chapter 6 for case examples) and may extend on occasion to an unconfirmed concern that medication for adults has been given to children. Often if he comes under pressure from the parents the GP will refer such families to a consultant paediatrician. Whilst a few of these families may be involved in more extensive and dangerous fabrications the majority are not. Many of these families are familiar to other professionals in the primary health care team, either because they are disorganized, chaotic families with poor parenting, or because the health visitor has noted a difficulty in building a rapport with the parent and has concerns about parental perceptions of aspects of the children's health.

The range of roles for primary care professionals is wide in these circumstances, some of which may never reach the level of substantial concern, some may be just at the threshold for harm, and others may cross it. In the last circumstance, it is very likely that secondary care professionals will be involved and these cases are discussed below. Social services may or may not have been involved and, if so, perhaps only for more ordinary parenting problems or poor care. Social services have rarely been involved with well organized families with very distorted perceptions. Both such groups of families usually have long-standing difficulties, either widespread and general or specifically related to health issues, and the long term perspective of the GP and primary health care team is invaluable in their management. For those families where concerns about health care use always remains at Stage 1 (i.e. of worrying about the unusual use of health care but never a confident identification of harm or significant factitious illness), the primary care team's role may continue for many years.

The roles of primary care professionals may be summarized as follows:

1. Monitoring the index child and their siblings' health and development and keeping their psychological health in mind.
2. Reassuring parents and resisting unnecessary health care if there is no evidence of physical signs to substantiate the parental report. Therapeutic work (see below).

3. Managing such families' demands and needs in the practice by preventing parents visiting different partners, thus ensuring health care requests are routed firmly to a single primary care physician.
4. Greater precision in record keeping than usual. Ensuring that notes make it clear when symptoms and signs are reported by the parent and when professionals themselves have made the observations.
5. Seizing available opportunities for the family to accept mental health and social work input if they have not done so previously (it is common to decline this).
6. Declining specialist consultation requests unless they are truly necessary and ensuring that any necessary or urgent specialist consultations are directed to a well briefed paediatrician who can then involve any other specialists, particularly surgical ones, only when a full appraisal has taken place.
7. Keeping in touch with other primary care and community professionals who may have information about the child's or family's health or functioning in other arenas. These other professionals can be actively involved in the recognition of factitious presentations, identification of other associated difficulties and awareness of family functioning. Collating different information may raise or reduce anxiety about complaints of illness that are being made and may therefore bring forward the need for a strategy or child in need meeting.

Therapeutic work at Stage 1
With the mildest forms of abnormal illness behaviour, including frequent consultation and persistent unsubstantiated complaints about a child (which are often a reflection of maternal or family mood or relationship problems or recent obvious stresses), the GP will be in a position to manage the situation himself. He will identify the difficulty as residing within the parent's perceptions, beliefs or responses, or within the relationships with the child, rather than being within the child's health. This is an important therapeutic task in these circumstances. If there is sufficient uncertainty about the child's health in the GP's mind to justify secondary paediatric assessment he can prepare the specialist for meeting the family. This may be by a phone discussion or perhaps a joint appointment with a paediatrician (community or otherwise) to prepare the specialist for a consultation which attends fully to the family's concerns but recognizes their preoccupations. In situations where the GP is confident about the child's state of health, he or she can prevent altogether the child entering the secondary paediatric system.

Stage 2: When harmful factitious illness is suspected – the information gathering stage
Cases where primary care management and the prevention of unnecessary health care have been unable to contain the parents' pressure for specialist consultations will probably be recognized as harmful in the secondary sector. This is usually so in severe cases of MSBP abuse which involve more gross fabrications or illness inductions. The major role of the primary care team is in adding to, corroborating and enlarging the pool of information about the family members and their functioning.

1. In both mild and severe cases, the GP has unparalleled access to trans-generational patterns, and to information about the family's social circumstances, their stability and contact with social services and their health care use. He or she also has access to notes and letters about past behaviour.
2. An important role at this stage is the corroboration of parental histories by scrutiny of general practice records including contacts with other services.
3. Attendance at any strategy meeting or child protection case conference (see Chapter 11) introduces a useful community perspective for hospital and social services staff.
4. In severe cases of MSBP abuse, usually identified or suspected by hospital staff, the GP is likely to be aware of the parents' and siblings' health and of their patterns of illness behaviour, provided he or she is the practitioner for the whole family. It is then possible to piece together parts of the puzzle that are more difficult for the paediatrician or other specialist to acquire.
5. In these circumstances, and with lesser degrees of persistence and exaggeration, the GP has the power and authority to curtail and regulate dangerous patterns of seeking further opinions during the assessment phase. The GP may firmly need to resist pressure, even when the family threatens to leave the practice. Therapeutic work (see below) may be possible even at this stage.
6. Last, but far from least, the GP is in communication with a web of primary care and community professionals, of whom the health visitor, school nurse and community paediatricians are perhaps the most crucial. These are professionals who may have information about home circumstances, family relationships, parenting skills and the performance of other children.

Therapeutic work at Stage 2

In order to use their powerful position for the good of children, GPs must not only recognize and manage maternal (or paternal or family relationship) difficulties, but also the presentations of children, which are one manifestation of these. He or she must be skilled in the identification/discovery of parental psychopathology, mental health service contacts and psychosomatic presentations in adults (Gask, 1992): of course in this area, GPs, who work across the age range, will have a significant advantage over paediatricians. A GP can make links him or herself between the parent's history and current state and the concern about a child, and can then use their knowledge and relationship with the family to help the parent to see the connection. This is a more difficult task with families at Stage 2 than at Stage 1 but it can be undertaken by those who are skilled (Eisendrath, 1989). In this task, GPs might be assisted by discussion with an experienced child mental health specialist with expertise in working with family systems. In such a situation, there is the potential for child and adolescent mental health service liaison with primary care.

Stage 3: Judgement of harm and risk, child protection and legal proceedings

At this stage, in cases of serious risk of harm, the primary responsibility for the child's health and well-being is probably being shared between the family and other professionals or may be with social services entirely (see Chapter 12 for further discussion of these issues). Occasionally, if the family is remaining together whilst a comprehensive assessment takes place, the GP or his representative may be a very important member of the core group who monitors the health of the child and siblings.

In the more common situation of separation of the child from the suspected MSBP perpetrating parent whilst full assessment and decision making takes place, the GP's role shifts to a focus on the mother, father and siblings if they remain at home. Especial vigilance may be necessary in three quite different areas:

1. The parent, probably the mother, is likely to be extremely disturbed and to demonstrate difficulty with the boundary of self and non-self for all her children. She may well be persistent in fabrication of illness, especially if she has carried out severe illness induction. Other children, especially siblings, may risk becoming victims of factitious illness. Whereas the GP may be aware of this risk (which should of course have been considered at the strategy meeting or case conference) if there have already been exaggerations or inductions in siblings, the risk may not be apparent if, for example, the current victim is an only child. The author is aware of one such mother who, when separated from her own child, then involved herself in fabricating illness with friends' and neighbours' children. Awareness of these connections puts the family doctor or other primary care professionals in a unique position to protect other children.
2. The perpetrator herself may show extreme reactions when factitious illness is recognized and confronted: anger, self-harm and gross somatizing presentations are all commonplace. The GP is obviously vital in helping the mother and alerting other professionals (from accident and emergency departments, mental health and other medical specialties to which she may present) to the sources of her behaviour. It is useful at this stage to involve a psychiatrist or other local mental health specialist who is independent of the child care issues, to help the mother if she will permit it.
3. Third, the father or other family members registered with the practice may also present in the course of the crisis and may merit input in their own right as their awareness of the problem increases.

Stage 4: Management and treatment

If this is judged to be safe following child protection or legal proceedings, after a period of assessment (and hopefully treatment) a reunited family will be living in the community. This situation requires a tightly organized core group of key primary care professionals, with GP, health visitor and school nurse communicating closely to monitor progress and identify further fabrications or stresses that might trigger these (see Chapter 13, p. 288). The majority of these activities and roles are as described above under Stage 1 (numbers 1–7). Additional roles are:

1. Being in regular liaison, in the early stages at least, with personnel and any other professional engaged in treatment.

2. Liaising with a single nominated secondary or community paediatrician for assessment and investigation of any true or suspect intrinsic illness.

Naturally, level of concern will be higher in families where proceedings have taken place. It should be the case that this increased concern is balanced by the provision of substantial resources in these cases to assist, support and monitor the family's progress.

Conclusions

If primary care professionals are to fulfil these numerous roles in relation to factitious illness and MSBP abuse, awareness of the problem is a prerequisite. The skills involved in most of the tasks outlined are also those that are, *par excellence*, the strengths of good primary care professionals. An area for development is the establishment of models of liaison and communication between primary care and community paediatrics, child mental health professionals and secondary paediatricians. There need to be opportunities for discussion of such difficult cases and the approaches to their management, including perhaps on occasions, joint professional consultations face to face. Such developments require a willingness to change behaviour patterns, flexibility, mutual respect, and adequate time and professional resources to try out new health care services. A difficult case is sometimes the spur that is required to initiate change.

Summary

This book's aim is to convince health care professionals that an understanding of how Munchausen syndrome by proxy abuse occurs will bring benefits in all their consultations. In essence, we wish to increase understanding of the way in which the health care system may be used to harm children, rather than benefit them, and the way in which health workers may become the unwitting instruments of this harm. We believe that an understanding of parents and of consultations, combined with good basic skills in history taking (Donald and Jureidini, 1996) and observation, are the keys to early recognition of these situations, to ensuring that children receive appropriate health care, to the prevention of further harm, to the protection of children from abuse, and to the design of training for health workers which creates thoughtful, skilful and non-judgmental professionals. Understanding the range and nature of parents' behaviour is also key to the development of child protection systems. These should integrate the skills of all children's professionals to support families, to prevent abuse by the health care system and to foster children's development in the best way possible.

References

Asher, R. (1951) Munchausen syndrome. *Lancet*, **ii**, 339–341.

Bools, C.N., Neale, B.A. and Meadow, S.R. (1992) Co-morbidity associated with fabricated illness (Munchausen syndrome by proxy). *Archives of Disease in Childhood*, **67**, 77–79.

Bools, C. (1996) Factitious illness by proxy: Munchausen syndrome by proxy. *British Journal of Psychiatry*, **169**, 268–275.

Burman, D. and Stevens, D. (1977) Munchausen family. *Lancet*, **ii**, 456.

Day, D.O. and Parnell, T.F. (1998). *Munchausen by Proxy Syndrome: Misunderstood Child Abuse* (Day, D.O. and Parnall, T.F., eds), pp. 47–67. Sage Publications.

Department of Health (1989) An Introduction to the Children Act 1989. HMSO.

Dine, M.S. (1976) Tranquilliser poisoning: an example of child abuse. *Paediatrics*, **36**, 782–785.

Donald, T. and Jureidini, J. (1996) Munchausen syndrome by proxy. Child abuse in the medical system. *Archives of Pediatric and Adolescent Medicine*, **150**, 753–758.

Eisendrath, S.J. (1989) Factitious physical disorders: treatment without confrontation. *Psychosomatics*, **30**, 383–387.

Eminson, D.M. and Postlethwaite, R.J. (1992) Factitious illness: recognition and management. *Archives of Disease in Childhood*, **67**, 1510–1516.

Fisher, G.C. and Mitchell, I. (1995) Is Munchausen syndrome by proxy really a syndrome? *Archives of Disease in Childhood*, **72**, 530–534.

Gask, L. (1992) Training General Practitioners to detect and manage emotional disorders. *International Review of Psychiatry*, **4**, 293–300.

Gray, J. and Bentovim, A. (1996) Illness induction syndrome: Paper 1. A series of 41 children from 37 families identified at the Great Ormond Street Hospital for Children NHS Trust. *Child Abuse and Neglect*, **20**, 655–673.

Horwath, J and Lawson, B. (1995). Conclusion: affirming, challenging, linking and developing practice. In *Trust Betrayed? Munchausen Syndrome by Proxy, Inter-agency Child Protection and Partnership with Families* (Horwath, J. and Lawson, B., eds), pp. 210–218. National Children's Bureau.

Levin, A.V. and Sheridan, M.S. (1995). *Munchausen Syndrome by Proxy: Issues in Diagnosis and Treatment.* Lexington Books.

Meadow, R. (1977) Munchausen syndrome by proxy – the hinterland of child abuse. *Lancet*, **ii**, 343–345.

Meadow, R. (1985) Management of Munchausen syndrome by proxy. *Archives of Disease in Childhood*, **60**, 385–393.

Morley, C. J. (1995) Practical concerns about the diagnosis of Munchausen syndrome by proxy. *Archives of Disease in Childhood*, **72**, 528–529.

Pickering, D. (1964) Salicylate poisoning: the diagnosis when its possibility is denied by the parents. *Acta Paeditrica*, **53**, 501–504.

Pickering, D. (1976) Salicylate poisoning as a manifestation of the battered child syndrome. *American Journal of Diseases in Children*, **130**, 675–676.

Rogers, D., Tripp, J. and Bentovim, A. (1976) Non-accidental poisoning: an extended syndrome of child abuse. *British Medical Journal*, **1**, 793–796.

Schreier, H.A. and Libow, J.A. (1993) *Hurting for Love, Munchausen by Proxy Syndrome*. Guildford Press.

Sigal, M., Gelkopf, M. and Meadow, R. (1989) Munchausen by proxy syndrome: the triad of abuse, self abuse, and deception. *Comprehensive Psychiatry*, **30**, 527–533.

Southall, D.P., Plunkett, C.B., Banks, M.W. *et al.* (1997) Covert video recordings of life threatening child abuse: lessons for child protection. *Pediatrics*, **100**, 735–760.

Taylor, D. C. (1992) Outlandish factitious illness. In *Recent Advances in Paediatrics* (David, T., ed.), pp. 63–76. Churchill Livingstone.

2

Background

Mary Eminson

Introduction

This chapter is mainly concerned with gaining an understanding of Munchausen syndrome by proxy (MSBP) abuse and the reasons why this troubling phenomenon should be so prevalent today. Initially the problem is defined as addressed in this book, and different ways of defining MSBP abuse are reviewed, including the approaches taken by the international classifications ICD-10 (World Health Organization, 1992) and DSM-IV (American Psychiatric Association, 1994). Having then considered the extent of the problem and such evidence that exists of its epidemiology, there is an analysis of the circumstances which have allowed or encouraged it. This analysis begins with an examination of changes in the context of health care in nations with high technology medical systems. This is followed by an examination of the effects of emotional abuse, the mechanisms through which this may present with somatic symptoms, and the way this and other factors in these families and individuals may have an impact on the use of health care by different vulnerable groups. Case histories which illustrate a variety of different pathways leading to factitious illness by proxy and to perpetration of MSBP abuse are interspersed through this section. Finally, the existing clinical series will be reviewed in the light of the factors identified earlier.

Whilst seeking to shed light upon the pathways to MSBP abuse, to organize the existing information and, hopefully, to increase understanding of the behaviour, the aim is not to excuse, but to explain. It is unlikely that most of the human race can achieve empathy with the severe fabricators and illness inducers who have caused serious harm and even death to their children. These are individuals whom we cannot understand 'because we cannot empathize with the transgression of the basic and ancient taboo of child rearing' (Fisher, 1995): the basic task of child rearing being to protect and rear one's child, rather than to harm him or her. For those with less severe manifestations of fabrication or manipulation (e.g. exaggeration of symptoms or frequent consultation), the combination of knowing about an individual's background and the stresses they experience may lead us to compassionate understanding. Whether or not we can achieve any sympathy for the abusive parents, it is certain that our appraisal and judgement of situations will be better if our emotions are not too far aroused and if we can retain our humanity in dispassionate care of the families we meet.

The definition of MSBP and MSBP abuse

A variety of different ways of defining 'factitious illness by proxy' or MSBP will be reviewed here. In the literature there is frequent acknowledgement that children's factitious illness presentations constitute one of several different types of unusual parental behaviours in relation to their children's health in health care settings. These unusual behaviours are referred to in this book as 'parental abnormal illness behaviour' and 'abnormal consultation behaviours'(i.e. the tendency to consult for their children's health) and constitute one end of a spectrum of health care and illness behaviours by parents. Factitious illness presentations, whether of induced or invented illness, are not clearly distinguished from other types of parental behaviours which include zealous pursuit of medical treatment; 'mothering to death', 'doctor shopping', 'hysteria by proxy', 'masquerade syndrome', 'mothers with delusional disorder' and 'overanxious parents' are some of the titles used by Meadow (1995). On the other hand, the most extreme forms of factitious illness (suffocations, feeds of faeces) are also close relations of other grosser forms of abuse and neglect of children (Fisher and Mitchell, 1995),which involve direct physical harm ('shaken' babies, limb fractures, failure to thrive due to neglect): in other words, extremes of factitious illness also have much similarity with 'ordinary' physical abuse (all of which has some element of emotional abuse, too). Nevertheless, there has been a substantial effort to separate and define either the perpetrators of factitious illness or the acts of fabrication into much more specific categories. These other ways of defining the issue and their advantages and drawbacks will now be reviewed.

Definition by motivation

In many accounts of MSBP abuse there are efforts to describe the psychological make-up and motivations of parents who behave in these ways towards their children, in a medical setting. Indeed there are those who would *define* the disorder by the motivation of the abuse perpetrator (Meadow, 1995; Schreier and Libow, 1993). Meadow (1995) believes the term 'Munchausen syndrome by proxy' abuse should be reserved for the abuse itself, i.e. it is a description of what has happened to the child. He points out that the definition must rest firmly upon skilled paediatric (i.e. medical) opinion about the cause of the child's ill-health, that is, on a judgement about whether the illness is intrinsic or extrinsic, i.e. 'factitious'. The MSBP abuse label is then applied to factitious cases. Grounding of the phenomenon firmly within the paediatric evidence of an external cause of sickness is essential for good paediatric practice (especially when building a case for the legal arena) and is consistent with ICD-10 (see below). It also, helpfully, draws attention to the importance of paediatric history taking and diagnostic skills (Donald and Jureidini, 1996; Rosenberg, 1995) in recognition and assessment.

However, having begun his definition with the identification of factitious illness rather than an overlooked intrinsic disorder in the child, Meadow (1995) argues for restricting the term 'Munchausen syndrome by proxy' to those parents whose motivation is 'either the sick role by proxy or another form of attention seeking behaviour'. On the grounds that 'understanding the motivation of the perpetrator may be the key to understanding the abuse and formulating a policy for safe parenting and prevention of future harm', he views these perpetrators as a 'homogeneous group' for whom formulation and trial of treatment and therapy should be possible.

Other authors, particularly Schreier (1996) alone and together with his colleague Libow (Schreier and Libow, 1993), have also advocated a narrow conceptualization based on motivation. In their early work (Libow and Schreier, 1986) these authors divided parents into three broad groups: 'active inducers', 'help seekers' and 'doctor addicts', with 'help seekers' (who really want help for themselves) and 'doctor addicts' (who are attracted to the medical setting for the sense of importance and for the indirect nurturing through health care it provides) having a more positive prognosis if intervention takes place. 'Active inducers' have less easily established motivations. This analysis arises in part at least from the authors' psychodynamic formulations of mothers or perpetrators, for which their book *Hurting for Love* provides perhaps the richest examples, and is a stimulating source of this theoretical perspective on the area.

It is difficult, however, to be confident that the assumption that there is an identifiable group of parents whose motivation is the sick role by proxy can be supported in practice. Case reports (Loader and Kelly, 1996; Nicol and Eccles, 1985; vignettes in Chapters 8 and 13 of this book; Schreier and Libow's case examples) suggest complex psychopathology underlies these perversions. The limited descriptive literature of victims of parental abnormal illness behaviour supports this: relevant issues include attachment, the relationship between parent and child, the parents' relations with doctors and the child, and diversions from parental sources of distress (Joell Gregory, 1999).

A further major difficulty with definition by motivation is establishing motivation itself. Even for experienced mental health professionals, motivation is rarely easy to define, and is particularly in an area as complex as child abuse, likely to be concealed, mixed, ambiguous and changeable. (Some interesting examples of such mixtures are given in Chapter 7.) Motivation is even less susceptible to any form of scientific testing (for example, by standardized interview) than most psychological concepts. It is subject to multiple *post hoc* rationalizations especially if legal sanctions are imminent. Furthermore, it is quite risky to assume, especially in a group of parents whose defining characteristic is their dishonesty in relationships, that our normal explanations about behaviour are correct or that the parent will be truthful when describing their motives. It is certainly not evident when first meeting a child in the out-patient clinic that his mother's motivation for being there is unusual in any way; the time and skills required to make even a rough attempt at assessing individual parents' motivations in out-patient clinics is a substantial demand to make on paediatricians. It is suggested that this is not a useful way to identify and define factitious illness perpetrators, despite the importance of such theorizing for understanding.

This is not to say that there is *no* utility in attempting to identify subgroups of MSBP abuse perpetrators, particularly if this enables professionals, as Meadow suggests, to define appropriate treatment approaches (see Chapter 13). Nor is it to deny that adopting the sick role by proxy may be a motivation of some perpetrators. In the present state of knowledge, however, limitation of the area of scrutiny to a single perpetrator group, so difficult to define in practice, seems premature and probably unattainable.

Broader definitions incorporating motivation

Schreier has also argued for inclusion of cases which involve fabrications in settings outside the health care system (based on similarity in motivation, but somewhat broader than adoption of the sick role). Case reports have been presented, including those involving other helping services (e.g. fire brigades) and public agencies such as child protection services, particularly where fake allegations of sexual abuse are concerned. Their inclusion in the category of MSBP is on the basis that this includes mothers whose motivation is related to building a 'manipulative relationship with . . . other professionals who occupy positions of power in society' (Schreier, 1996). This grouping would then include a set of parents who tell false stories in which their children are incorporated, whatever the setting of the falsification.

This broadening of the definition based on motivation has further disadvantages. It is essentially based on circumstances where the parent's motivation is apparently difficult to understand and seems contrary to assumptions about child rearing. (Although Schreier would include fabrications in the context of divorce which are relatively easy to understand as a way of seeking revenge upon a former partner.) It includes as unwilling participants, who may be instruments of harm, a very wide group of professionals (health care professionals, fire fighters, benefits agencies, law enforcement agencies, social services) whose training and work setting have little in common otherwise. So the inclusion of all in one class of 'unwitting agents of harm to children' seems unlikely to yield much by way of opportunity for common training, education or for prevention. Another disadvantage is that this will exclude from further study a large number of children and families where harm has occurred in a medical setting, but where the apparent parental motivation does not clearly fit the criteria, or is more obviously deviant. For essentially pragmatic reasons, Jones (1996) rejected the extension of Munchausen syndrome by proxy abuse into these other areas. The argument he advanced was for limitation of the label 'MBP' (as he describes it) to medical settings both because of the range of background problems and apparent motivations in perpetrators, but also because it would result in 'dilution of its (the term MSBP abuse's) present meaning' which was described as 'alerting paediatricians to risks and types of presentations in a medical context'.

Another concern is that limitation of study to one group of factitious illness perpetrators may distract attention from the facts currently available about judgement of risk. There is ample evidence from Meadow's own work of the lack of uniformity in perpetrator characteristics (Bools, Neale and Meadow, 1994). Previous and present behaviour, together with the extent of acknowledgement of what has occurred, are the best indicators of the current risk to the child (Oates, 1997), which must be considered by including a wide range of variables (discussed further in Chapters 9, 11 and 13). There is scant evidence that motivation has relevance in making these judgements and it is possible that it may complicate an already complex analysis by making the situation appear either more or less serious than the objective information can support.

Psychiatric classifications: DSM-IV and ICD-10

The existence of these abusive behaviours within a medical setting has misled many into thinking that because the behaviour happens near doctors it can be defined as a disease. The American habit of dignifying many behaviours with a diagnostic label has probably added impetus to this trend, as has the fact that some of the perpetrators properly fulfil diagnostic criteria for medical conditions: many suffer from personality disorders (i.e. lifelong difficulties) and also from psychological and psychiatric illnesses (e.g. depression and somatoform disorders).

DSM-IV: Definition by motivation again

Uncertainty about terminology has been maintained by the position of the DSM-IV classification (American Psychiatric Association, 1994). In this, 'factitious disorder by proxy' is identified, not in the main section, but in Appendix B, which consists of 'criteria, sets and axes provided for further study' – a list of twenty mainly psychiatric conditions. Research criteria for 'factitious disorder by proxy' are given. These criteria are identical to those for factitious disorder, except that the 'proxy' element is included. These are:

- Intentional production or feigning of physical or psychological signs or symptoms in another person who is under the individual's care.
- The motivation for the behaviour is to assume the sick role.
- External incentives for the behaviour (such as economic gain, avoiding legal responsibility, or improving physical well-being, as in malingering) are absent.

This categorization, if adopted, would clearly allow the perpetrator to be given a DSM-IV psychiatric diagnostic coding and provides the basis for 'definition by motivation'. It also has the effect of 'medicalizing' a behaviour which has none of the characteristics of a disease to justify this. It is difficult to provide an intellectual justification to support a category of this type, which is almost without parallel in this coding system. Similar confusion arises around some of the somatoform disorders: in the category of factitious disorders, there is an attempt to distinguish different motivations for producing or mimicking illness in oneself, some of which will be deemed 'illness' and some not. The reasons for this confusion are uncertain but there is a moral flavour about them which is distasteful but which will not be explored further here. The situation is summed up in the following quotation:

'If it is a situation or parental behaviour (a fabrication) that has come to be known as Munchausen syndrome by proxy or factitious illness by proxy then logically there

cannot be a disease or illness entity, or a condition, or even a syndrome called Munchausen syndrome by proxy or factitious illness by proxy that perpetrators have. Instead perpetrators have various psychological, psychiatric, and environmental "pathways" leading to a behaviour of fabricating illness in a child.'
Fisher and Mitchell (1995)

ICD-10: Maltreatment syndromes to define the aetiology of the child's illness

The other international classification system, ICD-10 (World Health Organization, 1992), which is explicitly a descriptive and atheoretical classification, adopts a clear position in relation to the child victim: that a factitious illness caused by another person is not a diagnosis classified as such on axis one, which defines the child's health state NOT its aetiology, (axis two and axis three relate to learning and cognitive capacities.) However, axis four (medical conditions) contains a section (T74) for 'maltreatment syndromes' where an extrinsic cause of an illness identified on axis one is coded: factitious illness is coded in the section on 'injury, poisoning and certain other extreme causes'. This is consistent with Meadow's position that the initial definition of this area must be of the nature and source of the child's illness. Thus for example a child injected with insulin by his mother would have an axis one diagnosis of 'hypoglycaemic coma' and on axis four, a coding of 'maltreatment'. When considering the classification of the perpetrator, MSBP abuse or factitious illness by proxy is not included amongst potential psychiatric diagnoses: thus the confusion between a behaviour and an illness is avoided. Factitious illness *in the perpetrator herself*, as well as any of the other psychiatric disorder categories she might suffer, can of course be used if appropriate.

Definition by harm: a spectrum of parents' abnormal illness and consultation behaviours

The author's paper (Eminson and Postlethwaite, 1992) did not propose a definition of this area but attempted to point out the dimensional nature of parents' desire to consult for their children, which could be set against the 'objective' need for consultation as defined by doctors. It was suggested that it was useful to define three broad groups of parents:

- Those who could distinguish their child's needs from their own and put their child's first.
- Those who were sometimes impaired or variable in putting their child's needs first, due to a variety of factors (psychological, social etc.).
- Those who were unable to put their child's needs first and instead put their own needs ahead.

Thus an inability to put the child's needs first was a uniting factor, which brought together, at one end of a spectrum of parental competence, those parents who were neglectful of their children's health care by under-consulting and undertreating, with those parents who were over-zealous in fabricating symptoms where none existed. Implicitly this conceptualization defined parents by their capacity to be 'good enough' parents and took a child protection perspective, defining the area of potential abuse as the extent of the discrepancy between the parents' behaviour and an objective view of the child's health needs. This is summarized in Figures 2.1 and 2.2.

This categorization is based on two assumptions. The first, already alluded to, is that the behaviours are at one end of a spectrum or continuum of parental behaviours towards children in a health care setting. The second assumption is that as much may be learnt from comparing MSBP abuse perpetrators with those who are only on the brink of harmful fabrications (i.e. where unusual and abnormal illness behaviour does not amount to abuse) as from comparisons within the group of perpetrators of serious abuse.

The spectrum of factitious illness

As a result, the boundary of this book is clumsily defined by the term 'abnormal parental illness behaviour and consultation behaviour in a medical setting': this includes those who have harmed their children and those who have not, but are at risk of causing harm by factitious presentations of children in such medical arenas. Factitious illness by proxy (MSBP) is used here to include induced illness (suffocation, poisoning) and invented symptoms (false or exaggerated histories and reports). The criterion for inclusion in the category Munchausen syndrome by proxy abuse is that harm has occurred, from the factitious presentation, to the child who is the victim. 'MSBP abuse' is shorthand to include all kinds of harm, physical and emotional, and to indicate that the medical system has been used as the instrument to cause the harm: that the triad of a health care system, a dependent child and a parent to present the child to the health care system with invented symptoms or fabricated signs, is involved. The harm usually occurs through the combined actions of the perpetrator and the health care professionals, rather than directly from adult to child as occurs in most abuse.

Within the boundaries of 'abnormal parental illness and consultation behaviour in a medical setting' is a very mixed set of factitious illnesses presenting in extremely wide-ranging ways. This book includes discussion of the entire range of the 'abnormal illness behaviours' of parents for children, i.e. to include abnormal parental perceptions and beliefs about the child's health or illness, consultation patterns (usually, but not necessarily, very frequent), limitations of the child's activities on account of supposed illness, and unnecessary pressure for investigations and treatments. Such abnormal illness behaviours range in their effects from harmless to harmful. Any of the 'abnormal illness behaviours' may cross the threshold for harm and therefore merit the label 'MSBP abuse'; many will not. Active illness induction is defined as the extreme end of abnormal illness behaviour, obviously clearly harmful. This is not to argue that an individual perpetrator will show the whole range of behaviours, or necessarily move up or down the scale. It is only a categorization of behaviours. It is not novel to suggest that there is a good deal in common between what Taylor

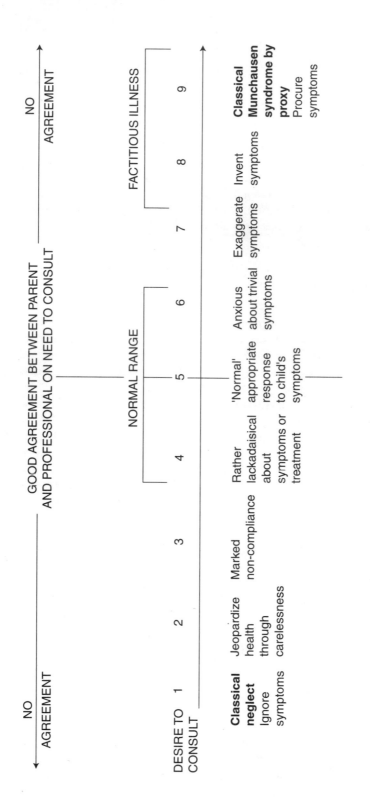

Figure 2.1 Parents' desire to consult for their child's symptoms

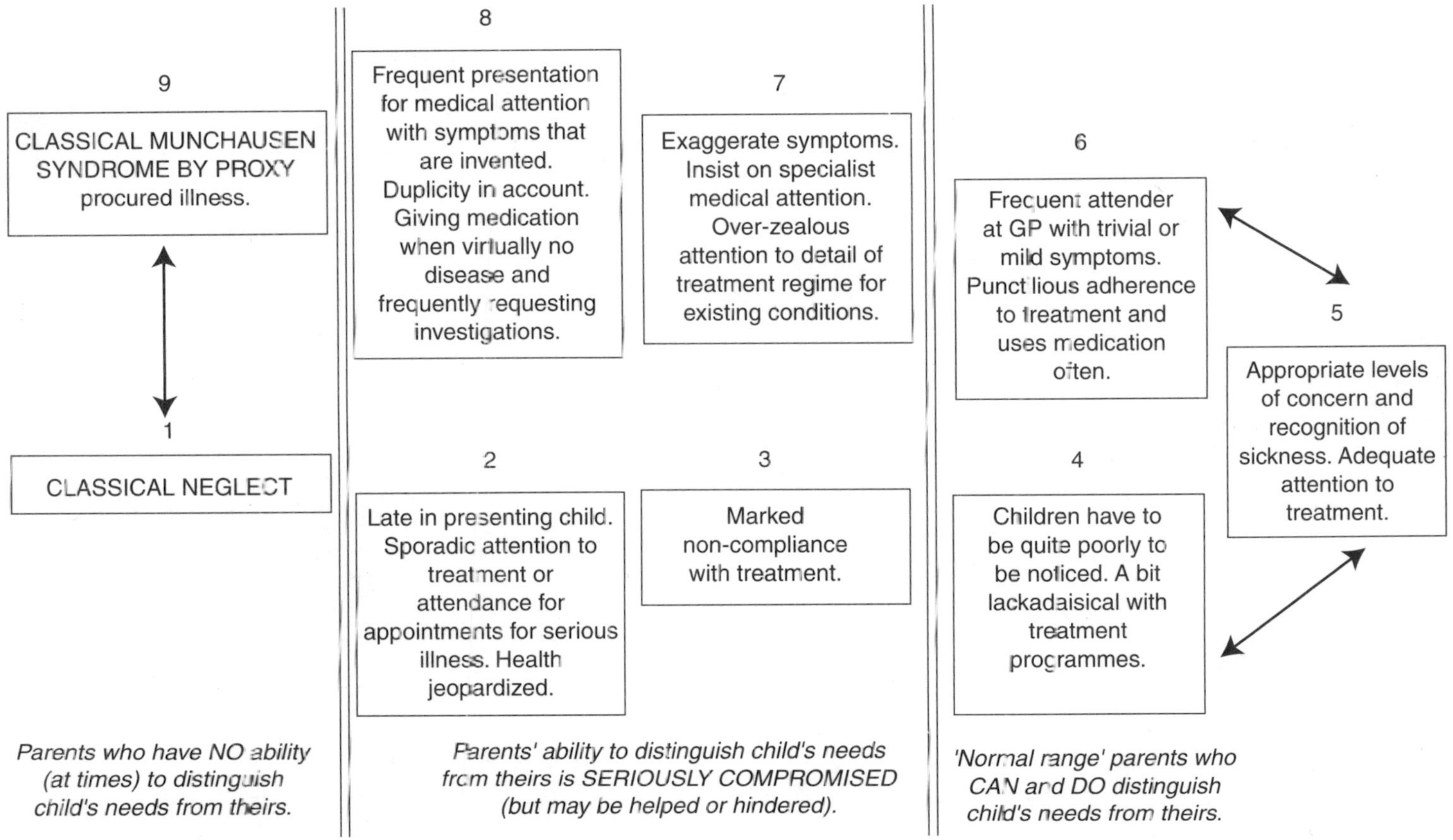
9
CLASSICAL MUNCHAUSEN SYNDROME BY PROXY procured illness.
1
CLASSICAL NEGLECT
Parents who have NO ability (at times) to distinguish child's needs from theirs.
8
Frequent presentation for medical attention with symptoms that are invented. Duplicity in account. Giving medication when virtually no disease and frequently requesting investigations.
7
Exaggerate symptoms. Insist on specialist medical attention. Over-zealous attention to detail of treatment regime for existing conditions.
2
Late in presenting child. Sporadic attention to treatment or attendance for appointments for serious illness. Health jeopardized.
3
Marked non-compliance with treatment.
Parents' ability to distinguish child's needs from theirs is SERIOUSLY COMPROMISED (but may be helped or hindered).
6
Frequent attender at GP with trivial or mild symptoms. Punctilious adherence to treatment and uses medication often.
4
Children have to be quite poorly to be noticed. A bit lackadaisical with treatment programmes.
5
Appropriate levels of concern and recognition of sickness. Adequate attention to treatment.
'Normal range' parents who CAN and DO distinguish child's needs from theirs.

Figure 2.2 The spectrum of health care seeking by parents for their children

(1992) called the 'hands on tampering' of directly induced illness and other 'outlandish factitious illness', as he described sicknesses promulgated by parents' beliefs and supported on occasion by 'fringe medicine'. These sicknesses included strongly promoted invalidity because of imagined allergens in one case, and the tendency for a little boy to swallow inedible and dangerous objects being labelled as 'pica syndrome' in another. Taylor pointed out both the interference with child development and other kinds of harm, as well as the difficulty of challenging the situation within child protection legislation. He also pointed out the discomfort it causes to contemplate harm in so many consultations.

Defining 'harm' may appear easy when a physical assault has occurred through the parent's own actions, such as poisoning or suffocation. It is also easy to recognize when a physical assault (an operation, an intrusive investigation, treatment with powerful medication which is unnecessary) has been carried out by doctors because they have been grossly misled by an inaccurate history or results from a specimen which has been tampered with. Identifying harm becomes progressively less clear the further one travels from these situations. How harmful is it to a child that his mother produces gravel from the family's garden path and claims he passed it in his urine? Is this more harmful or less harmful if the doctor fails to consider this as a possibility? Is the mother more guilty if the doctor carries out a cystourethrogram? How damaging is it to have numerous blood tests, all of which demonstrate normal results, or to be taken to a number of different doctors in order to be examined, physically or psychologically because of a false account of symptoms? How often does this need to happen over a period of time for it to be judged as harmful? How harmful is it to a child to be encouraged to adopt a sick role when objective measures suggest no limitation of a normal lifestyle is necessary? Is it bad for children if their parents claim they have autism and need special schooling, when medical and educational specialists consider this label to be inappropriate and think a more normal environment could be maintained? It is suggested that judging the 'critical threshold' of harm in certain circumstances may be very difficult, and hence the boundary between harmful and harmless, between abusive and non-abusive, is difficult to draw, with many grey areas in defining this type of abuse.

Thus the spectrum of factitious illnesses discussed here includes, at one extreme, a mother suffocating her baby whilst observed on covert video surveillance (severe directly induced illness), and at the other extreme, a mother bringing her child frequently to a GP with complaints of unverified symptoms. When suffocation occurs in hospital (illness induction) the harm is immediate and obvious, is both physical and emotional, and the involvement of the medical or health care element is only because the suffocation takes place in a hospital ward. Clinical series (Southall *et al.*, 1997) suggest that the parents who commit these acts do indeed have more in common with physically abusive parents than do some other groups of Munchausen syndrome by proxy abuse perpetrators. Some would suggest excluding these cases from the MSBP arena because of the differences from more indirect, medically induced harm (Donald and Jureidini, 1996; Meadow, 1995). However, for the purpose of this book this type of abuse is included within the MSBP abuse canon because it shares its medical links with other types of factitious illness.

In the case of a mother bringing her child frequently to a GP with unverified complaints, there is no harm, unless the doctor treats and investigates the child unnecessarily. In between two ends of the spectrum of harm represented by these examples is the next case, which illustrates circumstances where factitious illness is invented not induced and which, in the author's opinion, rests on the threshold of abuse and harm.

Simon, a healthy, intelligent eight year old, was an only child brought up by parents who were legally separated but lived close to each other. Over three years Simon's mother presented him increasingly frequently to the GP and then at the local hospital, pressing firmly for investigations for his symptoms which she described as 'not being with it', 'having a banging in his head', temper outbursts, 'pain in his penis', tiredness and many more. Mother believed these symptoms arose from brain damage sustained at birth. Specialist opinions at different hospitals regionally and nationally were sought by local paediatricians and a large number of neurological and urological investigations undertaken; these had largely normal (but occasionally borderline) results. Reassurance did not halt the mother's search for more opinions. Increasingly Simon was kept from school on account of 'his' symptoms and he became more withdrawn, with a fall in his academic attainments. Interviewed alone, he was extremely quiet and inhibited about speaking to any professional about himself or his home life or his symptoms: it was difficult to be confident of what he experienced.

Does the reader deem the account given to be what they would judge as physically harmful and reaching criteria for 'abuse'? Clearly the details supplied make this difficult to judge. All the investigations were carried out by doctors or at their request, and this included much time in hospital, numerous blood tests and scans of various kinds. Whilst clearly the responsibility for all the harm rested with the mother, most of the physical harm in this case was caused to Simon by the medical profession, there being no evidence that his mother induced any symptoms. The psychological harm (being kept from school and peers, infantilized, told how he felt, being inhibited from speaking freely, being told he was ill: the tangible results being a withdrawn child with poorer school attainments than expected) was caused directly by the mother.

Awareness of the potential for harm in medical investigations of this kind, and a facility in thinking out the threshold for harm in such a case, will help both in understanding and making judgements about circumstances more clearly damaging. The aim of this book is to alert clinicians to presentations at this level, on the assumption that this is a point at which, for many children, more extensive harm can be prevented, either by a constructive refusal to carry out further investigations or by other means.

Within this broad definition of MSBP abuse have been included all factitious illnesses in children where health care personnel are involved and harm has occurred. Logically this may include those cases seen in the context of custody and access disputes, where one parent alleges *sexual abuse* by the other and demands medical examination of the children, with no corroborating information of any kind. This takes us also into the psychological arena where the history constitutes much of the evidence of a child's disorder and where it may be particularly difficult to tease out objective evidence of a child's functioning: a situation discussed more fully in Chapters 5 and 8.

Advantages of this definition of MSBP abuse

Defining the area for review in this way has, it is contended, clear advantages. First, it narrows the focus to those aspects of MSBP abuse which concern those who work in the health care system in the broadest sense. Attributes of health workers and health care environments which have, albeit unwittingly, permitted or failed to prevent such abusive behaviours are discussed later in this chapter. It is argued that the greatest potential for reduction in MSBP abuse lies with increased awareness amongst health care professionals.

This 'broad' approach considers the fabricating parent to be defined by her or his behaviour. The assumption is that the behaviour may be provoked, maintained or prevented by a variety of different personal, familial and professional, social, psychological and practical factors. This places the perpetrators of MSBP abuse within our current understanding of abuse.

Definitions: wider implications and uses of categorical and descriptive methods

The importance of arguments about the definition of this area is far from purely intellectual. To grasp that this behaviour is a manifestation of a sociological and cultural phenomenon in which doctors are incidental participants, rather than a disease in which the medical diagnostic role is central, enables the use of a very different set of explanatory mechanisms and research techniques in this arena. This is not an 'all or none' situation, where a perpetrator has the capacity to produce factitious illness in their child, and all other parents do not. It is a behaviour on which doctors may have a powerful effect by their own actions: there may be minor degrees of the phenomenon and these may be managed well or ill, depending on skill and awareness. Perhaps the best analogy is with the likelihood of crimes, such a burglary and theft, which may be affected by whether the opportunity for the crime is afforded. The numbers of these crimes will be influenced by security precautions, independent of the urges of the would-be thief.

Implicit in the discussion so far has been the idea that for a classification system to be useful, its purpose must be established, as well as evidence that the categories are robust and reliable in various ways. The critique and suggestions advanced so far have been based on the assumption that medical methods of categorization of disease have little place in the definition of this behaviour, and that both for prevention and for definition of the behaviours and their prevalence it is better to adopt different (sociological and child protection) approaches. For understanding (and possibly for treatment) of individuals who perpetuate such behaviours, a medical (psychiatric) diagnostic classification combined with analysis informed by both psychodynamic and systemic models may be useful. Another area of importance is further study of the outcomes of individual children and perpetrators in various different circumstances, considering legal, child protection, medical and psychological outcomes. More research which helps in understanding how mothers' perceptions of their children become distorted may assist an analysis of the behaviours, and help in prevention and in treatment. Grouping case examples for future research and study of outcomes may be achieved by combining various measures from different theoretical perspectives: for example, the examination of perpetrators using rigorous measures of psychological and psychiatric categorization with measures of their offence. Another method would be to review personality and temperamental variables, together with the co-existence of psychiatric illnesses such as a somatization disorder or depression in groups of perpetrators of different types of harm. Whilst some studies of this kind have taken place (Bools *et al.*, 1994) such work is in its early stages. It is hampered by the limitations of existing instruments examining personality characteristics and the limited evidence of the reliability and validity of some questionnaire measures as predictors of behaviour. An important issue in this regard, in view of the over-representation of somatoform disorders in MSBP abuse perpetrators, is the current debate about whether extreme cases of preoccupation with somatic complaints (for oneself) may be better described as personality characteristics or disorders, rather than as discrete psychiatric illnesses (Bass and Murphy, 1995). The latter is currently the case in the psychiatric classification DSM-IV (American Psychiatric Association, 1994) and ICD-10 (WHO, 1992).

For the more severe and physically abusive perpetrators, the utility of clear descriptions of perpetrator psychological functioning might be to study these in combination with knowledge about the legal categorization of the type of crime committed by the parent, to produce a two-dimensional table of perpetrator characteristics by severity of offence. This would give some measure of the persistence with which harmful health care seeking behaviour is pursued by the abuser. This would require the collaboration of forensic psychiatrists and psychologists with paediatricians, lawyers and child mental health professionals, for further substantial studies in this area. There are other combinations of categorizations that would be useful in other areas of this subject: most complex of all are those which need to be brought together in order to make decisions about treatment, and which require a comprehensive assessment integrating many perspectives and categorical schema (see Chapters 11 and 13).

Summary: the area included in this book

Despite the many case reports and clinical series giving accounts of victims, we remain at a very early stage in understanding the pathways which lead parents to perpetrate Munchausen syndrome by proxy abuse. Early papers (Meadow, 1977) suggested particular parent characteristics, such as a 'good' mother, much admired on the ward with a typical background of work in nursing or medical fields. As larger case series (Bools *et al.*, 1992 and 1994; Rosenberg, 1987) broadened understanding, this stereotype was replaced by a confused picture, some parents with much evidence of other abuse problems and with a history of substantial personal and familial difficulties (including child deaths) in the family, but other mothers with a more functional facade which when cracked (i.e. a comprehensive history acquired) revealed a history of deception, of abuse and somatization on their own account as well as for their children. As awareness has increased, so has the awareness of connections with other sorts of maternal psychopathology (Schreier, 1996; Welldon, 1988), but this has threatened to draw attention to one aspect of the triad (the parent/perpetrator) to the detriment of awareness of this as a systemic problem involving a parent, a child and a health care system. More recently a variety of more complex systemic explanations, including interactive and interlocking historical, social, psychological and relationship variables, have been advanced (Gray and Bentovim, 1996; Jones and Ramchandani, 1999; Loader and Kelly, 1996; Fisher, 1995) which highlight similarities to the background factors relevant to other forms of abuse. From the evidence to date no single characteristic of parents, either current or historical, seems likely to prove to be a litmus test to identify factitious illness. In these circumstances, the author argues for a broad approach which includes the study of all those whose children's illnesses are exaggerated, fabricated, invented or induced; all those whose responses to their child's health seem discrepant from the view of a trained health care professional (Eminson and Postlethwaite, 1992). This allows the inclusion of a wide range of parents with a variety of motivations, and includes those whose concerns are because of anxiety, or mental illness, or previous failures or mistakes in medical care. Keeping all of these parents and children in the frame, limiting it to the health care setting and defining as reaching criteria for MSBP abuse those whose behaviours are deemed harmful to their children will, it is believed, provide the best opportunity to study all the routes (and roots) to the behaviour. This inclusive approach should ensure good evidence of all the background factors and provide a heterogeneous group of parents who may present the material for a variety of assessment and treatment protocols as well as more theoretical study of parents, their behaviours and the impact on children. Not enough is yet known about the pathways, or the motivations, or the outcomes for children, to exclude anyone from our study.

Epidemiology

It will be apparent that the intention to include all who harm their children by factitious illness presentations in a health care setting makes it difficult to define the size of the problem. There is no doubt that the extent of the behaviour merits attention. Whilst undoubtedly less common than other forms of child abuse, MSBP abuse has now been described widely in countries with 'Westernized' medical systems (USA, UK, Canada, Australia, Israel, New Zealand) and sporadically but increasingly in other countries and continents (Meadow, 1985).

Fabrications of every type have been reported, involving tampering with every organ system and most forms of medical technology (Rosenberg, 1987). Consistently women (usually biological mothers) are reported to carry out this form of abuse far more than men (Meadow, 1982; Southall *et al.*, 1997; McClure, David and Meadow, 1996). Even when tightly defined criteria have been used (disability or illness fabricated by an adult in a child, non-accidental poisoning and deliberate suffocation of children), as studied from notifications of paediatricians over a two year period between 1992 and 1994 (McClure *et al.*, 1996), the figures for different regions of the UK and Republic of Ireland varied from 0.1/100,000 to 0.8/100,000 children under sixteen years, which difference the authors attribute at least partially to under reporting. This study suggests that one occurrence per health district per annum in the UK, on average, may be a fairly accurate estimation. However, more recently doubt has been cast upon the accuracy of the reported figures of children dying as a result of 'cot death' (sudden infant death syndrome) with the suggestion that far more than previously recognized may be due to suffocation (Meadow, 1999). Doubt must then be cast even further upon the prevalence figures above.

If such extreme forms of harm as non-accidental poisoning and deliberate suffocation are hard to measure accurately, and these are the forms of fabricated illness in which the role of the medical profession is only in recognition and not at all in contributing a part of the action, how much more difficult is recognition of less harmful fabrications. Suffocations and poisonings must be the tip of the iceberg. Developing a more accurate picture has to rely not only on agreement between paediatricians about the factitious nature of a child's illness, but also on agreement about the severity of the harm that has ensued if it is to be recorded as abuse. This, in turn, relies upon consistency of judgement between child protection case conferences throughout the country, as well as equivalent levels of notification. Further complexity is added if one subscribes to the view, as the author does, that aspects of our health care system have a role in the elaboration of the behaviours; for if this is the case, the prevalence may be increasing. Perhaps accurate measurement will always be impossible.

On the assumption that professional recognition is an important variable, and as a first step in gaining an estimate of the extent to which professionals recognized these behaviours in their broadest form, a study of professionals was carried out in one health district of 65,000 children and adolescents under sixteen years (Watson, Eminson and Coupe, 1999). This was an attempt to examine the extent of worrying parental behaviours, and to bridge the threshold of harm on the assumption that clear-cut cases of factitious illness are unusual and that there is little agreement about the threshold where 'abuse' begins. The method was to request from health and social work professionals confidential nomination of cases seen in the previous two years defined in the following way: where 'concern that excessive seeking of health care (excessive and unnecessary consultations, imaginary or exaggerated illnesses) or abnormal illness behaviour (unnecessary use of medication or hospital appointments) by the parent on behalf of a dependent child (up to sixteen years) caused you to consider whether significant harm was occurring to that child'. Fifty-eight children were identified from forty-two families. This is equivalent to eighty-nine per 100,000 children who are reported to have experienced parental abnormal illness behaviour over a two year period. Fourteen children were on the child protection register as 'at risk' (usually for reasons other than factitious illness) and in four cases, care proceedings were pending. The most serious and harmful cases were, as expected, nominated by more than one professional. General practitioners did not identify cases which they judged to have crossed the threshold of harm and they had not themselves involved social services on any occasion; when in doubt they had referred the family to a paediatrician. It is not suggested that comprehensive identification has been achieved by this small study, although it would be surprising if identified severe and harmful fabrication had not come to light, in part because of the stability of personnel involved. This suggests the broad pattern of behaviours (disturbed and distorted consultation behaviour by parents for children) is commoner than previously recognized.

This study further reinforces the dimensional view of factitious illness by proxy, with a large unseen 'iceberg' of parental excessive or discrepant health care seeking in relation to children, surmounted by a 'tip' of clearly more severe factitious illness. The study cannot shed further light on the perpetrators of severe abuse. Prospective collection of such data in a defined geographical area, with clear operational definitions of the concepts involved, is an obvious next step.

A framework for understanding the occurrence of MSBP abuse

What framework should be adopted to help in making sense of this pattern of behaviour? The author favours a systemic understanding of the situation of abnormal parental illness and consultation behaviours, much as illustrated in the biopsychosocial formulation of Fisher (1995), whose simple diagrammatic summary of possible influences, both distal and proximal to the abuse, is summarized in Figure 2.3. This is consistent with the developmental/ecological model of the aetiology of abuse as outlined in Figure 13.1. These explanations begin with an individual who may have a variety of biological vulnerabilities, including temperament and intelligence, on which early experiences act to affect later personality development and in turn interact with family factors and experiences, past and present. This individual with their 'predisposing factors' enters a set of relationships or culture which may provide new risks and opportunities in the form of children, relationships and health care systems. A variety of triggers may act on this situation to precipitate the behaviour.

The narrative approach described by Loader and Kelly (1996) is also illuminating. They suggest that the fabrication of illness in one's child is 'the end point of a particular human story': this serves as a reminder that the stories are examined always with the benefit of hindsight. In the out-patient clinic, in paediatric wards, in the literature and in court, only those cases are seen where earlier and later factors have combined to produce the end point, the fabrication. How are the early stages of these narratives to be examined, before any fabrication has occurred?

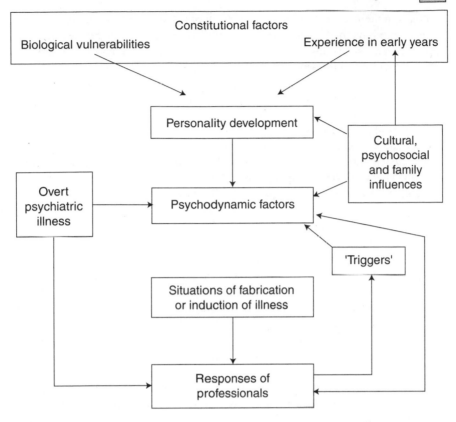

Figure 2.3 Factors and triggers leading to fabrication or induction of illnesses. (Reproduced from Fisher, G.C. (1995) *Munchausen Syndrome by Proxy. Issues in Diagnosis and Treatment* (Levin, A.V. and Sheridan, M.S., eds), Lexington Books)

The evidence from existing case series is that there is no single 'risk factor' or 'personality' or particular early experience which will inevitably produce an MSBP abuse perpetrator. These case series and meta-series (Rosenberg, 1987; Gray and Bentovim, 1996; Bools, Neale and Meadow, 1994) are broadly consistent in the picture they present of the backgrounds and early lives of individual perpetrators. Their early experiences were often emotionally abusive, sometimes there was sexual abuse, the family life was in some cases disorganized and sometimes cold and uncaring, and some perpetrators had heavy personal experience of illness. The personality characteristics of many included being untruthful, sometimes massively so, and the psychological problems of the perpetrator mothers included somatization, anxiety, depression and self harm. Their personal difficulties included marital problems and difficulties with relationships generally.

These characteristics of mothers are all common ones, far more common than is factitious illness in even its mildest form; any socially disadvantaged population has many members who possess several factors. Clearly these factors are not sufficient in themselves to explain the pattern of behaviour, for there will be many women who have had such experiences without going on to fabricate illness in their children. Nor is any single factor necessary to produce an MSBP perpetrator, with factors and influences relevant to one perpetrator being missing from the biography of another. It is crucial to emphasize that in the existing state of knowledge, it is the interaction between various distant and proximal factors which produces the 'setting conditions' for factitious illness in one's child. For each perpetrator of harm, and those whose actions do not cross the threshold for harm, the ingredients and their interaction will differ.

Nor indeed should it be assumed that the natural history of this behaviour is uniform. There are those who begin by fabricating illness in themselves and then begin also to do so in others as soon as they have a dependent child to be the focus or victim. They may continue for many years, whereas this is not the case for all perpetrators. Those who produce verbal fabrications do not all go on to induce illness directly in their children. What is clear is that social and cultural influences upon this behaviour are very strong, for there is an enormous preponderance of female perpetrators and also a huge bias of ascertainment in high technology Westernized medical systems (Brown and Feldman, 1999; Rosenberg, 1987). This is a behaviour carried out predominantly by women in wealthy countries with abundant health care.

There are several different ways to study this. One way is to consider the various biological, psychological, social and cultural issues as they impinge on the ability to care for children. Such a developmental/ecological model for child abuse is especially useful when considering intervention because it serves as a framework to examine the areas and processes to be considered in treatment and prevention of future harm (see Table 13.1). A second way is to examine this as a biographical narrative, looking first at those factors which will have affected the mother in infancy, childhood and so on. A third way to produce a meaningful account of the relevant factors and influences is to begin with the common setting (the hospital or health care system) and move outwards to examine why this is the place where abuse occurs. This is done by studying those who use health care systems for themselves and their children, in particular those who are at high risk of abusing their children. By taking this third approach, the analysis begins in the same place as the intended reader: from within the health care system.

The 'bargain' between parents and doctors: assumptions and realities

In the introductory chapter a triad was described as 'necessary for MSBP abuse to exist'. This triad involves a doctor (who stands for the resources of the health system), a parent to present the child and a dependent child to 'carry the illness'.

Assumptions of 'the bargain' and of health care workers

Exploration of the beliefs of health care providers is the starting point for study of the phenomenon of MSBP abuse. Most of those who work in Western medical systems, especially those who work with children, do so within a belief system that assumes health care happens when parents bring children to medical settings because the parent notices something is wrong with the child's health, and that the parent gives a faithful account, as far as they are able, of what symptoms the child has experienced. The health care worker, in accordance with their belief about their own role, sees him or herself as entering a contract to bring to this situation both their own knowledge and skill about the range of diseases which might explain this set of symptoms, and also the technological might of medical science in carrying out investigations and bringing forward treatments. Invasive investigations are justified in the search for disease; a physical cause for a symptom or a rare illness must not be missed. There is an implicit bargain here: that parents bring children who are sick and tell the truth about them and that doctors bring expertise and technology and act to do their best for children.

Assumptions about mothers

Underlying this are our assumptions about mothers. Mothers continue to hold the primary parenting responsibility for most small children in our society. The common-sense view is that women care for their children and will sacrifice themselves if necessary for the well-being of their offspring: the basic task of child rearing. So there is an assumption that in the setting in which health care workers see mothers (in a surgery, clinic or ward), when a mother is acting as historian and advocate for her child, that she will be giving a truthful history as far as she can and will be acting in the best interests of her child, not of herself.

Even in the best of circumstances, this is always and has always been an oversimplified account. Some complexities are woven into the underside of the bargain.

Real parents

Parents have always noticed some children's ills more than others, have turned a blind eye to sickness when they had to pay for medicine and money was short and they were preoccupied, and have favoured some genders of children (usually boys) in some cultures more than others (female foetuses are aborted in those cultures more often than male ones). In the West, girls with major chronic illness handicaps still die more often than boys. In a study of the chronically sick (Pless et al., 1989), survival to age thirty-five years was highest for those males from non-manual class homes (95 per cent survival) and lowest for females from manual class homes (only 85 per cent survival). Parents have pursued heroic treatments for some children and not others. Every hospital clinician has observed with surprise and disapproval the inconsistent caring which is evidenced at its most basic level by mothers' visiting children in hospital in patchy and insensitive ways. Parents' ambivalence (or the way their caring resources may be overwhelmed or exhausted) is seen in their failure to give treatments which are life saving. For example, probably the commonest single reason for loss of a child's renal transplant is failure to take immunosuppressive treatment subsequently (Ettenger, Rosenthal and Marik, 1991). For further examples, one has only to study the popular press to see that parents derive immense personal gratification very evidently from their child's or children's ill-health and its treatment.

Real doctors

On the other hand, doctors have always worked for money as well as for the good of their patients, have always relished the gratitude of patients as well as the pleasure of bringing health, are as vain as any other group in society and like to get it right in the eyes of colleagues and the world. Doctors consider, probably in common with most of the population, that identifying a rare physical disease is more satisfying and prestigious than finding a common psychological ailment or social problem. Gray and Bentovim (1996) write of the great difficulty of persuading doctors referring children to Great Ormond Street of the factitious nature of their patients' illnesses, despite overwhelming evidence.

Doctors also enjoy the psychological rewards afforded by medical practice with its inevitable hierarchy of knowledge, skill and power: a hierarchy which favours those with the greatest physical power in their hands. With certain notable exceptions, and often for good reasons, paediatricians have been focused on children and less interested in parents themselves and their social and psychological circumstances. These truths about parents and doctors have not prevented the basic facts of 'the bargain' being honoured for much of the time and 'good enough' medicine being dispensed.

Changes in children's health care and their impact on 'the bargain'

Increased medical contacts

The first change to note is that at the time of writing the contact in Western societies between children and health care professionals is enormously increased by comparison with fifty years ago. Whilst the 'bargain' and the individuals within it may have altered little in this time, the context in which it operates has undergone radical change. Visits to primary care have more than doubled between 1955 and 1981 (see Table 2.1). Contacts with secondary services have also risen. It seems unlikely that those growing up in the 1950s received as much secondary care as a sample of Salford secondary school children in 1989, of whom 77 per cent of a random sample of 206 eleven to sixteen year olds had been patients at the local children's hospital (this excluded birth records) (Eminson, personal communication). Paediatric hospital admissions have continued to rise inexorably from the 1950s onwards. Medical admissions at Edinburgh's Royal Hospital for Sick Children increased steadily from 1500 in 1950 to 4500 in 1993, whilst average length of stay fell from twelve to just over three days (Forfar and Arneil, 1998). In the North West of England, paediatric hospitalizations in those under fourteen years rose from 27.9 per 1000 population in 1974 to 46.9 in 1984. Medical (as opposed to surgical) admissions of children under one year made the greatest contribution to this rapid rise (North West Regional Health Authority, 1988). Further evidence is offered by examining survival of children, by comparison with fifty years ago: children survive with extreme prematurity, with renal disease identified before birth, with the majority of childhood leukaemias, with major gastric malformations – all closely involved in receiving substantial amounts of health care for much of

Table 2.1 Consultation rates in primary care per 1000 population of children and young adolescents between 1955 and 1992

Age (years)	1955–56	1971–72	1981–82	1991–92
0–4		7538	9815	9930
	6287			
5–14		3815	4159	4309

Source: Morbidity Statistics from General Practice, 1958, 1979, 1986, 1995.

their lives. Children who just about survived previously now survive longer and with better health, but as a result of more intensive and invasive treatments (e.g. children with diabetes, asthma or cystic fibrosis). There has been an accompanying massive growth in those specializing in the care of children, mostly doctors. A crude measure, the expansion of membership of the British Paediatric Association (founded in 1928), now the Royal College of Paediatrics and Child Health (see Table 2.2), is perhaps the most powerful significant single statistic: these are children's doctors and there are a lot more of them. There is no disagreement about the fact that these increases are of enormous positive benefit both to those children who survive who previously did not, and to those who now receive better care. My argument is that this has produced much increased contact between doctors and children and that effects incidental to the benefits may merit attention.

Higher stakes and increased risks
What else has been happening whilst this explosion in contact between children and health care has taken place? Some things have not changed: first, it remains primarily mothers who take responsibility for the care of children; second, children remain dependent upon adults to advocate their needs; and third, it is parents (mostly mothers) who bring them to doctors. As a result of the changes mentioned in the previous paragraph, contact between parents and the health care system has increased markedly: the juxtaposition of the two major forces, the parent and the doctor, in 'the bargain' of health care is much closer and much more frequent than previously. Leaving aside any changes in medicine or in doctors' approaches or ethics, this places the parental side of the bargain under greater pressure, and

Table 2.2 Specialists medical care for children: membership of the British Paediatric Association (now the Royal College of Paediatrics and Child Health) from 1940 to 1999

1940	1950	1960	1970	1980	1990	1999
92	138	309	522	1072	2361	4975

Source: Royal College of Paediatrics and Child Health.

parental skills in responsibility and advocacy are in greater demand. For doctors too, the potential of medicine and surgery to carry out invasive procedures was, for a long period, much more limited than it is today. A second key change is that nowadays the stakes being played for are higher than ever before. Medicines are more powerful, operations more heroic, and opportunities for intimate access to children's bloodstreams (through drips or central lines), to their gastrointestinal tracts (through gastrostomy buttons and other stomas and feeding tubes), to their renal tracts (through catheters and urinary diversions), and to their respiratory systems (through tracheotomies and ventilators) are more extensive than at any time in our history. These factors provide huge opportunity for care and for health and, on the other hand, enormous dangers. The potential exists for extraordinarily rapid and extensive manipulation and abuse if mistakes are made or if there is malign intent.

Certain medical specialties are especially vulnerable to manipulation of course, especially if parents lie. Gastroenterology and urology and their surgical side are especially obvious victims, for reported problems of failing to thrive, of vomiting and of passing urine uncontrollably are all hard to dispute. These functions and their distortions are likely to be heavily affected by psychological and developmental factors and, in studying them, doctors must rely on reported history. This may be an unacceptable notion to some doctors and parents: each for different reasons may succumb to an urge to find an 'intrinsic' cause for reports of symptoms, and to act to 'resolve' the problems rather than to reflect on the complaint. Investigations like urinary flow and pressure studies are highly vulnerable to belief and without substantial norms which take into account psychological factors (the most powerful factors after all). Such 'new' disorders as 'pseudo-obstruction' can prove a fertile ground for active gastroenterologists egged on or threatened by parents with an agenda and many complaints.

Increased involvement of parents in care

A third significant change is the access that parents have to their children once they have entered the health care system. Until about twenty years ago parents handed their children to nurses once the hospital threshold was crossed and, as a result, a trained and relatively impartial workforce tended to the administration of treatment, the observation of symptoms and signs and decisions about suffering and surgery. (The exceptions to this professional standard, such as Beverley Allitt, the nurse who in 1993 was convicted of murdering a number of children in her care, are so unusual as to be noteworthy.) Previously, when children were in hospital, parents were sent home and access for visits was limited. In 1948, on being admitted to the Royal Manchester Children's Hospital for plastic surgery to her palate, an eight year old was told her parents would not be allowed to visit for a fortnight, to 'let her settle'. Children were sometimes abandoned into hospital care by neglectful parents, but leaving aside these unusual circumstances, the arena for parents was much more circumscribed once they entered either out-patient or in-patient care. The contexts of these hospital visits have changed out of all recognition. In response to a growing recognition of the adverse effects on children of parent–child separations (Robertson, 1970) and the beneficial effects of parental presence in reducing fears and distress, parental access to children in hospital has steadily increased. Pressure from groups such as the National Association for the Welfare of Children in Hospital (NAWCH) has ensured that parental presence in the paediatric wards, often throughout the twenty-four hours, is now axiomatic. Indeed the parent's role in carrying out much of the care of the children, completing their charts and making observations of them, is now relied upon in many units. The child patient's notes are often freely available in the ward for parents or others to inspect and contribute to, rather than closeted in an office. There is a greater openness between parents and ward professionals, especially nurses, who are not infrequently on first name terms. Thus access for parents has increased markedly and they are now much more active participants in an environment where these same parents have an important role. These changes in practice have much to recommend them but some of the results may not be those anticipated and hoped for when they were introduced.

Changes in parent–professional relationships

A fourth difference in circumstances from fifty years ago, is the security of the arena within which doctors operate. The climate in which we work is one of much greater concern about litigation than previously. This is a realistic concern, in that litigation in all areas of life (not just medicine) has increased, and where defence against possible future criticism is used as a rationale for investigations. The result has been an alteration in the balance of power between parents and doctors in favour of parents. The distance between all professionals and 'health consumers' has diminished.

In the same period, the trust placed by members of the general public in their doctors has declined and the respect afforded to doctors has diminished. The percentage of patients in the USA willing to use the family doctor as a source of 'local health care information' declined from 44 per cent in 1984 to 21 per cent in 1989. Twenty-six per cent of patients said they respected doctors less now than ten years ago (Gallup poll in 1990 quoted by Shorter (1992)). All British doctors will be aware of similar trends here. In the UK, the 'Bristol' cases where parents trusted surgeons' skills, which were then found wanting, may have proved a watershed in this respect. So when parents, in their more powerful position, request or demand investigations, the possibilities for unnecessary and intrusive acts by doctors upon children, and the pressure which doctors feel to undertake these investigations, are much increased. The vignettes described later in this book ('Unexplained vomiting', p. 134, 'Gastro-oesophogeal reflux investigations' p. 134, and 'Unnecessary intrusion' p. 135) give examples where doctors are viewed by their colleagues as having been recruited to harm children by intrusive and (in the judgement of the authors) unnecessary care. The GPs in the epidemiological study described earlier felt they could not refuse investigations or referrals if patients demanded them for their children, however healthy those children were deemed to be by the GP. A simple case example is offered here.

An apologetic referral

A three year old boy was referred to a specialist renal clinic by a secondary paediatrician. The child had suffered a single urinary tract infection with lower urinary tract signs. A DMSA scan and micturating cystourethrogram (MCU) were normal. The referral letter apologized for referring the patient and also commented that the MCU was not justified using guidelines operated in the referring department, but had been performed to try to reassure the mother. In the out-patient clinic routine detailed discussion about the benign but sometimes troublesome nature of lower urinary tract infections only seemed to increase the mother's 'anxiety'. She was invited to write down her concerns and bring them to the next out-patient visit. She arrived at the next visit with five pages of questions.

Comment

This boy was referred 'apologetically' to a specialist service. We are told he had already had a micturating cystourethrogram against the protocol of the unit, 'to try to reassure the mother' in addition to a less invasive procedure. Thus the three year old received a physical assault and unnecessary radiation with normal findings. The 'apology' is presumably because the doctors deemed both this assault, and the referral, unnecessary. Thirty years ago such an investigation would have been, for a three year old child, the provenance only of a specialist service and probably rather unusual for them. The modern opportunity to irradiate a three year old without any medical rationale, and inflict distress and physical assault upon his genitalia using the justification of improving his mother's mental state, was not at that time available. When the technology and skill to carry out such procedures are more widely available, the opportunities for abuse also become more widespread. It is necessary for all paediatricians to become as skilled in their management of the mother's so-called 'anxiety' in the consultation, as in management of the renal tract disease. They must be confident they can evaluate objectively the need for investigations to manage the child's condition, rather than acting in response to the expressed maternal concerns. In this case, the label of 'anxiety' has been applied by the paediatrician to describe what he thought the mother was feeling. Perhaps she was anxious, she certainly left the doctors feeling under pressure. The referring doctors in this scenario seem to have felt extremely uncertain about their position if they refused what they saw as unnecessary investigations. (No investigations were necessary so this child was in effect physically abused.)

Thus the original 'bargain' of health care has come gradually to be translated into another one: because doctors assume parents are truthful in their account of their children's symptoms and behaviour, if parents continue to complain about their children, doctors must continue to investigate and treat. This continuation is synonymous with physical investigations and treatment.

Summary of changes with an impact on the 'bargain' of health care

To summarize: there has been an increase in the contact between children and health care in primary and secondary settings, with many more admissions, contacts and treatments; there has been an increase in medical activities and power to intrude; a decrease in doctors' power and confidence to disperse these health care resources and treatments as they see fit; a greater sense that parents' demands and preferences take precedence; and an increase in access for parents to hospitals, wards and health care. The result is to bring parents, doctors and children closer together, more intimately, more often. This places the 'bargain' under new pressures. This would be unimportant if all parents were balanced in their judgements and perceptions of their child. But assumptions about parental universal beneficence were always false and parents with a more complex personal agenda and ambivalence about their children are now in the health care arena much more often than before. Parents are in a much more powerful position in relation to doctors than ever before; it is a novel and exciting position for those who have perhaps been relatively powerless, to find themselves in with those formerly so powerful, the medical profession. Most importantly, parents are in the driving seat in demanding that investigations and procedures be carried out, with the sense that this is their right, an entitlement. But doctors are no better equipped than fifty years ago to talk to children themselves, or to understand parental psychopathology, which has previously been largely an irrelevance or a nuisance at best, something to be left to social workers or psychologists perhaps. Doctors are in a much less powerful position than fifty years ago to deny parents the things they ask for. Perhaps it is not surprising that more parents simply take the opportunities this affords to meet their own needs rather than their children's in these circumstances. The health care system then becomes a place where parental psychopathology can be displayed and in which doctors can be trammelled.

Parents at risk of exploiting the changed 'bargain'

The previous section outlined radical changes resulting in the appearance of an opportunity for parents to be more present and more powerful in a health care arena. Which groups of parents might be most at risk of using this opportunity in unexpected and unwelcome ways? To address this question it is necessary to review briefly what is known about the risk factors for child abuse generally, and the effects of emotional abuse.

Risk factors for abuse

Most readers will be familiar with the factors that predispose to abuse of chidden, and many such factors are, of course, interrelated. Most of these factors should be considered at any consultation between paediatricians and parents about a child, especially a child who is too young to contribute meaningfully to the substance of the consultation.

1. **Characteristics of the parent's own childhood.** A childhood characterized by abuse and neglect, a failure to acquire compensatory positive experiences in care, at school or with other adults.
2. **Parents' enduring characteristics.** Low intellectual ability, personality disorders, long-standing drug and alcohol dependency.

3. **Factors which affect the skills a parent develops.** Having depression or other psychiatric problems (which produce distortions in the way the child is viewed), being insensitive to the child's needs, immature, extremely young (which makes it difficult to put the child's needs first), being brought up in a culture and history of violence.

4. **The physical environment.** Poor housing, debt, a neighbourhood culture of violence and fear.

5. **The parent's social supports.** Lack of partner or an unhelpful partner, unemployment, lack of supportive friends or neighbours, lack of close relationships with one's own family. One result of these is another factor: lack of respite from the child.

6. **Immediate or proximal triggers in the family situation.** Factors which make the parent disinhibited and irritable such as; substance abuse, tiredness, a recent argument, low mood.

7. **Characteristics of relationships with the child.** Problems developing normal attachment, an unwanted pregnancy, premature birth, early separations and lack of biological connection, i.e. being a step-parent.

8. **Characteristics which increase the likelihood of this child becoming a victim of abuse.** Having special needs or chronic illness, having a frequent or high pitched cry and a 'difficult' temperament – this involves irregularity of biological functions e.g. being slow to settle into a sleeping/waking pattern, having intense mood expression (often negative), slow adaptability to change, displaying negative withdrawing responses to new stimuli.

This set of risk factors does not automatically create an abusive parent: it remains a set of vulnerability factors which may interact to result in child abuse. As ever, this will depend upon an interlocking set of circumstances which will end, on any particular day, with 'good enough' parenting or, conversely, with physical, sexual or emotional abuse of the child, depending on trigger factors, strength of feeling and a variety of extraneous circumstances including available supports. Which of these parents might be most vulnerable to the new invitations offered by the changes in the health care environment? Not all these parents at risk have an equal likelihood of abuse of an 'MSBP' type which includes exaggeration of symptoms, invention of symptoms, fabrication and induction of illness (directly, by poisoning or suffocation, or indirectly by allowing doctors to carry out unnecessary treatment). Broadly speaking, parents at risk are most likely to reproduce the experience they had themselves: those who were physically abused risk physical harm to their children; those sexually abused have the most difficulty with establishing appropriate sexual boundaries. Those who are emotionally abused will be at greatest risk of acting in an emotionally abusive way to their children.

Types of emotional abuse and effects in childhood

One of the many problems of emotional abuse is that it is the least visible and least well-measured form of harm done to children. It produces adults who themselves have more subtle difficulties with relationships than may be evident in those who have had more major and grossly physically distorted experiences. Those who are emotionally abused and also have social and educational disadvantages, particularly those who are limited intellectually, have several extra layers of problems. This will make for substantial difficulties in relating to adults and to one's own children. Garbarino, Guttman and Seeley (1987) described five types of emotional abuse, all of which are seen very commonly in mild forms.

1. **Isolating.** The adult removes the child from normal social experiences, preventing him/her from developing friendships and making the child feel that he or she is alone in the world.
2. **Terrorizing.** The adult bullies the child or mounts a campaign of verbal or physical attack that makes the child believe that the world is capricious and hostile.
3. **Rejecting.** The parent abandons the child physically and/or psychologically, or rejects the child's legitimate physical and emotional needs.
4. **Ignoring.** More passive and neglectful than rejecting, ignoring refers to a parent who deprives the child of essential stimulation and responsiveness by virtue of parental incapacity and/or self-preoccupation.
5. **Corrupting.** Parental behaviour that trains the child to be socially deviant, antisocial, or otherwise unfit for normal social experience qualifies for this term.

Of course, leaving aside the elements of physical assault, the first four of these, especially terrorizing, rejecting and ignoring, characterize the experience of a child who is subject to MSBP abuse, when their parent imagines or fabricates ill-health.

Responses to emotional abuse

There is every reason to think that emotional abuse is experienced equally by boys and girls, but the way the two sexes respond is likely to be affected by biological, cultural and social factors which mediate to alter likely ways the effects will be shown. For both sexes the effect of severe emotional abuse is to produce individuals who are lonely, who find it hard to trust others, who are used to capricious emotional responses and as a result rarely show their own feelings directly, who have difficulty knowing what they are feeling because they have so often been told what they must think, do and feel (rather than asked), and who have therefore been encouraged to ignore their own distress, mental and physical. It is difficult to grow up being truthful if one comes from such a background. It may be difficult to know the cause of physically distressing bodily sensations experienced. Some grow up with a great drive to take power over others, perhaps those who have experienced more of the terrorizing and ignoring. Some grow up with uncertainty about the boundaries of 'themselves', perhaps because they have dissociated from and split off some parts of their own intolerable feelings and experiences as children. They may then experience similar difficulties with the boundaries of their children and their bodies. One of the characteristics of some of those whose own needs have been ignored in this way is that they develop an urge to care for others: to do to others that which was not done for them, i.e. nurturing care, which also involves power too. For women particularly this is an acceptable role in our society and is accompanied by a habit of denying their own feelings, and instead acting as carers and feeling useful and fulfilled through looking after others. Many jobs open to women in this society, such as nursing, health care assistant and foster carer, allow this role to be fulfilled. It goes without saying that many less damaged individuals choose the same path. Becoming a mother oneself is, of course, another version of the same solution.

A proportion of these emotionally abused children will come from families where the vocabulary available for feelings was itself truncated and diminished; at its most extreme this is known as 'alexithymia' (no word for feelings) (and, of course, it is found in families that are not abusive as well as those that are). This tendency to have trouble finding words for feelings will be exacerbated by general cognitive difficulties. In some such families it seems that physical symptoms (which may themselves be due to the experience of emotional distress but not recognized or acknowledged as such) are experienced and expressed with greater ease than emotions. Physical symptoms may elicit a response from a parent or partner, and in some families may bring about affection and care. At its extreme, this is known as 'conditional caretaking' – affection given for physical complaints which is not delivered if emotional distress is present or shown directly. Children in 'alexithymic families' and in those which have different constellations but which are emotionally abusive and neglectful, continue to want and need the ordinary attention, care and affection of adults. Many will experience and complain of physical symptoms and receive attention as a result; even so the child is probably not properly nurtured emotionally but a pattern has been established. The child will be attentive to what elicits care and affection from their parents.. (They will perhaps be described as 'manipulative' when doing this at school.) Coincidentally, some may also receive more extensive hospital treatment themselves, providing an even richer learning experience of the positive and nurturing effects of health care. However, it is the author's impression that even without such an experience, both substantial and trivial, bizarre and commonplace psychosomatic and factitious presentations are extremely common in emotionally abused children and young people. Some of these children, both boys and girls, will also intermittently experience common psychiatric symptoms of anxiety and depression, which themselves are associated with an increase in the experience and reporting of somatic complaints with or without an abusive history (Goodyer, 1996). Such young people may demonstrate self harm with overdoses but also sometimes cutting and scratching, or other non-specific physical problems, sometimes mixed with eating disorders or bulimia, demonstrating how one may have problems in trusting one's own body, and in responding to its signals. They will demonstrate a pattern of difficulty in confiding and use of their somatic complaints as a way of signalling emotional distress (but usually without the capacity to develop a relationship based on a more honest exchange). This can occur up to and including a level of dissociation or dislocation from one's body to such an extreme degree as may also be found in the somatoform disorders. These include multiple pain syndromes, numerous unexplained physical complaints and also factitious illness such as damaging and picking at skin, eyes and other wounds. The term 'young people with somatic focus' broadly describes this very disparate group.

Long term effects of emotional abuse in those who develop a somatic focus: somatoform disorders, emotional disorders and relationship difficulties

As emotionally abused young people with somatic focus start to grow up they present to services in a variety of ways. The characteristics of patients (adults) with severe somatoform disorders, of whom a substantial minority are men, is that they coerce attention from health care professionals by presenting with symptoms whilst not seeming to experience more than temporary relief from the diagnosis, treatment and operations they receive. Their somatic presentations are, to a mental health professional, a way of presenting their distress about them-selves, but one that is highly dysfunctional because the resulting physical care fails to assuage the distress. There are many different degrees and forms of pres-entation with unexplained physical complaints. The most extreme of these are the factitious illnesses, of which the eponymous label 'Munchausen syndrome' is used as shorthand for those who are persistent in their invention of symptoms, their presentations 'demanding' medical and nursing care, with fabricated histo-ries and signs which justify their 'need' for health care demands. Most such patients angrily deny emotional distress and many reject psychological explana-tions and help. The patients in turn elicit anger and frustration from health care professionals. To read some of the descriptive accounts of 'Munchausen syn-drome' patients by Asher (1951) and Blackwell (1965) is instructive, as one gains a sense of the isolation but also the persistent drive which accompanies this dys-functional pattern of behaviour. These accounts, and more recent ones (Rosenberg, 1995), paint a picture of an underlying pattern of psychosomatic and relationship problems which may be long-standing, but, within this, the pattern of hospital attendance and health care seeking may be triggered (or interrupted) at any time by other psychosocial stresses, such as marital conflict and breakdown.

Whilst an extreme picture has been presented here, there is a wide range of pat-terns of response to emotional abuse in those with a somatic focus – from the extreme picture above, to much milder forms in individuals with a tendency to somatize distress, particularly at times of stress and when psychologically vul-nerable. The much commoner milder presentations include those with depression, anxiety or other mental health problems: these are individuals who have received enough positive parental care or compensatory experience to be relatively intact in their awareness of their own body, although this may become distorted at stressful times.

The risks for children emerging from both greater and lesser degrees of child-hood emotional abuse, in addition to the constellation of somatizing symptoms and problems, include becoming a young adult with particular difficulty in close relationships, especially with honesty, confiding in another person, and in acknowledging feelings (especially negative ones such as anger). Friendships and other relationships, when formed, may be superficial and lack deeper levels of trust. These problems will produce difficulties when forming intimate partner-ships.

Severe disturbance as an outcome of a combination of emotional abuse, psychosocial disadvantage and disrupted attachments

The picture painted so far is one which includes the most extreme examples of emotional abuse, often combined with other forms of abuse, which will themselves give their most extreme effects in those who are disadvantaged socially and intellectually and who have also received disrupted childhood's with parental relationship breakdowns, periods in care, and grossly disrupted attachments. Not all of these people display somatization as a response, but they are likely, if they become parents, to display their difficulties through their children. They are the group of parents who will display the first, the earliest, the grossest, most physical forms of abuse (including MSBP abuse, usually directly induced) in their foetuses or babies. If the pattern is not interrupted early it will probably continue. The more disturbed the individual, the earlier the problems are likely to appear. These adults have enormous difficulties in relation to their own bodies and lives, exhibiting gross somatization sometimes, disrupted relationships and failure to complete education. Their parenting difficulties (difficulty with the bodies of and relationships with their children) are also displayed extremely and immediately, even during pregnancy, but certainly quickly thereafter. They will use a variety of primitive and undesirable child rearing practices, including putting their hand over a child's mouth to stop it crying (Van der Wal *et al.*, 1998). Being a parent is almost incidental to their severe difficulties in all aspects of life. A formulation of the difficulties of Vanessa, a mother perpetrating MSBP abuse, is now presented. Vanessa's is a typical case of a young woman who was vulnerable to committing abuse either in or out of a health care setting. The child became a conduit for the feelings and behaviour of his mother, feelings expressed in other ways before and after the child was available to be a victim of them.

Vanessa was the eldest of four children of a forces family. Temperamentally, from very early on she was strong willed and had intense reactions including severe, unchanging jealousy of her fifteen month younger sister, and was very oppositional with a cruel streak. Vanessa's mother found it hard to manage the children and hard to like Vanessa; there were several house and country moves because of father's postings and as a result Vanessa's mother lacked the support of her own family. The marriage had difficult periods when father drank heavily. Vanessa grew up hostile and argumentative, with aggressive antisocial behaviours at home and school and problems with friendships; her parents used harsh and punitive methods to try and coerce her into compliance.

From the age of twelve Vanessa began running away and social services were involved; Vanessa dropped out of school, took overdoses and cut herself on occasion, spent time in foster care, and became involved in petty crime and possibly prostitution, with her whereabouts unknown to her family for periods of weeks at a time. She did not consult doctors frequently but occasionally had dramatic and unusual symptoms. When Vanessa was fifteen she became pregnant (the father was unknown) and family relationships improved briefly, with mother becoming more sympathetic to Vanessa, who returned home more often whilst simultaneously preparing to live independently in a flat.

Following the birth of a normal baby son, Vanessa stayed at her parents' home. When the baby was ten days old Vanessa said she noticed he had had an episode when he went pale and blue around the lips and stopped breathing; they rushed to hospital. There were no evident ill-effects, no cause was found and reassurance was offered. Over the next few weeks there were numerous 'apnoeic attacks' and the baby was kept in hospital more and more, his attacks puzzling the staff. After initially appearing to enjoy being in hospital, where she stayed in the hospital parents' accommodation, Vanessa became more unpredictable in her moods and behaviour, she stole from other parents and set fire to furnishings. Hospital staff, who had not been suspicious about the nature of the early 'apnoeic attacks', came to dislike Vanessa and to be concerned about her parenting of the baby, who was finally removed from his mother at four months of age, having sustained a fractured femur. Whilst never confirmed, it seems very likely that Vanessa had suffocated the baby to produce the 'apnoeic attacks'. Vanessa, whilst on bail for the assault on her son, became involved with a young man in committing a violent crime.

Commentary on the case example

Vanessa's background was a deprived one both socially and emotionally: factors in her and in the relationships seem to have resulted in Vanessa becoming the most disturbed of all her siblings. With small children close together, far away from her own family, unsupported, with a husband who drank heavily, Vanessa's mother had great difficulty providing a warm and non-judgmental nurturance. She may have been depressed and certainly blamed the children for her own unhappiness. Early relationships in the family followed a textbook example of patterns of physical and emotional abuse which produce conduct and relationship problems in the children. The parenting was punitive and cold, there were early problems between Vanessa and her mother, with attachment difficulties, and later there were critical, coercive parenting strategies and interactions characterized by scapegoating, aggression and impulsive decision making.

Temperamentally Vanessa was strong willed all her life and had intense reactions. She must have been a very difficult child to parent. At school Vanessa could not be contained emotionally, made few friends, had difficulty achieving academically, acted out against others and met no adult figure who warmed to her. Despite problems at home, some children can establish a source of successful relationships at school, but this did not occur. Vanessa's problems with friendships during middle childhood start to indicate pervasive relationship problems with family, siblings and other authority figures.

The breakdown in the family when Vanessa entered adolescence gives a measure of the severity of the problems. Social workers were also unable to make trusting relationships with Vanessa; children's mental health professionals were involved but the parents were reluctant to try to change and Vanessa could not be engaged. Vanessa would have met criteria for a conduct disorder in adolescence, with antisocial and impulsive risk taking behaviours (self harm, overdoses) in her early adolescence suggestive of severe relationship difficulties and a wish to pursue excitement and novelty (substance abuse), and little concern about how other people feel and think. She had mood swings, with a mixture of anger and misery. Later in adulthood Vanessa met personality disorder criteria. This history contains no significant element of somatization.

For such a young person, providing the care needed by a small baby must have been very demanding, and major parenting problems were (quite accurately) anticipated. There was no obvious immediate trigger for Vanessa's cruel behaviour to her baby: only the existence and demands of the baby in a situation where an extremely vulnerable young woman was living with her family. Vanessa probably suffocated her baby to produce the apnoeic attack at ten days, having for once an obvious recipient for her frustration and fury, and being obliged to spend her time in care of the infant. She was quite incapable of imagining how the baby might feel. Whether this first episode was factitious or not, it produced a drama in which Vanessa was a central and important figure, and quickly removed her from her parents' home to an alternative and nurturing environment. The sequence seems to have been a satisfying one, for it was frequently repeated. Did Vanessa simply enjoy her power over the baby? Was the baby punished for being so demanding of Vanessa's time, for reminding Vanessa of how powerless she felt herself in childhood, for being difficult to comfort? Was he a thrilling toy to frighten and then to bring back to life, or an incidental object who enabled Vanessa to enter an arena where she had a satisfying role to play which met her needs? The hospital seems likely to have been simply an incidental place where these problems were manifest, an escape route rather than an active choice.

Risks for the future

Vanessa never acknowledged her abusive acts to any significant extent. The early severe injury and the suffocations, together with her denial, antisocial acts and difficulties in relationships with anyone, make it unlikely she will be able to parent a child safely. The courts removed her baby permanently and Vanessa went to prison for her other offences.

Long-standing somatization, factitious illness and factitious illness by proxy: the drive to somatization for oneself and one's children

The effects of a well organized, stable background characterized by emotional deprivation, problems in family communication about feelings, including 'conditional caretaking' in some cases, may in the context of certain relationship and temperamental variables, lead to long-standing somatization in a child, with profound effects when the child becomes a parent. Ways in which this may proceed along a pathway to factitious illness and MSBP abuse are now explored.

Emotional abuse is certainly no respecter of class or intellectual ability boundaries, and when it occurs in families that are stable, better organized and with greater educational attainments, we cannot expect that the individuals emerging will appear to be so obviously dysfunctional as in the preceding example. Indeed, those from less disorganized families will merge, with many less abusive variants, actually and apparently, into the rest of the population, who have not received such an abusive early life. As a group, when becoming parents, such individuals will seek to resolve their own psychological discomforts in the best way they can, but the same mechanisms (somatization and caring for others) may be used to attempt resolution of their feelings following their emotionally abusive childhood. It is to be expected that the more intellectually capable of such individuals will find themselves in caring professions such as nursing. Not only does the job provide the psychological solution of care for others as a proxy way of caring for oneself, but the social and peer group contact involved in training and working as a nurse (for example) provides automatic companionship and easy access to relationships which are, as has been described, otherwise so difficult. A superficial level of friendship is much easier to maintain within a group of colleagues who naturally associate because of unsocial hours and similar interests. The other psychological advantage of roles such as nursing is the power entailed over patients, their families, even over doctors. For this is the other element in emotional abuse: that the child is a victim and this too may have its inevitable consequence in adulthood, of the former victim coming to identify with the (psychological) aggressor. But such individuals who have struggled to resolve and cope with the impact of an abusive childhood in the best way they can, bringing with them an individual mixture of traits and experiences, will still be vulnerable when the level of demand rises (psychological demand is referred to here). Parenting one's own children is, of course, the most psychologically demanding task faced by most people in their lifetime.

When those with an emotionally abusive background (whether or not combined with other forms of abuse and attachment difficulty) become parents themselves, they are inevitably handicapped by their problems, including their distorted, inaccurate perceptions of themselves and their bodies and their uncertainties about the boundaries of their own feelings and responsibilities. Many continue to use attendance at health care as a way of eliciting care for themselves. The existence of a child provides extra stresses (and results in difficulties in managing the children's behaviour: itself a cause of increased consulting in primary care) and extra opportunities to elicit care through attendance with children. Given that it is women who give birth to children (and who indeed, in severe cases, use their foetuses' bodies whilst pregnant to display their extreme difficulties through obstetric factitious symptoms) and women who also deliver most of the care of children, it is not surprising that it is women who mostly use their children as a way to gain care for themselves, or to gain help in coping with a variety of worries and concerns (Kai, 1996a and 1996b). This simple fact may explain most of the preponderance of women perpetrating MSBP abuse, although other possibilities exist.

The first group of parents described, i.e. poor, unsupported and socially disadvantaged families (such as Vanessa's) contains those with the greatest vulnerabilities to become abusive. They are also the group with the greatest use of secondary paediatric care for their children (Spencer, Lewis and Logan, 1993). This paper demonstrated that hospital admissions for such families are seen to serve both a social and a medical purpose: that hospitals are asked to provide support and care for poor and inadequate parents. So the parents at greatest risk of abusing their children will probably have opportunity to experience this environment in hospital at times when they are under the greatest stress. For some of these parents, then, the hospital is a place where coincidentally the same behaviour is displayed as at home, such as for those restless and uncomfortable people whose parenting and relationships with adults are under the most severe stress, as in Vanessa's case (see earlier vignette). But for other parents, with more specific emotional and developmental distortions, other specific aspects of the hospital environment may be important. For those with the highest levels of emotional abuse in their own pasts, and the greatest tendency to emotional cruelty to their own children as a result, the hospital provides special opportunity to act out their difficulties in a particular environment, which already provides a 'solution' to their sense of discomfort with their child's body and their need for care and attention.

Which of these vulnerable parents, coping with difficulty with their children, might be especially likely to find seeking health care an attractive proposition to which they might be drawn? Perhaps we should consider a less direct intentional motive or purpose, where the parent might learn by experience the benefits of such a course. Obviously those who have already demonstrated their preoccupation with their own health, and who have displayed their own psychological difficulties through abnormal illness behaviour, would be prime candidates to learn quickly that psychological benefits accrue from health care given to their children as well as themselves. So parents who are frequent attenders in primary and secondary care, and those with somatization disorders are likely to derive the same gratification from health care attendance for their children as they do for themselves.

There are many factors which may exacerbate such difficulties or may trigger a bout of presentations. Amongst frequent attenders in both primary and secondary care there is an excess of parents, especially women, who have psychiatric problems, particularly anxiety and depression. Anxious and depressed parents are themselves more likely to experience and report more somatic symptoms (Craig *et al.,* 1993), and are more likely to present their children at health care facilities (Bowman and Garralda, 1993). Any psychiatric difficulty, be it anxiety, depression, eating disorders, personality difficulties or substance abuse, makes it more likely that a parent will have difficulty managing their children, who are in turn more likely to have behaviour difficulties (Oates, 1997; White and Barrowclough, 1998; Cooper and Murray, 1998; Bates and Bayles, 1988; Wooley, Wheatcroft and Stein, 1998). All of these variables, i.e. parental depression and anxiety, children's physical ill-health and children's behaviour problems, increase the likelihood of health care attendance, although most of these will not reach an abusive threshold. It is to be expected that paediatric wards will contain a population heavily weighted with both parents and children with emotional, behavioural and relationship difficulties as well as those who are poor and socially disadvantaged.

For all of them, a period of hospital care may provide warmth, respite and distraction. Another characteristic of the group of vulnerable, potentially abusive parents is their difficulty within relationships generally, so that they are often single or in unsupportive relationships. Their interpersonal relationships are often unrewarding, in part because their own early experiences have damaged their capacity for attachment (Ney, 1994; Garbarino and Ebata, 1983).

The case example of Jean (below) combines many of the known vulnerabilities for 'classical' MSBP abuse including a mixture of induced and invented illness, with a stable family, a history of emotional abuse and somatization, and problems managing children's behaviour – clear predisposing factors and triggers to episodes of fabrication. It illustrates the pathways and transactions in the development of MSBP abuse.

Jean was the younger of two children, was born and grew up in the north of the country, a plump, shy girl, with few friends. When she was seven her mother was found to have a rare disease, after a year of mysterious symptoms and many trips to doctors. The parents were devastated and decided to move back to the area the mother came from, in the west of Britain, so as to be closer to her family of origin. Jean and her brother moved into a local school where they were subjected to much teasing and ridicule because of their accents. Jean's older sisters adapted quickly, adopting a local accent, but Jean withdrew into herself and seems to have made little connection with either children or teachers at school. Her father was a powerful, intrusive man who ran a small business and dominated all aspects of the family's life, whilst the mother's illness deteriorated quite quickly. She and Jean never had a confiding relationship, and Jean was also distant from her sisters who emigrated to Australia and did not keep in touch. Jean's mother died when Jean was ten and her father remarried quickly thereafter.

In early and middle childhood Jean was not taken to doctors frequently, and there is no good account of whether she experienced numerous physical symptoms at home. From the age of twelve onwards she was seen very frequently by her GP, initially with upper respiratory tract infections, and then with other pains, and trouble with her ear, fainting and many other non-specific symptoms. At the age of fifteen she went on a school canoeing trip. Much later Jean said she was raped by one of the boys on this trip. This was not reported at the time, but Jean sprained her knee and, on return from the holiday, complaints about her knee brought numerous consultations at the GP, A & E and orthopaedics: objectively there were no abnormal findings. Jean stayed away from school for a great deal of time and started hanging about the town where she lived, on the edge of a crowd of other young people, drinking a bit but still with no firm friendships.

Leaving school at sixteen Jean had no qualifications, and no future college or career plans. She never had a job for more than a few days. She continued to be a frequent consulter of her GP: her doctor sometimes tried to talk to Jean about her mood, wondering if she was depressed, but Jean never confided well. Jean's major recreation was spending evenings at the local pub and there, when she was eighteen, she became friendly with one of the other regulars, Daniel, who was a single man living with his dominant and powerful mother and working as a gardener. Despite the opposition of both their parents, Jean and Daniel moved in together and married when Jean was eighteen and Daniel twenty-seven. Jean was more intelligent than Daniel, who was a quiet and extremely unassertive man. Jean was always dominant in the marriage (i.e. Daniel reproduced the power relationships he had previously had with his mother). Jean and Daniel later reported that the sexual side of their marriage was never enjoyable.

Their first-born child Adrienne was a healthy girl, bottle fed. Within a few days of her birth Jean was having difficulty with the baby. She would apparently not feed well, was constantly posseting and vomiting and cried a good deal. The health visitor was worried by the way Jean fed and managed her. Adrienne was admitted to the local hospital several times because of feeding problems. Jean was very friendly with the nursing staff, who also recognized that she had problems. Jean's facade as a competent mother seems to have cracked during an admission when Adrienne was about nine months old. Jean left the hospital ward and came back having been drinking, was abusive to the nurses and at one point threatened to take an overdose. Later it turned out that Jean and Daniel were getting on very badly at this time and Jean eventually told the nursing staff she was considering leaving her husband. The concerned paediatrician, recognizing there were problems in Jean herself and her mothering of Adrienne, referred Jean to an adult psychiatrist (whom she refused to see) and the whole family to child psychiatry. Jean and Daniel were outraged with these suggestions and went to only one appointment, after which Jean criticized and denigrated the services. After this crisis period, which covered two or three months when Adrienne was nine months old, the family returned home. Three weeks later, Jean announced she thought Adrienne had had a fit, she was transferred to hospital and the stories of convulsions continued. No convulsions were ever witnessed by a member of staff or another adult, although Jean told complex stories which suggested that neighbours, friends, family members and other parents on the ward had witnessed fits. Adrienne was eventually started on anticonvulsants after appropriate investigations (all normal) and her 'seizure disorder' continued to be managed by the local paediatrician with some difficulty, with numerous blood tests, investigations, use of multiple anticonvulsants and frequent hospital admissions.

Christopher was born when Adrienne was three and he too was a difficult baby to feed. Within a few weeks his mother reported 'convulsions' in Christopher, and reports of Adrienne's 'fits' subsided although they never went away. Throughout Christopher's life he too was subjected to reports of convulsions, investigated, and given anticonvulsant treatment. Through the third year of Christopher's life there were increasing complaints about

Christopher's bowels, with worries about his having diarrhoea and constipation. The local paediatrician now became suspicious and Christopher was sent for a number of investigations to a more distant regional centre: all investigations proved normal. Eventually phenolphthalein derivatives (laxative components) were found in Christopher's stools and his mother, when challenged, acknowledged poisoning him on one occasion only. She denied inventing seizures.

Removed from their parents, both children had no seizures and were taken off medication. After a brief spell with foster parents the children were placed with their maternal grandfather and his wife. Jean initially lived at home with Daniel, who tried to share himself between his wife and his children. Jean buried herself in learning about computers; the marriage remained deeply uncommunicative and the couple were unable to talk about what had happened. When Jean was charged with the assaults on the children, relationships at home became so bad that she moved to a bail hostel, to which she subsequently set fire. Psychiatric assessment at this time made clear Jean's personality disorder and many depressive symptoms.

Commentary on the case example

Background factors

This case contains many classic elements including emotional neglect and conditional caretaking in childhood, Jean's own substantial somatization, family models of illness and the fabrications providing a solution to marital difficulties.

Emotional aspects of Jean's very early life and attachments are shrouded in uncertainty although in practical terms her family was stable and well organized. Jean's own early memories are vague and idealized. Jean's father was an extremely overbearing man, and her mother emotionally unavailable because of her illness and later, her death. It is probable that the scale of the family crisis when mother's illness was discovered was such that the children's emotional well-being was not really considered. Jean was quite profoundly emotionally neglected in childhood, and received harsh discipline. Conditional caretaking was certainly present in this family: being ill seems to have been a trigger for care. There is a strong impression that the family had a problem with communication about feelings.

Much later Jean said that her father had sexually abused her in childhood but, whereas such a claim merits careful assessment, Jean's limited acknowledgement of her own poisoning of the children, her problems with truthfulness generally and the fact that she made these statements at a point where family relationships had totally broken down (her father and stepmother having custody of her children), make it difficult to know exactly what weight to put on this allegation.

Somatization and other psychiatric issues

Jean's temperament in infancy and childhood is hard to assess but she was certainly shy and withdrawn and had a characteristic difficulty with confiding relationships. Despite good average intelligence, she certainly had great difficulty expressing feelings, in honesty and in openness in relationships.

Through her adolescence, during the course of which Jean's difficulty in confiding continued, her problems were demonstrated through marked abnormal illness behaviour, with low mood and temper outbursts. Jean might have met the criteria for one of the somatoform disorders at this point, and probably had depressive symptoms too. This is not an uncommon picture of psychiatric difficulties typical of emotionally neglected adolescents from such a background, which also facilitated somatization.

Marital issues and trigger factors

Jean and Daniel's relationship, which superficially seemed to present such a successful way for each of them to escape their family of origin, was a clear example of a profoundly unsatisfactory relationship. There was great difficulty in communicating about emotional and sexual issues. Jean's insistence on her control over the children and matters relating to them led Daniel to withdraw more and more; in fact, Jean found that the children often made her feel desperate and overwhelmed. Her father would interfere and tell her what to do and the difficulties would come to a head in a report of a significant physical symptom, thus resolving the marital or child management crisis for a while by hospital admission. Thus problems in the marital and family relationships produced many occasions when Jean would induce or invent illness to provoke a change of environment. The hospital, with a team which Jean knew very well, gave her the opportunity to demonstrate herself as a caring mother, while nurses praised her for her tenacity in caring for children with such difficult epilepsy. The elements included outwitting the professionals, punishing Adrienne and Christopher for being so hard to manage, and escaping her husband, father and her own inadequate self, as well as playing a valued role in a hospital setting to reinforce that pattern.

Prognosis

The beginnings of acknowledgement in this case led to strenuous efforts by professionals to help Jean. Unfortunately the extent of the interlocking difficulties mitigated against this: the extent of Jean's personality difficulties and her inability to work with mental health services became more evident, as did her dangerousness. Daniel's passivity was extreme and he was unable to make changes to be sufficiently protective of the children or assertive with his wife. The premature placement of the children with Jean's parents prevented the necessary work on these relationships and discouraged honesty in family work. As a result, reunification was impossible and the risk remains high for any future children of Jean's.

Intermittent factitious illness by proxy: less damaged parents who are vulnerable to perpetrating abuse in circumstances that foster it

Many parents in poor social and emotional circumstances are known to use health care to provide bolstering and reassurance for their own functioning (Kai, 1996a and 1996b). Many also employ a variety of child rearing practices which include highly dysfunctional methods of quieting children, even occasionally using techniques such as brief suffocation of a crying infant (van der Wal, *et al.*, 1998). Much is known about those whose skills in managing their children are more limited. Vulnerability factors include learning difficulties and limited support, as well as the psychological vulnerabilities such as depression, which are also risk factors for increased use of health care. There is even some evidence that there is a link between parents who fail to be reassured by normal investigations of their child's headaches in a paediatric neurology clinic and those who have had significant losses, such as early loss of their own parent (Gulhati and Minty, 1998). It is relatively easy, then, to see a pattern which produces extra risk of factitious illness in a typical parent already at some risk of perpetrating neglect and abuse: such parents were abused to a degree themselves in childhood, often in care, young, single, poor at problem solving, unsupported or poorly supported by partner and family, with relationships characterized by impulsive acts and changes. Now, faced with the overwhelming demands of a small child, the mother finds herself frequently in the environment of a hospital. It is simply the case that most of those finding themselves in this position and responsible for children are young women. If they did not have small powerless children to provide the focus for their actions, they might continue to demonstrate them through somatic symptoms and somatoform disorders, or to seek to resolve their difficulties by other analogous situations, even looking after animals or children perhaps. The health care system is an attempt to meet many of their own needs for validation, warmth, importance and distraction. There will be many more or less serious and life threatening uses of the health care system by this group, which will certainly not all involve harm. They often show bouts of consultation and somatic focus on the children coinciding with periods of stress in other relationships. Continued problematic child rearing skills will continue to be displayed by these parents, some of who even provide the symptoms which justified the attendance and/or admission. Their ability to separate their needs from their child's will vary but may be extremely poor; this is often accompanied by an over-involved relationship with the child, who the mother treats as an extension of herself. In certain circumstances, perhaps linked to issues in their own past, or a particular child, they may be caught up in more complicated dramas involving over-use of medication, invented symptoms and relentlessly pushed investigations.

The case example of Jennifer illustrates this third group of parents, characterized by intermittent and varied forms of abnormal illness and consultation behaviour, also often neglecting necessary prescribed treatment for her children. Here there is a serious risk of MSBP abuse in the more disturbed or if caught up in a dangerous game with the medical profession.

Jennifer is the middle of three children who grew up in rural poverty in Lincolnshire: although neither intelligent nor articulate she was well aware of tensions in her parents' marriage in her childhood. She was frightened of her mother's unpredictable temper and in middle childhood had a long hospital admission, with a period of several enjoyable weeks in a convalescent unit, following an appendectomy. She probably always expressed emotional distress somatically, through aches, pains and complaints. When Jennifer was ten, her mother suddenly left home taking the children with her, to Jennifer's total shock and surprise. They moved in with the local butcher, with whom mother had evidently been having a clandestine affair. Relationships with her father were abruptly severed after an initial period of terrifying violent disputes between the adults. Jennifer did badly at school, often presenting there with physical complaints. She remained wary of her mother in whom she did not confide. The presence of a local air base presented the opportunity to meet many young men and at eighteen she met and quickly married Brian, moving with him to his distant home town.

Brian's family was large, close knit and disorganized, with an intrusive mother and sisters. Jennifer felt welcomed but nervous and then criticized. Brian left the airforce and took up a job driving long distance lorries and so was often away. They had three children: Jennifer found the middle one, a boy, James, very difficult. Her own parenting skills were adequate to cope with the other two who were quite placid girls. After initial feeding and sleeping difficulties, Jennifer began to present James frequently to the GP with complaints about vomiting and diarrhoea, mixed with complaints about his behaviour. Gradually the nature and force of the complaints increased and admission was arranged to the local hospital, after which Jennifer took to sudden presentations at the paediatric ward. Her accounts of James' symptoms at either out-patients or on admission were dramatic: there were many symptoms, differing and new at each visit, symptoms which were incredible to an experienced paediatrician, particularly as the child never had significant physical signs. James was usually quiet and a bit pasty, but often became lively on the ward, where nurses could see his mother could not manage him. The paediatrician resisted further investigations after the initial stage, despite constant complaints.

After a few months, a referral to child mental health services was made. Jennifer was offered regular appointments after an initial session when she came with all three children, who were healthy and active and hard for Jennifer to manage. Brian never came. In these appointments Jennifer seemed to develop some rapport and talked with emotion about her childhood. She began to acknowledge links between her feeling overwhelmed, James' naughty behaviour and her worries about his health, which would culminate in a trip to hospital. She admitted almost any symptom would do as the excuse, though some seemed genuinely to preoccupy her, i.e. there was a mixture of deliberate fabrication, helpful distraction and true anxiety or abnormal health beliefs. Brian remained a shady figure about whom her account was vague, despite extensive efforts to persuade her to bring him and other family members to appointments. Negotiations with the GP, health visitor, paediatricians and child mental health professionals ensured shared understanding of the pattern and led to an agreed management plan for presentations: identification of named doctors for James, basic physical examination when he was presented, followed by reassurance and immediate discharge.

The situation was managed for six months successfully, with far fewer presentations. Suddenly the presentations ceased and Jennifer no longer came to her psychiatric appointments. She had left Brian and moved in with a man down the road, following her mother's pattern. The family remained registered with the same GP. Hospital attendance ceased; only occasional visits to the GP have taken place for the last two years. There is no evidence of presentations elsewhere and school reports for all three children are unremarkable.

Comment

This is a further example of a mother with an emotionally neglectful childhood including a 'classic' experience of hospital care as nurturing and positive by comparison with cold, capricious, frightening and distant parents. Jennifer's cognitive limitations are typical of those who readily present somatic symptoms as a way to signal their emotional distress: her vocabulary for feelings was very limited. These same cognitive limitations curtailed her skill in presenting a truly worrying history for James to tantalize doctors, so that her deceptions or exaggerations could be seen through without much difficulty. Although economical with the truth (largely through fear of being disapproved of), unlike Jean, she did not reach criteria for a personality disorder. There were limits to how far she went in putting her own needs ahead of her children's and there is no reason to think she ever went beyond verbal fabrications and exaggerations. She was quite a frequent GP attender on her own account with physical and psychological complaints, but this too was manageable by the GP without referral. Her capacity for trusting relationships was greater than that of either of the previous cases although still limited. The dramatic reduction in presentations when Jennifer escaped from her marriage is impressive, but will this pattern reappear should the new relationship run into trouble?

Because this case did not involve social services and formal child protection procedures, many aspects are less definite than in more harmful circumstances (whether Jennifer currently somatizes on her own account, other perspectives on the relationship with Brian etc.). It is speculation only to assume that as the relationship with him became more uncomfortable, she escaped more often through presentations of James; the precise triggers within her own life and current family relationships were only starting to be discussed when she ceased to attend.

*Power in the medical arena: factitious illness by proxy as the main
evidence of severely disturbed attachment and manifested in pursuit of
medical care and treatment for children*

Next in this category of less ostensibly vulnerable parents who may display
abnormal illness behaviour for their children, including factitious illness and
abuse if the circumstances foster this, are a group of persistent fabricators and
exaggerators: those parents, mothers usually, whose functioning and circumstances appear superficially to be less pathological than any of the three groups
already described. They are not characterized by any of the major social, intellectual, psychological and financial handicaps of those who are easily identified
as vulnerable parents (such as Vanessa and Jean in their different ways) nor the
obvious risk factors and triggers of Jennifer and her ilk, although the mechanisms
are the same. For these, less instantly obvious candidates, we must scrutinize
more of the psychological (and less of the social) aspects of both the 'bargain' and
the way in which this has changed. It is also necessary to scrutinize the group of
more able but emotionally neglected and abused parents who may well have
seemed to make adjustments through working in 'caring' capacities. Here again
we must predicate some profound disturbance in the parent if he or she pursues
factitious illness routes for her child to the extent of, say, allowing or encouraging unnecessary operations or injecting with insulin. But the assumption that profound disturbance will be obvious has been one of the major mistakes made by
paediatricians, for it has prevented the recognition of how subtle and well hidden
the difficulties may be.

For this group of often intelligent, apparently competent parents it is difficult
to adduce scientific evidence to support the case – a relatively easy task for the
less able and competent parents. Innumerable anecdotes (McKinlay, 1986;
Schreier and Libow, 1993; Meadow, 1982) provide speculative evidence and theorizing arising from situations where mothers' reactions to doctors' failures to
find a cause for their child's illness were not the expected ones (anger and disappointment instead of relief that the child was well). In other words, the mothers'
responses and their behaviour seemed incongruous. Other authors in this book
(see Chapters 8 and 13) speculate that this has more to do with the relationship
between the mother and her child, and in turn, that relationship should be studied
in the light of the mother's own early relationships. Whereas all the previous
group of vulnerable and abusive parents are apparently more prevalent today,
simply because of the increased availability of primary and secondary hospital
care and its use as a form of social support, this group of parents does not appear
to need social support and their difficulties are better hidden. Nevertheless, they
too find it difficult to relate to, to manage and keep an appropriate boundary for
their child, often being enmeshed yet also lacking empathy. All sorts of attributions about their child's behaviour will be used, labelling difficult behaviour as
illness or as a psychological disorder. The parent continues to have difficulties in
adult relationships too, being untrusting and hard to get to know, but sometimes
with a sense of strong suppressed emotion or unpredictable mood swings. They
also use a variety of games and roles to distract themselves from their discom-

forts and naturally, if they have children, these will be used as pawns in the game; pursuit of a particular theme will be at the expense of other interests and well-being for child or family. Depending on the severity of the difficulties, the scenario of the child and their health problems (heavily involving doctors and other professionals who are, or are not, playing the roles which the parent needs) will play a central role in the parent's life, especially when other roles such as the marital one are problematic and unrewarding. Sometimes the mothers seem to play the role of saintly parent to a sick child, sometimes relentless pursuer of a diagnosis. On all occasions the parent needs allies in the form of medical practitioners who are caught up in the content of the presentation instead of studying the process and the child. A characteristic this group shares with the first one is that if recognized as having difficulties and referred to mental health services, these parents may remember little of their childhood or they may present it in an idealized form (Crittenden, 1988). This should not be viewed necessarily as further dissembling but recognized as a psychological defence to protect the parent from being overwhelmed by unpleasant memories of her past.

A 'real life' example was given by Julie Joell Gregory in the *Sunday Telegraph* (1999) describing her mother's long-standing search for medical treatment for Julie from age three onwards, although 'she never actually injured me in order to have a reason to take me to the doctor . . .'. This account includes a well organized search (ultimately unsuccessful) for open heart surgery, but Julie received cardiac catheterization, invasive investigations of bladder function, a tonsillectomy, treatment for migraine, restricted food intake, innumerable investigations and tests and medication. Although the mother's background is not explored, the daughter mentions that her father's only active intervention was to prevent a similar sequence happening to Julie's brother. Many interrelated aspects of the mother–daughter–health care professional relationship are mentioned: excitement, romance, power and control, cruelty, the daughter feeling sorry for her mother, incongruous reactions. Gregory describes herself now (aged thirty) as having been 'short changed by my mother (an extraordinary understatement – author's comment) . . . any contact with her is traumatic, and I see and speak to her rarely'. The mother 'is incapable of understanding that she has done anything wrong'.

Parents with major mental illness

A final group of parents is better researched in terms of their known distorted perceptions about their children: those with severe mental health problems such as schizophrenia, very severe psychotic depression and eating disorders, and severe obsessive compulsive disorders. This group includes sufferers from any illness in the course of which perceptions and cognitions about the environment and the people in it are severely distorted; the majority will have some difficulties in the relationships with their children (Rogers, 1992). At the very severe end of the spectrum are: (1) parents with very severe personality disorders – parents who cannot readily be distinguished from the socially vulnerable group who have suffered severe abuse, for severe early abuse is an important aetiological factor in personality disorder; and (2) those with severely thought-distorting illnesses such as schizophrenia – their difficulty is obvious, for example when a parent's delusions prevent them from appropriately perceiving and thus from rearing and caring for their child. It is relatively easy to understand how such parents, distorted in their view of their children and handicapped by their illness, may present to medical facilities their fragmented or over-inclusive thinking processes in which their children are central. Again, it is necessary for a doctor to be caught up, to fail to recognize the source of error and/or to be misled, for harm to occur. For this group, it is unlikely that changes in the provision or frequency of care, or the changes in access to doctors for health consumers has made a significant difference to the numbers of children presented. Here, the potentially fatal combination is that of the doctor's powers to intrude on children and the potential failure to resist the parent's persistence, and as argued earlier, both of these have changed. It is likely that the size of this group of perpetrators will have changed little in the last fifty years if this thesis is correct, but they may create substantial demand and great harm in the individual case and perhaps have been allowed to do so more, as doctors fail to resist them.

Simon, described earlier (p.27) to illustrate the threshold of harm, was an only child. His maternal grandmother was powerful and cold and his mother's early history is really unknown. There was no family history of mental illness. After university and further training, his mother married and gave birth to Simon, following a difficult painful delivery; he was taken back to hospital a few days later because of worries about his feeding. Mother returned to work after a few months but her health visitor had already noted her incongruous and cryptic remarks and seeming out of touch with reality at times. When Simon was four, mother developed a fixed belief that her husband was having an affair (he was not) and then she started to believe Simon had brain damage. She then pursued this as described previously, by insisting on multiple medical opinions and investigations.

The mother's delusions and disordered thinking were very obvious to anyone psychiatrically trained but she refused psychiatric treatment repeatedly and could produce a functional facade. Using her high intelligence she mounted successful verbal attacks on other professionals, such as teachers, or doctors who opposed her. The father remained passive to action despite Simon's missing school and being taken to more and more hospital appointments. After numerous hospitalizations of Simon, a child protection conference registered him as 'at risk of emotional abuse'. The mother fled with him to another part of the country. Over the next year the situation was monitored closely. The mother's mental state deteriorated and she talked of an elaborate plot to poison and torture her and Simon. The risks of her killing Simon and committing suicide were deemed sufficiently high for intervention and she was sectioned under the Mental Health Act (1983). Within a week she ceased to speak of her delusional preoccupations and has concealed them successfully subsequently, suggesting the fragmented thinking of a personality disordered patient rather than a frank illness (depression or paranoid psychosis). She now receives no psychiatric treatment. Simon lives with his father and has regular contact with his mother. He is very quiet and passive but he and his father do not wish, at present, to pursue any therapeutic work for him.

Clinical studies of MSBP abusers: evidence to support the hypotheses and patterns described

In the previous section the links have been made between Western medicine in paediatric settings and vulnerable parents whose needs are satisfied by their presence in those settings, with their children, for reasons other than organic, 'true' illness in their child. Case histories have been used to illustrate some of the most common factors and pathways to this form of abuse with several broad groups of parents who might display factitious illness in different circumstances. If the factors are relevant as hypothesized, parents who have been identified in clinical case series should also demonstrate a range of backgrounds with the psychological components and mechanisms described.

Such systematic retrospective studies are hard to find, as the substantial literature on factitious illness contains many single case reports and short series, which tend to concentrate on the content of the paediatric presentation and, understandably, report details of the parents only from the perspective of the paediatrician, who rarely has access to a comprehensive psychiatric assessment of the parent and family. Furthermore, by the very nature of emotional abuse in its severest forms, many of the most damaged parents deny, or say they cannot remember, their childhood experiences; they may not be of a mind or in a position to co-operate with psychological and psychiatric assessments.

Induced illness in young children

Southall *et al.* (1997) describe thirty-nine cases in which covert video surveillance (CVS) was used to investigate suspicions of induced illness in children aged between two and forty-four months (median nine months); abuse was confirmed by CVS in thirty-three cases. Thirty children experienced documented intentional suffocation; poisonings and a deliberate fracture were also observed in addition to a variety of other forms of emotional and physical abuse, often including frightening and/or ignoring the infant. The children had forty-one siblings, of whom twelve had died suddenly. Both male and female parents and stepparents are included with, it appears, the male perpetrators being involved in a more direct physical form of MSBP abuse. A strong impression of sadistic cruelty is created in this paper, with the parents' abuse captured on video appearing to be merely a sample of abusive behaviour which was occurring in the index child and other siblings virtually continuously; the authors express the view that the hospital setting made no difference to this. Twenty-three of the parents were said to suffer personality disorders and several had somatizing presentations but few had other psychiatric symptoms; not all agreed to assessment and not all assessments were available to the authors. Several possible reasons are advanced for the absence of other psychopathology. Unfortunately, there is limited information about the early experiences of the perpetrators in this series. At least four had long periods in care, and two were adopted and rejected. Their behaviour is reported however: some had major disturbances, psychosomatic presentations and self harm during late middle childhood and adolescence, but scrutiny and independent corroboration of the early histories has obviously not been possible. This void is frustrating because the information base here is otherwise very rich.

It is concluded that this series does provide support for the theory that the most disorganized, intellectually limited, severely damaged parents brought up in physically and emotionally abusive households are likely to be most at risk of these early primitive and systematic cruelties secondary to parental attachment disorders. In such scenarios the children and hospitals are almost incidental victims (as in Vanessa). Somatization disorders are not universal and when present are often of the most desperate, attention seeking kind. It is not yet possible to draw further conclusions about the combination of individual temperamental traits and early experiences which may have laid the ground for later influences to mould these very disturbed fabricators of stories and inducers of illness. Comprehensive longitudinal case studies, including studies of children removed from abusive backgrounds, will hopefully provide answers in the longer term.

In order to examine whether assumptions are correct about pathways to less immediate and direct physical MSBP abuse, it is necessary to examine cohorts of less severely abused children.

Mixed cases of induced and invented illness

Bools, Neale and Meadow (1994) carried out the only systematic study to date which used standardized instruments to interview nineteen mothers; these included the Clinical Interview Schedule (Goldberg et al., 1970) to identify psychiatric diagnoses, and Tyrer's Personality Assessment Schedule (Tyrer et al., 1995; Tyrer and Alexander, 1988) to study aspects of personality. They also reported on the lifetime psychiatric histories for their nineteen interviewed subjects and a further twenty-eight not interviewed, to give a total of forty-seven mothers in the study. Although a very mixed group of perpetrators, including those who had invented symptoms in addition to directly procured sicknesses, twenty-five mothers (and twelve of the nineteen interviewed subjects) had either smothered or poisoned their child as a part of their fabrications (i.e. there was evidence of severe abuse). It must be emphasized that this cohort were part of a clinical series of 100 known at that time to Meadow because of his expertise in this area. Those approached and interviewed were, the authors speculated, 'a sample of mothers with relatively less disordered psychopathology', but from a child protection perspective over 50 per cent had carried out direct and severe physical abuse. Varying lengths of time had elapsed between the abuse and psychiatric assessment (between fifteen years and a few months), so that there were amongst the sample those who might with some credibility claim to have changed. Striking in this study is that seventeen of the nineteen reached criteria for a personality disorder, with fourteen achieving high scores on five or more of the categories of personality disorder used. Although there were some disagreements between the clinical assessment and the questionnaire in terms of which disorder was the most significant, discrepancies usually occurred when another reliable informant (partner or family member) was not available for interview. The commonest predominant personality disorders selected were 'histrionic' (eight) and 'borderline' (five). Three of the nineteen had diagnosable psychiatric illnesses currently (one suffered an eating disorder with anxiety, one a recent psychosis and one hypochondriasis), but as a group they had numerous psychological problems in their histories. Sixteen had displayed substantial self harm with overdoses and cutting, eight were substance abusers and fifteen had a somatizing disorder: these somatoform disorders were a mixture of factitious illnesses (fabrications of haematemesis, ante-partum haemorrhage, and renal stones) and chronic physical complaints with no organic basis, usually stretching over many years. At the time of interview, eleven had significant psychiatric symptoms which often included physical symptoms without evident intrinsic cause.

The backgrounds of these mothers contained the factors anticipated in producing abusive parents with a health system focus. Four had generalized learning difficulties and one a specific arithmetic learning difficulty. Fifteen had suffered emotional neglect or abuse in their own childhood, of whom two had also experienced both physical and sexual abuse and four had experienced either physical (two) or sexual (two) abuse. There was other evidence of disruption and disturbance in these women's childhoods, including being in the care of the local authority, attending special school and having severe problems in adolescence. The larger cohort of forty-seven (which included the nineteen interviewed) had their case notes scrutinized for psychiatric symptoms and, of these, thirty-four were deemed to have a somatoform disorder (as before, a mixture of fabrications and preoccupation with ill-health), of which the commonest occured in a group of nine mothers who had factitious seizures without an organic basis.

Mixed series without smotherings (i.e. without early, direct and physical abuse)

Gray and Bentovim (1996) reported a series of forty-one children from thirty-seven families identified at Great Ormond Street Hospital. Although the parents were not interviewed using standardized assessments, both the psychiatrist and psychiatric social worker had extensive clinical interviews and present a careful, conservative estimate of what they label 'key, substantial family issues'. This does not extend to personality assessment of the parents but does include psychiatric diagnoses where evident or volunteered from the history. Learning difficulties are not mentioned. As one would expect from a series collected from a tertiary specialist centre, the clinical accounts are dominated by presentations with puzzling discrepancies, such that the children were usually referred (having been seen at between one and five hospitals previously) in order to exclude rare diseases. Smotherings, if identified, were referred elsewhere and were not included here. The authors identified four patterns of presentation, although with overlap of families into more than one category on occasion. These were:

- Allegation of a symptom of a worrying nature (fifteen cases).
- Failure to thrive through active withholding of food (ten cases).
- Active administration of substances or active interference with the child during the course of medical treatment (eleven cases).
- Alleged highly allergic children receiving insufficient amounts of food (five cases).

No particular associations were found between child and family characteristics and any of the patterns of presentation; all social classes were represented and all except one family were white. Thirty-five per cent of the families contained siblings who had also been abused. The patterns of social circumstances and patterns of psychopathology, whilst not including psychiatric assessments of parents, replicate those identified in the previous series (Bools, Neale and Meadow, 1994; Rosenberg, 1987), but a particular strength of this study is in the information gathered about parental difficulties in managing their children.

'These parents seemed to have been intolerant of the ordinary behaviours of their young children but had not sought or received help to enable them to cope with their parenting roles. It could be hypothesized that the difficulties they experienced as parents may relate to their own poor childhood experiences.'

The authors also stress two issues of interest in relation to the genesis and maintenance of these problems medically: the common pattern of mothers (in half the cases supported by fathers) to demand extensive investigations, and the families' patterns of 'denying problems'.

'The parents dismissed relevant details of their past histories and presented an idealized picture of their own care as a child although frequently it had been less than optimal. When the professionals tried to substantiate the histories given, the parents' concept of reality began to be exposed as being at variance with other known information about the child and family. Not surprisingly there was tremendous resistance to professionals trying to explore other major dysfunctions and often significant information was not known. The way in which these families functioned resulted in it being very hard to understand the reasons for their current problems.'

These three series lend support to the view that those parents who commit the severest forms of physical abuse on the youngest children will be found to have substantial abnormalities of personality on systematic assessment, and histories of severe disruption and abuse, together with psychiatric illnesses including self harm, substance abuse and abnormal illness behaviour. Those with apparently more skill in promulgating a presentation which convinces doctors of the presence of illness (i.e. the second and third group and some of the persistent and less florid parents in the fourth group) do seem to be those with more subtle difficulties in relationship to their children, with more confused and 'boundary-less' perceptions of their child. There is more denial, perhaps even dissociation, from their own difficulties (early and late). The parents indeed may often conceal their pasts including psychiatric histories.

If, as hypothesized, paediatric settings simply provide an exquisite opportunity for displays of the difficulties of the most substantially disturbed parents, for which their children are merely the conduit, we may anticipate that less highly technological societies will identify the less highly refined forms of MSBP abuse, such as infants suffocated at home and a range of presentations at such medical facilities that exist with the use of medicines or equivalent to sedate children with troubling behaviour. It may also be assumed that the most intellectually able parents may be the most subtle in their use of health care facilities to meet their own needs, the most able at concealing their enormous difficulties in relationships and parenting, and the most likely to have distorted views and beliefs about their child, as in the Great Ormond Street series. These same parents are also, perhaps, the most difficult to identify and the most likely ones to evade child protection systems and to become embroiled with doctors in high technology solutions to non-organic problems. The Great Ormond Street series also suggests these doctors may find this very hard to accept. Of course, it is unlikely that systematic evidence of these points will be found.

These three series do suggest that frankly deluded parents (as is the case of those having a psychotic illness which involves substantial and more pervasive discrepancies from the perceptions of others) form a small component of MSBP abusers. Clearly much more research is required to examine the interaction between early temperamental traits, early experience and ways of processing this, before primary prevention at this level can be achieved. Until such an enormous body of work takes place, and until child protection processes improve substantially, secondary prevention will remain the role of health care workers.

In addition to examples in other chapters of this book, a further well explored case example which illustrates how such a case may be constructed within a narrative framework is given in Loader and Kelly's paper (1996).

Conclusions

In this chapter factors have been explored which have brought together a growing and powerful force, the Western medical system, to bring it in close apposition to a substantial group of emotionally abused, mentally unwell and vulnerable parents. It is suggested that many aspects of the difficulties experienced by such parents (and such people even if not parents) make them obvious candidates for involvement in health care systems. These have changed and grown extensively so that the system is readily available for those who wish to use (and abuse) it to solve aspects of their own difficulties. Although aspects of the context of this close apposition have changed as a result of social and political changes since the NHS began (e.g. parents' power and choice, parental access), the health care professions and doctors particularly do not seem to have grasped the implications this might have for their work. For parents who have difficulty putting their children's needs first, the impact of these changes is to offer a huge range of opportunities to meet their own needs in the medical system. These are parents for whom 'the bargain' between parent and doctor was always stretched and distorted. It breaks easily under the pressure of the opportunities provided by a panoply of investigations, treatments, operations, medications – all provided largely on parental 'say so' alone.

To summarize the problem in this way is to emphasize the dual responsibility for tackling this epidemic. Of course, parents must put their children's needs first. But this trite statement is a meaningless exhortation: surely it must be assumed that these parents are already doing what they can; that if they could be better parents, they would be. These are vulnerable individuals whose adverse experiences and distorted perceptions are very hard to influence. So responsibility has to be grasped by the health care system, and most firmly grasped by those who are most powerful in clinical decision making within this system, i.e. the medical profession.

It is suggested that much can be done in this regard. Awareness is crucial: not only of the problem of MSBP abuse, but a much greater awareness of human nature and of the use of the body and of one's children and their bodies for psychological purposes. The second key is in good history taking: an issue which has been brought into the centre of the arena recently (Donald and Jureidini, 1996). The third issue should be axiomatic, and it is good medical practice. By this we mean a constant comparison between the objective state of the child's physical health and the history provided, so that evidence is always clearly established before any invasive investigation or treatment is undertaken. There should be a constant consideration of a possible factitious cause as well as an intrinsic one. Finally, courage is required on the part of doctors: courage to cease to investigate, to remember that 'common things occur commonly' (poor parenting being much commoner than rare diseases, and psychological explanations including mistakes and invention are legion) and courage and humility to pause before undertaking heroic medical and surgical interventions in order to consider that the doctor might be perpetrating an unnecessary assault upon a child. These four elements should not be unattainable. The first and last are perhaps the most difficult, especially because it has not formerly been a feature of the medical culture in its highest echelons to step back, to pause and consult with colleagues and team members, and to undertake considered appraisal of parents. For many good reasons, the medical profession has valued those with the courage to act, swiftly and decisively, and most obviously, surgically. For many reasons this readiness to act and intervene may need to be tempered whilst the best aspects of 'active' medicine and surgery are retained. It is not new to call for these elements (awareness of abnormal illness behaviour and associated somatoform disorders, good history taking, good balanced diagnostic skills combined with reflection, open communication with colleagues and a willingness to consider a range of explanations and opinions) to be given a central place in British medicine. Unfortunately, the need becomes more urgent all the time.

References

American Psychiatric Association (1994) *Diagnostic and Statistical Manual of Mental Disorders*, 4th Edn. American Psychiatric Association.

Asher, R. (1951). Munchausen's syndrome. *Lancet*, **i**, 339–341.

Bass, C. and Murphy, M. (1995) Somatoform and personality disorders: syndromal comorbidity and overlapping developmental pathways. *Journal of Psychosomatic Research*, **39** (4), 403–427.

Bates, J. and Bayles, K. (1988) Attachment and the development of behaviour problems. In *Clinical Implications of Attachment*, (Belsky, J. and Nezwarski, T. eds), pp. 25–259. Erlbaum.

Blackwell, R. (1965) Munchausen at Guy's. *Guy's Hospital Reports*, **114** (3), 257–277.

Bools, C.N., Neale, B.A. and Meadow, S.R. (1992) Co-morbidity associated with fabricated illness (Munchausen syndrome by proxy). *Archives of Disease in Childhood*, **67**, 77–79.

Bools, C., Neale, B. and Meadow, R. (1994) Munchausen syndrome by proxy: a study of psychopathology. *Child Abuse and Neglect*, **18**, 773–788

Bowman, F.M. and Garralda, M.E. (1993) Psychiatric morbidity among children who are frequent attenders in general practice. *British Journal of General Practice*, **43**, 6–9.

Cooper, P.J. and Murray, L. (1998). Postnatal depression. *British Medical Journal*, **316**, 1884–1886.

Craig, T.K.J., Boardman, A.P., Mills, K. *et al.* (1993) The South London somatisation study. I: Longitudinal course and the influence of early life experience. *British Journal of Psychiatry*, **163**, 579–588.

Crittenden, P. (1988) Disturbed patterns of relationships in maltreating families: the role of internal representational models. *Journal of Reproductive and Infant Psychololgy*, **6**, 183–199.

Donald, T. and Jureidini, J. (1996) Munchausen syndrome by proxy. Child abuse in the medical system. *Archives of Pediatric and Adolescent Medicine*, **150**, 753–58.

Eminson, D.M. and Postlethwaite, R.J. (1992) Factitious illness: recognition and management. *Archives of Disease in Childhood*. **67**, 1510–1516.

Ettenger, R.B., Rosenthal, J.T. and Marik, J.L. *et al.* (1991) Improved cadaveric renal transplant outcome in children. *Pediatric Nephrology*, **5**, 137–142.

Fisher, G.C. (1995) Etiological speculations. In *Munchausen Syndrome by Proxy. Issues in Diagnosis and Treatment* (Levin, A.V. and Sheridan, M.S. eds). Lexington Books.

Fisher, G.C. and Mitchell, I. (1995) Is Munchausen syndrome by proxy really a syndrome? *Archives of Disease in Childhood*, **72**, 530–534.

Forfar, J. (1998) Demography, initial statistics and the pattern of illness in child-hood. In *Forfar and Arneil's Textbook of Paediatrics*, 5th Edn (Campbell, A.G.M. and McIntosh, N. eds), pp. 1–15. Churchill Livingstone.

Garbarino, J. and Ebata, A. (1983) The significance and cultural differences in child maltreatment. *Journal of Marriage and the Family*, **15**, 773–783.

Garbarino, J., Guttman, E. and Seeley, J.W. (1987) *The Psychologically Battered Child: Strategies for Identification, Assessment and Intervention*. Jossey-Bass.

Goldberg, D.P., Cooper, B., Eastwood, M.R. *et al.* (1970) A standardised psychi-atric interview for use in community surveys. *British Journal of Preventive Social Medicine*, **24**, 18–23.

Goodyer, I.M. (1996) Physical symptoms and depressive disorders in childhood and adolescence. *Journal of Psychosomatic Research*, **41** (5), 405–408.

Gray, J. and Bentovim, A. (1996) Illness induction syndrome: Paper 1. A series of 41 children from 37 families identified at the Great Ormond Street Hospital for Children NHS Trust. *Child Abuse and Neglect*, **20** (8), 655–673.

Gulhati, A. and Minty, B. (1998) Parental health attitudes, illnesses and supports and the referral of children to medical specialists. *Child Care, Health and Development*, **24** (4), 295–313.

Joell Gregory, J. (1999) What mummy did to my body. *Sunday Telegraph*, Review Section, Features, p. 4. 18th July.

Jones, D. (1996) Munchausen syndrome by proxy: is expansion justified? *Child Abuse and Neglect*, **20** (10), 983–984.

Jones, D.P.H. and Ramchandani, P. (1999) *Child Sexual Abuse: Informing Practice from Research*. Radcliiffe Medical Press.

Kai, J. (1996a) What worries parents when their preschool children are acutely ill, and why: a qualitative study. *British Medical Journal*, **313**, 983–986.

Kai J. (1996b) Parents' difficulties and information needs in coping with acute illness in preschool children: a qualitative study. *British Medical Journal*, **313**, 987–990.

Libow, J.A. and Schreier, H.A. (1986) Three forms of factitious illness in chil-dren: When is it Munchausen syndrome by proxy? *American Journal of Orthopsychiatry*, **56**, 602–611.

Loader, P. and Kelly, C. (1996) Munchausen syndrome by proxy: a narrative approach to explanation. *Clinical Child Psychology and Psychiatry*, **75**, 57–61.

McClure, R.J., David, P.M., Meadow, S.R. *et al.* (1996) Epidemiology of Munchausen syndrome by proxy. *Archives of Disease in Childhood*, **75**, 57–61.

McKinlay, I.A. (1986) Munchausen's syndrome by proxy. *British Medical Journal*, **293**, 1308.

Meadow, R. (1977) Munchausen syndrome by proxy. The hinterland of child abuse. *Lancet*, **ii**, 343–345.

Meadow, R. (1982) Munchausen syndrome by proxy. *Archives of Disease in Childhood*, **57**, 9298.

Meadow, R. (1985) Management of Munchausen syndrome by proxy. *Archives of Disease in Childhood*, **60**, 385–393.

Meadow, R. (1995). What is, and what is not, Munchausen syndrome by proxy. *Archives of Disease in Childhood*, **6**, 534–538.

Meadow, R. (1999) Unnatural sudden infant death. *Archives of Disease in Childhood*, **80**, 7–14.

Morbidity statistics from general practice 1955–56, Vols I–III. Studies on Medical and Population Subjects, 1981–82. Series MB5 No. 1, HMSO. 1979; 1986; 1995.

Neale, B., Bools, C. and Meadow, R. (1991) Problems in the assessment and management of Munchausen syndrome by proxy. *Children and Society,* **5**, 324–333.

Ney, P. (1994) The worst combinations of child abuse and neglect. *Child Abuse and Neglect*, **18**, 707–714.

Nicol, A. R. and Eccles, M. (1985) Psychotherapy for Munchausen syndrome by proxy. *Archives of Disease in Childhood*, **60**, 344–348.

Oates, M.R. (1997) Patients as parents: the risk to children. *British Journal of Psychiatry*, **170** (32, Suppl.), 22–27.

Pless, I.B., Cripps, H.A., Davis, J.M.C. and Wadsworth, M.E.J. (1989) Chronic physical illness in childhood: psychological and social effects in adolescence and adult life. *Developmental Medicine and Child Neurology*, **31**, 746–755.

Report of a Working Party on the Hospitalisation of Children (1998) North West Regional Health Authority, May 1988.

Robertson, J. (1970) *Young Children in Hospital*, 2nd Edn. Tavistock Publications.

Rogers, M.L. (1992) Delusional disorder and the evolution of mistaken sexual allegations in child custody cases. *Journal of Forensic Pathology*, **10**, 47–69.

Rosenberg, D.A. (1987) Web of deceit: a literature review of Munchausen syndrome by proxy. *Child Abuse and Neglect*, **11**, 547–563.

Rosenberg, D.A. (1994) Munchausen syndrome by proxy. In *Child Abuse – Medical Diagnosis and Management* (Reece R.M., ed.), pp. 266–278. Lea and Febiger.

Rosenberg, D.A (1995) From lying to homicide. The spectrum of Munchausen syndrome by proxy. In *Munchausen Syndrome by Proxy. Issues in Diagnosis and Treatment* (Levin, A.V. and Sheridan, M.S., eds), pp. 13–37. Lexington Books.

Schreier, H.A. and Libow, J.A. (1993) *Hurting for Love: Munchausen by Proxy Syndrome.* Guilford Press.

Schreier, H.A. (1996) Repeated false allegations of sexual abuse presenting to sheriffs: when is it Munchausen by proxy? *Child Abuse and Neglect*, **20**, 985–991.

Shorter, E. (1992) From paralysis to fatigue. A history of psychosomatic illness in the modern era, pp. 319. Free Press. Quotes Gallup poll commissioned by the American Medical Association quoted in *New York Times*, February 18, 1990, pp. A21.

Southall, D.P., Plunkett, C.B., Banks, M.W., Falkov, A.F. and Samuels, M.P. (1997) Covert video recordings of life threatening child abuse: lessons for child protection. *Pediatrics*, **100** (5), 735–760.

Spencer, N.J., Lewis, M.A. and Logan, S. (1993) Multiple admission and deprivation. *Archives of Disease in Childhood*, **68**, 760–762.

Taylor, D.C. (1991) Outlandish factitious illness. In *Recent Advances in Paediatrics* (David, T. ed.), pp. 63–76. Churchill Livingstone.

Taylor, D.C. (1996) Parental persuasion to sickness. *Association of Child Psychiatry and Psychology Occasional Papers*, **12**, 13–16.

Tyrer, P., Alexander, J., Cicchietti, D. *et al.* (1979) Reliability of a schedule for rating personality disorders. *British Journal of Psychiatry*, **135**, 163–167.

Tyrer, P. and Alexander, J. (1988) Personality assessment schedule. In *Personality Disorders and Diagnosis: Management Course* (Tyrer, P., ed.). Wright.

Van der Wal, M.F., van den Boom, D.C., Pauw-Plomp, H. and de Jonge, G.A. (1998) Mother's reports of infant crying and soothing in a multicultural population. *Archives of Disease in Childhood*, **79**, 312–317.

Waller, D.A. (1983) Obstacles to the treatment of Munchausen by proxy syndrome. *Journal of the American Academy of Child Psychiatry*, **22**, 80–85.

Watson, S., Eminson, D.M. and Coupe, W. (1999) Personal communication.

Welldon, E.V. (1988) *Mother, Madonna, Whore. The Idealization and Denigration of Motherhood*. Free Association Books.

White, C. and Barrowclough, C. (1998) Depressed and non-depressed mothers with problematic pre-schoolers: attributions for child behaviours. *British Journal of Clinical Psychology*, **37**, 385–398.

Wooley, H., Wheatcroft, R. and Stein, A. (1998) Influence of parental eating disorder on children. *Advances in Psychiatric Treatment*, **4**, 144–150.

World Health Organization (1992) *The ICD-10 Classification of Mental and Behavioural Disorders. Clinical Descriptions and Diagnostic Guidelines*. World Health Organization.

The doctor – the opportunity for abuse: presentations in out-patients

Robert J. Postlethwalte, Martin Samuels and Mary Eminson

'If there is a justification for continuing to treat Munchausen syndrome by proxy (MSBP) abuse as a specific form of child abuse, it is the special role that the medical system plays in its genesis and maintenance. Several authors have drawn attention to the role of physicians and nurses in the exacerbation and perpetuation of MSBP. We believe that we must go further and examine the role of the medical profession in the genesis of MSBP. For example, Morley argues that poor history taking contributes to the misdiagnosis of MSBP. We contend that poor history taking is central to its etiology.' (Donald and Jureidini, 1996).

'Of all the diagnostic aids available, a well conducted family interview and a thorough history are the best imaging procedures available. While the quality of the picture depends on the interviewer's skills, no other technology can provide as clear an appreciation of the child and family, their problems, and the psychosocial backdrop against which the problems have developed.' (Goldbloom, 1992).

The paediatric clinical assessment

In the preceding chapter the thesis was advanced that changes in 'the bargain' of health care have taken place. 'The bargain' was summarized as: 'Parents bring children who are sick and tell the truth about them and ... doctors bring expertise and technology and act to do their best for children'.

Whilst acknowledged as always an oversimplification of the truth, it was asserted that changes in health care systems and power relationships within them have increased the risk that this 'bargain' will be perverted more often and more dangerously than in the past. The new 'bargain' then becomes: 'Parents bring children pretending they are sick/or having made them sick (in the induced illness case) and persuade/cajole/bully doctors into using their expertise and technology to harm them further by unnecessary medical care (or failing to notice when the cause of the child's illness is extrinsic, in the case of induced illness)'. These changes are seen as the most significant single explanation for the presence of substantial amounts of MSBP abuse.

The remedies to this situation were summarized as: (1) awareness of MSBP abuse specifically but also of somatization, illness behaviour and parental psychopathology; (2) good history taking; (3) good medical practice; and (4) courage to reflect on one's own practice, and to question and discuss, with colleagues, whether investigations, interventions and treatment are truly necessary and advisable. This chapter is concerned with ways in which the second of these, good history taking, can be developed and enhanced by a knowledge of the first point.

The majority of paediatric consultations are straightforward, with ready agreement between the parents and the clinician about the nature, severity and management of the clinical problem. In other words, the old 'bargain' holds true for much of the time. However, this book is concerned with the occasions when this agreement is lacking.

If clinicians are to be alert to circumstances where other factors are operating, this implies a change in approach to consultations. This approach would include from the outset the possibility that a broader range of aspects of the consultation process is relevant in the formulation of hypotheses about the presented problem. This chapter is largely concerned with out-patient paediatric encounters and routine emergency and planned admissions in ordinary paediatric wards. This will be the place where the majority of factitious illness, as defined in this book, will present. The invented and exaggerated stories, the parent persistently seeking investigations and treatments and sometimes inducing illness through the use of proprietary medication or the patient's or parent's own medication will be seen; the whole range of parenting capacities, motivation and relationships will be met in this setting. By and large presentations of severe induced illness due to physical assault on tiny children will present more urgently and, although the principles of the approach described here are entirely applicable, such patients require a different, swifter pace of assessment: this is described in Chapter 4.

Clinical encounters: making an assessment which integrates process, content and physical findings

The approach we describe to the clinical encounter is one which is characteristic of many of the best clinicians of any speciality (and it would be insulting to assume otherwise) but it is rarely given a central place when teaching about acute paediatrics. Attention to the detail of such matters is most central, medically, to the field of psychiatry. This is because, for psychiatrists, so much is to be learned from the process of consultation to add to what is learned from the content. The maxim: 'believe everything the patient says and believe nothing the patient says' encapsulates this. It does not mean that all patients are liars. It means that all the other information, everything except the words the patient says, gives the clinician the opportunity to put the patient's utterances in to context. 'Everything' includes the letters about, phone calls from, the look, smell, sound, speed, dress, companions, intellect, affect and response of the patient. This includes the way they approach other staff and the impact that they have upon the doctor, i.e. how the patient makes the doctor 'feel'. Psychiatrists and other mental health practitioners add together and align the two sets of information all the time: everything the patient says and everything else that they learn about the patient. For psychiatrists the role of physical examination is rarely central after initial assessment. For other doctors, the balance of what is learnt from verbal content is almost always weighed together with the physical findings in the child as well as all the other information from the consultation and history. It is important to be sophisticated and non-judgemental in weighing up the three types of information. If there are no explanatory physical findings to support reported complaints, then no other aspect has precedence, necessarily. All is of interest in formulating a case and must be integrated to draw up a balanced set of hypotheses. Crucially this prevents too heavy a reliance on one aspect, either of the history or of reported symptoms.

This balance of the physical findings, parental reports and all the 'process' and contextual issues prevents the oversimplified approach that can result in practitioners suddenly shifting from believing the parent's account as the literal truth, to believing the whole account is fictitious, just because of one factor. An example of such a sudden and unwarranted shift in the field of MSBP abuse is the over-reliance on particular issues in the history as 'evidence' of fabrication in factitious illness by proxy. Thus, the 'discovery' that somatization disorders in parents are not uncommon background factors in severe factitious illness by proxy does not in itself prove the nature of a child's presentation: it is information to be weighed in the context of other aspects of the history, presentation and physical assessment of the child.

Assumptions of this chapter

It is suggested that paediatricians will need to develop an interest in these contextual and non-verbal issues for all consultations if they are to make sense of presentations where there is a lack of agreement between parents and professionals about the nature, severity and management of a clinical problem.

It is essential to point out that, when writing about the discrepancies between the medical or health care professional and the parental point of view, and when describing 'undesirable' behaviours by parents concerning consultations, in this chapter, perfection in medical attitudes, skills and practice is assumed. Discrepancies are described as if on each occasion, there is no other explanation but that the parental view and behaviour are distorted, difficult to understand or pathological. It must be made clear at the outset that, whilst this position is taken for the purposes of exploring the area, it is manifestly not the case. Quite apart from cultural and class differences which have an impact on such transactions (some of which are discussed in more detail in Chapters 8 and 9), all professionals must be aware that sometimes they have made a contribution to a consultation's failure to reach agreement satisfactorily. For example, when hurried, their impatience with a parent may have been apparent and the history taken too abruptly so that parents become defensive and silent; when tired, an inadequate history may be taken and too technical an explanation given in a way that discourages questioning and leaves parents unsatisfied; when overstretched, the parents one finds most difficult may receive less than one's best performance. There are huge strides to be made in health care professionals'(doctors' in particular) ability to attend carefully to parental presentations, to set up systems which enable parents to provide a narrative which is coherent to them but can be probed to make 'medical' sense too, and to reach an agreed 'contract' with the family about the nature and management of the difficulties.

Equally, impeccable standards in administrative and other hospital systems are assumed: for example, that appointments and letters generally are sent, that communication between specialists does occur as agreed. Finally, good medical competence is a prerequisite.

Whilst of vital importance, these are not the themes of this book, and it is assumed that any clinician reading this is aware of such possible failings and will have addressed them already. For the purposes of this chapter a 'good enough' doctor with adequate skills in a 'good enough' hospital is assumed.

Appraisal of non-verbal aspects of the consultation

Pressure and contact before the appointment

Patients usually arrive at medical facilities in response to letters, faxes and phone calls which justify the urgency of the contact in easily understood medical terms. There are generally two major components: the referring professional's assessment of the urgency of the case, and the family's concern and anxiety. The former may have several explanations (the GP may have had previous experience with this condition or with this family which leads him to be more or less concerned about this symptom or illness) and the family too may have a wealth of explanations for their behaviour. Of interest to note are the activities of families which raise their profile in the normally smooth routines of hospital medicine: repeated telephoning to insist on a particular professional or date; demanding appointments at particular times of day or places; unpleasantness to or bullying of administrative or junior medical staff. Conversely, parental lack of contact in the context of professional anxiety is equally puzzling. All these behaviours are stored as queries in the professional's mind, with answers to be sought when the consultation takes place.

Presentation at the appointment

The professional learns much from all aspects of the family's presentation, and records these as his or her impressions. This should be done in neutral, non-pejorative language, and in comparison with every other family he or she has met in similar circumstances. This is not a 'sheep or goats' distinction of 'normal vs. abnormal' and nothing diagnostic is recorded here. It is a record of vital contextual issues in the consultation and starts if possible with observations from the waiting room. Are the family numerous, noisy and untidy, clearly having imbibed on the way to the appointment, or are they silent, tense and well dressed? Who comes to the appointment? What is their cultural and ethnic background? Do professional and family share a first language? Variables include: level of cognitive capacity, verbal facility and education; familiarity with this illness and the language of medicine; and any unexplained discrepancy between the parents' mood, suspicion, anxiety, knowledge and interest in different areas. Does the parent become inexplicably withdrawn or angry? Are there areas of the consultation which seem particularly to raise the emotional temperature or create tension? All this is noted and compared with other families in similar situations. This is of interest, not a judgement.

Rapport with the clinician

What does the clinician observe about the quality of the interaction he has formed with the parent(s)? Has the interaction been tense and difficult or, conversely, is the mother too ready to agree to everything? Is there a real sense of a shared plan or more holding back, observing and lack of trust? Has the parent seemed tense and defensive or given relaxed expansive answers?

The rapport developed between parent and paediatrician and the paediatrician's theories about this are important, and so too is the congruence between the parental account, the level of concern, and the child's apparent state of health. This area is not one in which there are norms or standards or helpful questionnaires: again this is weighed in the context of the clinician's knowledge of parental behaviour.

There are many benign causes of incongruent parental presentations. Severe anxiety alone may produce great arousal and disinhibition in some parents, which can be understood if explored and will often reduce at later visits. Those with learning difficulties may also present unusually. A first step is to note any incongruence, recording it as a subjective impression in non-pejorative terms, with tentative hypotheses recorded as such with a query. This allows a check on such impressions, and whether they have changed, at each appointment. A comparison can be made with the feelings this parent arouses in other clinicians including non-medical staff. If the impression persists in circumstances where the illness is puzzling or difficult to manage, it should be respected and justifies caution before undertaking invasive investigations or treatments unless the evidence to justify them is clear-cut.

Communication between family members

Observations of the relationship between parent and child are particularly useful for trained observers. They include the extent to which the parent can attend to the child as well as to the clinician, the level and appropriateness of supervision given, whether the mother encourages the child to contribute to the consultation and how he or she responds to his/her mother or father. The language and emotional force in descriptions of the child and his health and behaviour are noted, as well as the child's responses (of all kinds) when his mother is talking about him; any skills or otherwise in managing the child are observed.

The child

What does the child play with while in the room and are age and development appropriate with this? Does the child respond when approached by the clinician directly and how wary is he/she? Can the child make a developmentally appropriate contribution to the consultation?

Examining illness and consultation behaviour: prevention of adverse effects of abnormal illness behaviour and promoting the identification of factitious illness

Theoretical background

Whilst building awareness of consultations depends on increased facility with observational skills as outlined above, this is only the first step in improving history taking. The second is to improve awareness and curiosity about the causes of discrepancies in consultation. 'Discrepancies' here alludes to all circumstances where agreement is lacking between parent and clinician about the nature, severity and management of a child's illness. In this chapter many possible reasons for the absence of such straightforward agreement are explored, with an analysis of how these may be understood and managed, and how much concern should be attached to them.

Experienced clinicians are well used to making sense of children's presentations and are familiar with a wealth of 'consultation behaviour' and 'illness behaviour'. These behaviours have several different elements: abnormal perceptions, abnormal beliefs, unusual patterns of consultation and patterns of pursuit of an invalid lifestyle, including the benefits thereof. The component 'consultation behaviour' is used to describe all aspects of parental behaviour related to the consultation for their child, with the exception of the physical examination and findings. 'Consultation behaviour' includes all that happens before an appointment (the letter, its urgency, the rate and frequency of contact between the family and the professional institution prior to the appointment), during the consultation (the processes involved in the transaction between the doctor and the family) and after the consultation (the extent to which an agreed plan is complied with by both parties, the behaviours of the family in relation to the treatment, the professional and to seeking other opinions). This area is presented and discussed here not because there is a lack of comprehensive information concerning consultations in paediatrics, Goldboom (1992) and Green (1998) provide excellent reviews of the paediatric clinical interview. However, this area is discussed in this chapter because of the need to illustrate all these approaches to the clinical consultation from the perspective of discrepancies between parents and professionals about the health needs of the child. In other words, the consultation is being reviewed from the point of view of all aspects of abnormal consultation and abnormal illness behaviour, including factitious illness and MSBP abuse, ranging from the mildest differences in interpretation between doctor and parent, to the opposite extreme of parental insistence on investigation or production of ill-health in a child.

The assumption of many inexperienced doctors is that the question posed when a parent brings a child to a consultation is merely 'what is the matter with this child?'. Yudkin (1961) suggested that when a child is brought to a doctor, two questions need to be answered: 'what is the matter with the patient?' and 'why is this child being brought for care at this moment?'. These ideas were explored in a paper entitled 'Six children with coughs, the second diagnosis'. In these six children, although the diagnosis was the same in all (recurrent respiratory infections), the answer to the second question, i.e. the agenda behind the consultation, was different in each. In one, the mother wanted support in a family argument about care of the child, in the second there was parental anxiety about tuberculosis, and so on.

In principle, the answer to the first question of 'what is the matter with the child?' lies in an objective professional assessment of the clinical story told by the parents, put together with a skilful physical assessment of the child. The answer to the second question lies in the understanding of why the parents are telling the story in this way at this time to this clinician. Yudkin encourages this curiosity and open mindedness about all aspects of the paediatric consultation, with attention to the process of the consultation as well as its content.

Waring (1992), building explicitly upon Yudkin's ideas but with his interest focused upon MSBP abuse and persistence in consultations, explored the concept of congruence. In the majority of paediatric consultations there is agreement between the reported symptoms and the clinical findings, and thus there is congruence between the parents' report and the doctors' findings, between parental persistence and child morbidity. Waring explored the incongruence existing when a parent 'is attaching much more weight to these symptoms than do other parents', i.e. when parental persistence and child morbidity were incongruent. He described this situation, if parents were persistent and no 'first diagnosis' or evidence of child morbidity was found, as one where the clinician needed to seek a 'second diagnosis', by which he meant an explanation. He constructed an algorithm to explore this situation, but emphasized that it could not be used until 'a history, physical examination, and probably some ancillary studies have been completed'. The algorithm assumes that parental persistence may well be appropriate in two situations, namely when morbidity is difficult to identify or when it has a psychological rather than physical cause (if there is a 'first' diagnosis but it is hard to identify). The algorithm's purpose is essentially two-fold: to alert clinicians to pathological causes of parental persistence (factitious illness by proxy under various labels) and to guide and assist physicians 'whose anger and frustration may occlude their view' of the possible explanations.

Eminson and Postlethwaite (1992) explored discrepancies between parental and professional formulations and actions over a wider area, which included under-persistence (neglect of treatment) as well as excessive persistence (frequent consultations and invented and induced symptoms). A diagrammatic way of presenting these discrepancies was used, suggesting that gross discrepancies are usually associated with severe parental problems in distinguishing the child's needs from their own (see Figure 2.1, p. 24), and less marked discrepancies between doctors' and parents' opinions and behaviour are due to less severe parental issues. A spectrum of behaviour with a variety of causes was proposed, with an assumption that severe discrepancies in over-treatment or exaggeration would be associated with other severe gaps in parental capacities too, i.e. neglect of various parental functions including treatment of illness. Figure 2.2, p. 25 summarizes this.

Causes of incongruity

The following section explores some of the common causes of incongruity in consultation behaviour that are met in many paediatric encounters. None of these is harmful *per se* although they may become so if pursued very persistently, or if they are not uncovered and are allowed to become the justification for unnecessary investigations or treatments.

Parents with limited cognitive ability

A common reason for parents giving a history that contains many incongruous elements is because of parental difficulties in knowing what is relevant, and their limited capacity in noticing relevant issues. It is worth remembering, as discussed in the previous chapter, that parents with many kinds of difficulties in parenting, which include being limited themselves, are more likely to present their children to doctors, and may perhaps be more likely to seek an illness explanation for their child's difficult behaviour. When faced with authority figures like doctors, such parents will not only report what are, in fact, irrelevant details, but when asked questions may 'embroider the truth' to fill a gap, rather than say that they do not know or cannot remember. Such parents are perhaps particularly likely to feel important through having a child who merits the attention of specialists. They may be reluctant to give up their place in this scenario. In addition, parents with such limitations are just as open as the rest of the population to the influences of the media in their focus on new or worrying disease, but may have difficulty in understanding some of the concepts presented. Therefore they may come with ideas about the cause of the symptoms which they have already incorporated into their own understanding, and so they will present the reported connections rather than the symptoms that they noticed at the outset.

Strong or unusual beliefs

This phrase is used to cover a wide range of reasons for incongruity, and the adjective 'unusual' is merely used to distinguish these ideas from those of the doctor. Beliefs about an illness may be arrived at by parents from a large range of historical, family and media sources, and parents will not necessarily reveal their beliefs either at the outset of the consultation or at any time unless it is comfortable to do so. Many parents faced with a child who is unwell will, of course, worry that there is a serious disease cause which doctors have not identified. The current media concerns will often figure highly. Thus, at the time of writing, meningitis is a major worry for many parents and numerous other examples could be given. Food allergy and 'ME' are currently used to explain many forms of physical and behavioural anomalies. 'Total allergy syndrome' was a 1980s example. In the psychiatric clinic, attention deficit hyperactivity disorder (ADHD) is the explanation advanced in many parents' minds for the behaviour difficulties of their children; dyslexia is a frequent equivalent in the educational domain. If the parents have arrived at this belief merely through recent media or neighbourhood exposure, this is usually explained quite early on.

Many aspects of the family's history contribute to the beliefs. Of course, if an earlier child has died or had a serious illness, or if this child has been ill with a significant problem in his or her life, this provides a focus for anxieties for many years to come. This is probably particularly true if parents feel guilty about those earlier illnesses; if they were slow to note them or feel that they were in some way responsible.

Strongly held beliefs and feelings about illnesses that run in the family are sometimes quite accurately held. It is always worth exploring the extent of significant illnesses in other family members and enquiring explicitly from parents whether they are worried about that issue in this particular child: what connection have they made with their child's circumstances? Family illnesses that doctors were slow to identify and which later 'came to light' seem to resonate loudly for some parents. Scepticism about medical competence is also exacerbated by popular press and TV reports, which 'fan the flames' for anxious parents who are slow to be reassured. None of these issues will necessarily be mentioned by parents. If this is the explanation, tension and pressure in the consultation often reduce if the doctor asks the parents if they have been worried whether he is sufficiently expert. The true level of his or her expertise, and its limits, can be discussed and what will occur if the doctor is uncertain and how he will acquire more expertise for them (rather than how they will search again).

Beliefs about aetiological events in the child's life may sometimes shade into the next category (another agenda) if a parent has attributed the cause of a child's illness or presentation to a particular time in their life or a particular experience. This may be used as the reference point for a very wide variety of different physical presentations. For example, a mother had an illness during her pregnancy but her husband refused to call out the doctor. Subsequently the mother gave birth to a child with cerebral palsy. She formed the belief that the brain lesion causing the cerebral palsy occurred at the time of her original illness, and used this as a point of grievance in arguments with her husband whom she subsequently divorced. Many other symptoms in the child were referred back to this illness during the pregnancy, with an attempt to make links and to make the husband 'responsible.' This mechanism is particularly prevalent in parents who have a child who has an obvious handicap and also where, as in this case, the mother felt guilty because in truth she could have called the doctor herself. Thus for children with epilepsy, parents will naturally search the narrative of the child's early life looking for an explanation for the appearance of this illness, wondering whether an immunization, or a pyrexial illness, was associated with a brain insult which caused the epilepsy.

Some parents hold somewhat more unusual beliefs about the cause of illness, including allergens in the environment, force field emissions from electrical pylons and beliefs about diet. Religious beliefs about the cause of illness may include beliefs about possession and black magic. Often parents are aware that these beliefs are statistically unusual and may therefore be reluctant to expose them to doctors who might belittle what is to them an important concept. It is axiomatic that such beliefs must be respected and are of interest for the impact they are having upon the parent's presentation of the child's symptoms. They are of concern only if pursuit of the belief is in some way harmful to the child. This does of course occur (as explored in Chapter 8 dealing with presentations in mental health settings), but many less harmful unusual beliefs are common and may lead parents to press for the investigation which they believe will elucidate the link.

Another agenda

This must be statistically the most important category and again includes a range of possibilities. 'Other agendas' include escaping from partners, diversion from one's own difficult life (arguments with family and neighbours), a way of gaining better housing and benefits, an excuse for not taking the children to school, especially when a prosecution for school absence is being threatened, an excuse for not going to work oneself, and an excuse for many parental failures, including not giving the treatment and not maintaining the agreed physiotherapy or splinting or diet, because of being too busy, tired, incompetent or distracted with one's own concerns. The more limited the parent's psychological, financial, social and intellectual resources, the more likely they are to use the available opportunities within the medical system to try and gain what they want from other arenas.

Less than ideal treatment previously

Many parents are concerned about their child's symptoms partly because they have indeed been treated less than ideally in another setting. Perhaps, even if the physical care was appropriate, their worries were not answered. Parents may see all doctors as sticking together and may initially be uncertain about admitting criticisms, whether justified or not, of another medical practitioner, thus not explaining this problem. It is not necessary to criticize colleagues in order to explore such concerns; they are usually evident from the way the parent speaks of the encounter and can be probed by asking questions such as 'Did you find this helpful?' This type of parental incongruence and persistence is likely, of course, to respond readily to thorough, sensitive medical attention and to quickly disappear when truly likely disease possibilities have been explored and considered and any illness managed appropriately. Often few investigations are necessary beyond a thorough airing of worries, concerns and the meaning of existing findings.

Another disease is truly present to explain the symptoms
This is usually the category the doctor selects most readily.

Case examples

The vignettes that follow include some examples of these common reasons for incongruence. In these and all the subsequent examples given in this book, an attempt is made constantly to weigh up both the history given by the parent, the morbidity in the child and the incongruence between them, but also the question of whether any harm is occurring from the incongruence noted. The way this chapter is constructed is to include examples that are clearly harmless to the child (although they may involve cynical manipulation of health care systems), those which approach the threshold for harm and those which clearly cross it. We recommend that *the question of harm arising*, as discussed in the previous chapter and in Chapter 9, *be considered as routinely as the physical state of the child.*

> Failure of previous medical help; learnt or inherent demanding style; high expectations
> A seven year old girl was referred to the out-patients with nocturnal enuresis. Before the out-patient appointment, three phone calls were received from the mother to confirm that the child would be seen by the consultant.

In this case there was incongruity between the mild clinical problem (nocturnal enuresis) and the frequency of contact before the consultation. During the consultation the explanation for this incongruity was established: the child had been managed at another institution for six months and was said never to have been reviewed by a consultant. Additionally, the family wanted action urgently as they hoped treatment would achieve dryness for an imminent family holiday. It is not clear why the first phone call did not satisfy the family.

> An over-attentive parent
> A three year old boy was referred to the renal clinic by a secondary paediatrician. The child had suffered a single urinary tract infection, with lower urinary tract signs. Appropriate investigations were normal. No more were judged medically necessary, nor was a referral to the specialist. In the out-patient clinic, routine detailed discussion about the benign but sometimes troublesome nature of lower urinary tract infections only seemed to increase the mother's anxiety. She was invited to write down her concerns and bring

them to the next OP visit. She arrived at the next visit with five pages of questions. The writing was very immature block capitals, the syntax was very primitive and simple words were spelt incorrectly; this was consistent with a superficial assessment of her intellectual abilities in the clinic. The questions were peppered with complex medical terms (endoplasmic reticulum, oxygen carrying capacity), which were spelt correctly. It was not clear at this stage, in this case, whether any harm was occurring but the risk of this was great because of the professionals acting on the mother's symptom reports and carrying out unnecessary investigations.

Clearly this mother's use of medical terms was incongruent with her level of intelligence and education, and she must have been copying them from some medical text or encyclopaedia. This does not, of course, mean that the illness itself was factitious – she might simply have been attempting, in a clumsy way, to communicate her concerns to the professionals. It is very difficult to judge the appropriateness of parents' knowledge. Zealous and flawless parents may have extensive knowledge about an as yet undiagnosed illness simply because it was mentioned in a previous consultation and they have access to the internet, but if there is no abnormal illness behaviour, they generally give up this possibility once the clinician has offered enough time in explanation. Understanding this mother and judging the level of concern must depend on a more extensive knowledge of the child and the parental persistence, and whether there were explanations for this in earlier experiences and beliefs.

Another agenda: escaping from a difficult home situation
Over a period of months an eight year old boy was repeatedly presented to the hospital for admission with a history of severe abdominal pain. On every admission his symptoms disappeared completely as soon as he was admitted. Mother always accompanied him to the hospital. There was no obvious relevant personal family history of note. Mother was a confident approachable woman who was in full-time employment in a solicitor's office. She seemed to readily accept that simple investigations were normal and that there was no identifiable pathology and that the situation needed managing pragmatically. She was not pressing for further investigations. The boy said very little.

The admissions continued. Although the boy seemed otherwise well adjusted and in full-time school, it was felt that child psychiatric review might be helpful in management of the illness in case there was a psychosomatic component: mother readily agreed to this. The psychiatrist, on being consulted by the paediatrician enquired about social stresses and supports. Why had the problems started now? Had anything changed? This prompted a review of the events around admission and with very little encouragement the mother revealed to the paediatrician her concerns about her husband whom she felt was depressed and occasionally threatened violence. This had been going on for many years but in the past when the situation had become too threatening at home she had escaped by going to her own parents. Her husband had often followed her there and frequently caused a scene. Following one of these episodes her own father had suffered a minor stroke which the mother attributed to the stress of the conflict. She was fearful that a further scene might give rise to much more serious consequences in her father and so her only route of escape from home was cut off. Social work intervention provided her with alternative refuge and the abdominal pain presentations ceased completely.

This parent was persistent in consulting but there was no incongruence in her response when her child 'recovered'. Most of the major risk and trigger factors for factitious illness were absent. In addition, a plausible psychosocial explanation was provided. Nevertheless, this scenario cannot be dismissed as harmless. The mother felt comfortable with her abuse of the health care system. As for the boy, it must be assumed that either he had been induced to lie about his symptoms or else he did experience pain when his parents argued, in which case this confident mother was slow to find a better solution to her child's distress than coming to hospital. This is clearly an example of where a little 'sleuthing' (Waring, 1992), which the paediatrician was slow to initiate, readily identified an important trigger factor for the abnormal consultation behaviour.

Limited intellectual ability and beliefs used as a simplistic justification for what are clearly parental failings

An ten year old boy with ureteric reflux was also very obese. At four consecutive out-patient reviews mother asked for re-explanation of the findings and persisted in her belief that the obesity was due to urine leaking back up the ureters and back into the bloodstream. The obesity was claimed to be due to the boy filling up with fluid in this way. The mother, who was of limited intelligence, remained convinced of this explanation despite repeated discussions. She was also insistent that the boy's failure to lose weight on a calorie-reduced diet was because of the urine leaking back into the body.

It is not unusual for parents to make sense of a child's symptoms by constructing a narrative which is biologically implausible to professionals, the 'leaking back up' had an obvious explanation. The family may abandon such muddled understandings after discussions with doctors but sometimes, as in this case, they persist and become a fixed belief. In this instance, the mother's limited cognitive abilities probably contributed to the persistence of her views, which also served to justify the boy's lack of response to the dietary advice offered.

The next level: the unresolved clinical problem

What happens when there is persisting incongruence between the story and the state of the child, or between parental requests for investigations and the state of the child? When clinicians have carried out the basic physical investigations necessary, reassured the parent appropriately and explored ordinary innocent reasons for incongruence, they will still often be faced by puzzling presentations with a need to tease out possible explanations. This will usually take place during a number of out-patient appointments, or possibly during an admission if there are abnormalities that are truly worrying and justify further investigations, but such admissions are usually brief. A logical approach to these clinical encounters at this stage is essential. First in this section, approaches to clinical problem solving are reviewed, with particular consideration of how factitious illness affects this. Second, areas of the history whose significance may be difficult to appraise are discussed. Case examples are used to illustrate these and hypotheses tested. Finally, a more critical, 'corroborating' information approach to the history is outlined for this stage in the management of unresolved clinical problems.

Approaches to clinical problem solving

There will be numerous explanations for clinical problems that are unresolved following the initial clinical assessment and further history taking. The problem may be 'unresolved' in the sense that the parent says the child still has symptoms and is still pushing for action whilst to the doctor the child appears well and no obvious and likely cause has been found. Alternatively, the child may seem unwell but the reason has not been elucidated. A third, extremely common, explanation, which will not be discussed in depth here, is that the child has a psychological problem, or the symptom is an indication of a relationship difficulty between parents and child. The explanations behind the majority of vomiting, feeding, wetting, soiling and pain complaints that are not due to obvious common physical causes lie in this area, but clinicians will seek advice from their mental health colleagues in these circumstances. An over-simplified view might be that, in these circumstances, when psychological and relationship problems have been ruled out or managed, and the clinical problem has still not been clarified, many clinicians fail to search widely enough for possible explanations. Their thinking favours the possibility that there is an organic disease they have not found, instead of including other possibilities such as parental anxiety, parental exaggeration and parental deceit to explain the problem. There is a tendency to consider factitious illness as diagnosis of 'exclusion' or ' last resort'. *Factitious illness should be considered in any unresolved clinical problems in childhood.* This might seem an extreme claim but is justifiable because factitious illness describes a spectrum of presentations ranging from mild exaggeration through to severe illness induction. Conversely, it is important to stress that, in an unresolved clinical problem, factitious illness is only one of the possibilities that may be more or less likely in different cases and in the same case at different times. If the method suggested so far is followed, the clinician will by this point already have a complex picture of the child and family. In this section, on the assumption that the clinician has already explored the structure and beliefs as outlined above, we examine three ways to tackle this situation. The first is to use an appropriate clinical problem solving method and these are discussed below. The second is to consider carefully some aspects of the background that may be relevant. These include maternal psychological problems, a history of children lost by death or reception into care, and a history of ineffective treatments. Methods to appraise these issues (if present) are offered. Third, a more critical approach to the complaints of symptoms is suggested, with an increased attention to corroboration of what the parent reports. Vignettes are again used to illustrate the situations, and frameworks given to assist understanding.

Oski, in discussing the diagnostic process (1994), describes four basic approaches to clinical problem solving.

1. 'Sampling the universe' refers to the ordering of laboratory studies in the hope that an abnormality will appear that will result in a diagnosis. Of course, no clinician reading this account has ever fallen prey to this, although they may know a junior doctor with a mild version! The risks of this approach are:
   - Children will be inappropriately investigated rather than their parents concerns being identified and addressed.
   - There will be no possibility of identifying factitious illness, as each new symptom or sign will elicit a further batch of tests. The more tests that are performed, the more likely (statistically) is it that a 'borderline' result, at one end of a normal distribution, will be found and used to justify both the complaint and more investigations.
2. Clinical algorithms are flow charts that help clinicians make decisions. A number of clinical situations have been captured successfully by algorithms but the majority have not. The first problem is that algorithms are only as useful as the range of possible situations considered. All begin with assumptions about the situation and these rarely include, at the outset, two crucial possibilities: that the report of symptoms is invented or exaggerated, or that the symptoms have an external (factitious) cause. As all subsequent 'branches' in the decision tree are based on these false premises, this quickly leads to more investigations and treatments whilst the overall picture is not reviewed. Indeed, algorithms used in this way are a charter for MSBP abuse. A second problem is that the questions generated require a simple yes/no

answer at each branch point. 'Maybe' or any other complex answer blocks progression of the typical algorithm. Many clinical questions cannot be answered so didactically.

3. Pattern recognition refers to the process by which a diagnosis is made on the basis of physical clues or 'linkage identification'. 'The seemingly intuitive diagnosis, often the hallmark of the older physician, is usually a result of linkage identification.' The obverse of this, the intuitive recognition that the pattern of illness does not fit in with a recognized pattern of illness, either in the way the illness presents or the signs and symptoms, should provoke a search for the reasons for this incongruity.

4. Hypothesis generation is the development of an explanation, or a series of explanations, for the patient's problem. It is an important technique for clinical problem solving and is particularly relevant to identifying factitious illness. The development of hypotheses distinguishes the problem solving process from mere data collection. Hypotheses are generated early in patient encounters. Studies demonstrate that the competent physician begins to generate hypotheses the moment the chief complaint is heard, and continues to do so as the remainder of the history unfolds. The formulation of tentative diagnoses serves to guide further enquiry. Thus the process of problem solving is an iterative one. Hypotheses are made initially from incomplete data. These hypotheses are used both to direct further enquiries and to review the original assumptions. This process is continued until the 'best fit' between hypothesis and the data is obtained. Common errors in the process include:

   – Available information is ignored in the generation of the hypotheses. The most important 'available information' is the current physical state of the child, but also includes information about other wider aspects of consultation and illness behaviour.

   – Selected facts or findings may be subsequently ignored because they are inconsistent with an existing hypothesis.

   – Physicians are loathe to generate new hypotheses after the initial list has been formulated.

The clinical problem solving principles set out by Oski may be modified to include awareness of a full range of consultation patterns, including all levels of factitious illness:

- Do not request investigations only because parents request them once basic investigations of all truly likely causes are complete.
- Always consider the harm the tests might do, including emotional and physical distress from the assault on the child. Balance the harm and the cost of tests against the information that may be gained.
- Frequently further investigations are justified by professionals on the grounds that the parents will be reassured by them. In the authors' view there is no evidence to support this assertion and reassurance should come from professional conviction based on professional skill, clinical acumen and confident advice.

Constructive refusal to carry out unnecessary investigations, with a full explanation of the reasons for this refusal, is a much better way to establish the nature of the parental discomfort. This may be lingering concerns about an illness or unreasonable persistence or lack of confidence in the practitioner, each of which will be managed differently.

- Include the parent's beliefs and behaviour in hypotheses about a clinical problem if the parent has presented the child. Study consultation behaviour discrepancies and incongruence so that aspects of parental functioning contribute to the formulation of hypotheses.
- Do not exclude the possibility of illness induction.

Areas meriting special attention in history taking: a maternal history of psychological problems and 'lost' children

There are important areas of the history that have significance in all paediatric clinical encounters, but which may be especially important in understanding why parental presentations are puzzling or incongruent. It is our impression that paediatricians receive little training about how to weigh up these important issues. All of these require careful study for, depending on careful appraisal, they may explain much about a puzzling clinical problem: their significance may be minor or a truly worrying sign.

Here two major areas are discussed: maternal psychological problems and a history of children lost by death or reception into care.

A maternal history of psychological problems

Paediatricians in their clinics and on the wards will meet parents who display a range of moods (anxious, depressed, tense, angry) together with parents who show little emotion or in whom the feelings displayed do not seem to fit the circumstances. Paediatricians will notice the extent to which the parent's mood, when relating information about the child, seems congruent with the account they give and the level of concern about the health of the child in front of them. In what circumstances should a paediatrician probe these issues further? What weight should be attached to a history of mental ill-health in the attempt to prevent factitious illness and in the elucidation of an unresolved clinical problem? If questioned about their own health in a way that explains the relevance of the enquiry to their child's problems, many parents will volunteer a history of mental ill-health in the past or present. Here, careful and sensitive enquiry will probably reveal how serious these 'difficulties' have been, usually measured by whether the problems have been treated, for how long, and by which professionals.

The first point to make is that the paediatrician should always be alert to these issues, not only for humanitarian reasons but because of the impact that maternal mental ill-health has on children. Parents with depression, anxiety, substance abuse, self harm and impulsive risk taking are very common in the population generally and are especially prevalent amongst hospital and health care attenders. This is not only because poor, unsupported parents (who are common in hospitals) have more mental ill-health than more wealthy, well supported families, but because depressed and anxious mothers are more likely to present their children (Wolkind, 1985; Garralda and Bailey, 1987). This is because they are anxious and concerned about their children and need more reassurance, because they may misperceive the seriousness of the illness, and because children are more difficult to manage if one is depressed (Cooper and Murray, 1998). Also, if the mother's depression or other mental health problem is long-standing, the children are more likely to have behavioural disturbance and may be more likely to complain of physical symptoms (Walker and Green, 1993). All of these factors make such parents more likely to bring children to both primary care and secondary paediatric clinics with a variety of complaints both psychosomatic and organic. Such depressed or otherwise disturbed mothers may find real support in the difficult task of child rearing from the sympathetic attention that nurses and doctors may give.

There is nothing specific to factitious illness in a background of psychological problems but, of course, the mother's health will be useful information, which the paediatrician should incorporate when making his formulation and plan. It will also help to explain the child's behaviour, the mother's ability to cope with advice and instructions, and her interpretation of what she has been told. Even when abnormal illness behaviour in relation to the child is not a concern, doctors will be aware that a depressed or anxious parent may find it harder to make decisions, may find an onerous treatment regime more difficult to comply with, and may feel unreasonably guilty or responsible for a child's ill-health or a failure of treatment. So more time and more support may be necessary for these mothers.

Parents with minor psychosomatic illnesses. Minor, less handicapping, more transient psychosomatic illnesses or illnesses with a psychological component such as irritable bowel syndrome are extremely common (even among doctors) and cannot be given great significance as risk factors for factitious illness. Such parents may be anxious, may for good reasons worry that the child has the same illness they experience, and may also have unusual health beliefs (for themselves or their child) that need to be explored if the consultation is to be successful.

Major mental illness. Parents who divulge a history of more major mental illness such as obsessive compulsive disorder and psychotic illnesses (i.e. those which seriously distort thinking) such as schizophrenia or very severe depression, do merit careful thought. The doctor must be aware that such an illness could be seriously interfering with the parent's perception of the child, his symptoms and their management. Here the question of rapport between doctor and parent must be assessed. If the parent seems to be in touch with events and communication with the doctor is unremarkable, it can be illuminating to ask simple questions about the parent's difficulties and whether these have ever had an impact on how the mother views the child's health and symptoms. If another family member is present, the question can also be broached with them subsequently. On the other hand, if the mother seems remote, preoccupied or is talking or behaving incongruently, the paediatrician will obviously wish to invite another close family member to attend a consultation, in order to check perceptions and how much these are shared. A discussion with a mental health professional in the interim may help to clarify the phenomena observed.

Substantial physical illness and those with somatization disorder. Of more frequent relevance to identification of factitious illness are those parents with histories of substantial physical ill-health. This area of enquiry should, of course, be routine earlier in a sequence of consultations but merits revisiting if there is a puzzling, unresolving clinical situation. When appraising such a history the following should be borne in mind: a substantial history of illness is usually associated with an account of understandable treatment from relevant specialists; operations leave scars; illnesses rarely vanish; common things occur commonly and have common causes; and common treatments will be familiar. Patients with somatization disorders (i.e. chronic or relapsing, severe, handicapping presentations with multiple unexplained physical symptoms and pains; hypochondriasis including factitious disorder with injuries inflicted to the skin, eye, cervix etc., and Munchausen syndrome where gross inventions are frequently reported) rarely volunteer them as such to their own physicians and psychiatrists, let alone to their children's medical attendants. If they could express their psychological distress verbally rather than physically, it may be assumed that they would. Such illnesses will therefore probably be presented as purely physical or will be 'forgotten' or lied about. So a history of substantial unexplained or unresolved physical ill-health must merit review ('believe everything the parent says and nothing the parent says') to establish whether a somatization disorder is present. *Permission to corroborate the details with the GP must be sought if there are any doubts or incongruities.* The more distorted the parent, the more likely it is that aspects of this history may prove to be pure fiction – but disturbance of this kind is not always obvious on superficial acquaintance.

A parent with a somatization disorder can be assumed to have difficulty with attributing the right significance and meaning to physical symptoms, for themselves and for others. If their illness has involved much elaboration and fabrication of ill-health (and this will almost certainly not be established at an initial interview), this merits special attention for the corroboration of any history or symptoms in the parent or their child. Their ability to form trusting relationships with professionals, to communicate directly about physical symptoms, and to treat their own bodies appropriately is, by definition, very impaired. The paediatrician must not assume that such parents are fabricating illness in their children, but in these circumstances congruence between the history and findings should always be checked meticulously, and any unexplained severe ill-health must be investigated with factitious illness included in the differential diagnosis in mind.

Personality disorder. Similar considerations apply when it becomes apparent that the parent has a personality disorder. As before, this is rarely volunteered, but often enough history of substance abuse, self harm, extensive emergency psychiatric contact and sometimes criminality and children in care will provide the clues to alert the clinician. *Although parents with either of these two forms of major difficulty (somatization and personality disorder) are at risk of providing distorted parenting, and their children are accordingly vulnerable to becoming a vehicle to signal parental neediness, equally, nothing prevents their children developing intrinsic illness.*

Lest doctors start to believe that all parental disturbance can be easily identified, it must always be remembered that many of the most damaged individuals, especially those from educated, well organized backgrounds, are able to present a superficially intact façade. Indeed, such parents are often reported as making particularly sociable, charming approaches to authority figures such as doctors whilst they manifest their own needs through their child. Such parents are likely to deceive many well intentioned clinicians and a constant testing of all hypotheses and possibilities for a child's presentation will be an important protection for the doctor from becoming an instrument of abuse.

'Lost' children

'Losing' children, whether through bitter dispute following family break-up, through removal into care by the local authority or through death, is a major life event for any parent and obviously one which has a significant effect upon the way they relate to other children. One of the most powerful causes of incongruity between medical assessment of seriousness and parental persistence in the consultation is a parental concern that the child might have serious illness, even a life-threatening one. A previous loss will, of course, have a profound effect upon the parent's relationship with professionals, whom they see as having the power to produce a similar loss for them with another child. In their eyes, this may be through professional lack of care in the case of illness, or through ascertainment of parental deficiencies, i.e. by reporting the parent to social services. It has been documented that most parents who witness their child having their first seizure fear that the child is actually dying or has died (Baumer *et al.*, 1981). This potential loss may produce a profound effect on parents which may distort their relationship with the child for some time afterwards.

For many parents the loss of a child by death brings guilt that they should themselves have done something more and on occasion of course this may be correct. Therefore the death of a child within a family or one known to the family clearly explains and is a powerful cause of some kinds of parental persistence. The vignette below illustrates this.

A five year old girl who had had episodes of nephrotic syndrome and had last received steroids six months previously was transferred to a regional centre with an encephalitic illness. Despite empirical antiviral treatment and inten sive care she died. No specific diagnosis was made. The precise relation-ship, if any, between this overwhelming infection and previous steroid therapy was unclear but the family always had a very strong belief that it was the previous steroid treatment that was the crucial factor in this tragedy.

Their other child, an eight year old boy, also had infrequent relapsing nephrotic syndrome. He had had two attacks of this, one at the age of two years and one at the age of four years, and had been previously managed adequately and appropriately in a District General Hospital. When the daugh-ter died, the family insisted on immediate review in the regional centre. Despite the boy never having a further attack of nephrotic syndrome, assess-ment by regional specialists was requested every time he was unwell over the next ten years. There were repeated concerns that he might be swollen from time to time and this required considerable discussion in out-patients. The concerns were always focused around the previous nephrotic syndrome and related symptoms and signs.

Although this reaction is perhaps slightly extreme in its persistence, the reason for parental concern was understandable. The anxiety was contained with appro-priate medical advice.

Although unlikely, it would be possible that an enthusiastic junior member of staff, unaware of this history, might have perceived the parental history with the second boy as being pathological. Indeed there was no doubt that this boy was over-protected and perhaps his development was less than ideal as a result – but this situation is essentially benign.

Deaths used to 'justify' extreme concerns being misused for the same purpose

A boy had been admitted to hospital fifteen times by the age of eight years. One admission had been due to a minor injury, then there had been a series of admissions because of reported chest problems. During this period the mother had also reported weight loss and vomiting, although the child was thriving normally. At the age of eighteen months the mother reported convul-sions, and these convulsions or apnoeic attacks were the reason given for five further admissions over the next eighteen months. As part of the review of the history, it was established that three different family members had died: one at the age of three days of extreme prematurity, one at the age of eleven months of hydrocephalus following neonatal pseudomonas meningi-tis and one at the age of three years with a malignancy. It was established that the reported convulsions were largely, if not entirely, factitious and the mother was confronted with this opinion. Follow-up was not kept and no more convulsions were ever reported.

The next admission was two years later with again a minor injury and then there were two further admissions over the next four years. Soon after this, at the age of twelve years, the focus changed to recurrent abdominal pain and vomiting; this was not confirmed on admission to hospital. No investigations were performed and the problem was contained subsequently by outpatient consultations.

There were no further admissions for another four years, when the child presented acutely unwell with neck pain, headache and nausea. Mother now gave a (false) history that three cousins had died previously of meningitis. Clearly both mother and son were understandably concerned that the current illness might be meningitis.

There were episodes of abnormal illness behaviour, factitious convulsions, exaggerated symptoms and false history giving in this family, but it was equally true that relatives suffered organic illness of which the mother was aware. At least initially it is possible that the consultations did relate to clear anxiety about previous deaths within the family, and this was the hypothesis that was pursued in the early years. As time went by, the illness presentation became very exaggerated. Whether the previous deaths in the family simply gave this mother a model for the presentations of her own child or served another function is not discernible. Other trigger factors were not looked for, unfortunately. Whilst it took a very long time for the mother's habits of fabrication to be recognized, by the time the boy was sixteen and the frequency of presentation had markedly diminished, there was no justification for an appraisal by social services. Nevertheless, the mother's notes and those of other family members should contain a summary of what has occurred and a high level of corroboration be sought for future complaints.

How, then, is the significance of a death in the family to be distinguished from more sinister circumstances where MSBP abuse has caused the death? Cot deaths are particularly difficult. Not only is there now evidence (Meadow, 1999) that far more of these deaths than previously recognized are from suffocation, but case series of MSBP abuse victims have made clear the grave and excess risks of infant death and abuse in these families (Bools, Neale and Meadows, 1992; Gray and Bentovim, 1996; McClure *et al.*, 1998). On the other hand, innocent loss of an infant by cot death can profoundly affect parents and increase their perception of the vulnerability of their children. It can distort their perceptions of the child's ill-health and, particularly if accompanied by severe depression in the mother, it can interfere with her parenting abilities and the nature of her rapport with professionals. The best advice that can be given in these circumstances is that professionals should identify children in the family who have died and, as carefully and precisely as possible, ascertain the cause of death. If he or she experiences unease and uncertainty, which may arise either because the way the mother describes the story does not seem to ring true or because the medical details seem implausible, the onus is on the doctor to verify the information with other sources, including GP and other hospital records.

A suspicious death

The mother of a twelve year old boy with nocturnal enuresis rang on three occasions before the out-patient review to check that the boy would be reviewed by a Consultant. A reason for these contacts was not identified during the consultation. The mother, who had six children, also reported a history of haematuria in a second child and of haemoptysis in a third child. She concluded the interview by reporting that she was consulting an orthopaedic surgeon that afternoon about a fourth child who had had a pain in the leg some four weeks ago which had lasted for twenty-four hours. Mother said she wanted to see an orthopaedic surgeon to exclude osteomyelitis, although she conceded that this was highly unlikely.

All treatments for enuresis were ineffective and at the next appointment there was pressure for further opinions for all the children. The mother was cheerful and seemed relaxed but made the clinicians feel uncomfortable. Father never attended the appointments and mother was disparaging of him as he performed manual work and she had been a teacher. During the review of the family history, a previous cot death two years before of a three month old baby was identified. Attempts were made to find out details about the cot death. It was discovered that a post-mortem had taken place, which the family had resisted, but the result evidently suggested that the death was not suspicious. However, the original GP, whose list the family had subsequently left, shared with the consultant his suspicions (which he had not expressed before but had thought since the death) that the cot death might have been caused by suffocation.

The concern of the GP at the time and of the consultant two years later was that the cot death felt suspicious. Concern in this instance was that it seemed highly probable that the death was due to the mother's actions. In the light of the post-mortem results, there was nothing to be done except to be vigilant about future abnormal illness behaviour and to alert the new GP to the concerns. The mother moved GP again soon after.

These vignettes illustrate the spectrum of relevance of previous deaths, ranging from the understandable extreme dependence on medical support that can arise as a consequence of the death of another child within the family, through to the much more sinister end of the spectrum where an unexplained cot death together with other factitious illness is highly suggestive of severe induced illness.

We move on now to the situation of having had children removed by the local authority – one that puts parents in a very particular light. It is most unusual for children to be removed for trivial failures in parental care, even though parents may, quite understandably, rationalize and minimize their own faults when sub-sequently explaining to professionals why they have lost their children. The identification of children lost into the care system will, except in the most bare-faced liars, be identified by simple questions about 'who lives in the family?' and 'have you any other children?'. This information would normally be obtained in a sequence of consultations when parents should be feeling well engaged and, presumably, with no reason for suspicion. Until proved otherwise, professionals would do well to assume that such parents have had substantial difficulties with parenting and this should increase the level of vigilance for all kinds of neglect or abuse. Denying the loss of children when enquiries have been made with genuine interest and tact is more pathological, but even this may be benign if, for example, the mother has concealed her past from a current partner if this partner is in the room. Checking the facts with the relevant social services department is, of course, mandatory should concerns arise about any form of abuse.

Corroborating the history and reported symptoms

One of the most important steps to take when there is persisting incongruity is to review the quality of one's information as well as its quantity. Critical appraisal of a wider variety of hypotheses about unresolved clinical problems includes the possibility that there may have been distortion in the account the clinician received. Many of the benign causes of incongruity have been explored earlier. It is prudent at this point for the clinician to move to different method of appraising information. This will include:

• Seeking clear corroboration from other sources for symptoms that are reported.
• Ensuring that the information that is received about the child's previous illness is corroborated.
• Checking other contacts with medical care by an examination of these records

The quickest method of acquiring this information is by contact with the GP and examining copies of correspondence that are in the GP notes. We are fortunate in the UK that the GP is still the source of most specialist referrals and will have letters in the patient's file from such contacts. It may also be appropriate to gain permission from the parents to ask the GP about the parent's history, again usually with the simple justification that one needs to understand the illnesses that they have suffered in order to judge whether they might have any relevance for the presentation of the child being reviewed. The illnesses of other children in the family can be considered also. This sort of search for corroboration is not at the level of scrutinizing all records. This may be reached later when concerns about harm and reports of suspicious of factitious illness have been received or reached onself.

The following vignette demonstrates a hypothesis testing approach at this stage with an unresolved clinical problem and incongruence.

An eight year old boy was referred for consideration of further investigations of haematuria. There had been an episode of reported haematuria two years previously. No urine sample had contained significant blood. Investigations including cystoscopy had been normal. The mother had been advised to bring the child back if the haematuria recurred but did not take up this offer for three years, at which point she reported that the haematuria continued persistently over the three year period. Mother was a confident, articulate individual who engaged easily in discussion in the clinic. Mother said she had not returned to the clinic because she had been reassured by the previous negative investigations.

On enquiring about the family history mother reported an uncomplicated appendectomy in her brother but no other family history of note. Later in the interview a chance question about family structure led to disclosure of a more extended illness history of the mother. She described herself as having had a 'rough year', culminating in hysterectomy which, according to her report, her medical carer said she had been 'lucky to survive'. She said she herself had been prone to bleeding, including some rectal bleeding, and she reported problems with bleeding related to the hysterectomy. Despite the life-threatening story, the mother seemed unconcerned when recounting these recent events. On direct questioning she indicated that she had worried that a similar bleeding tendency might account for the child's haematuria.

This prompted revisiting of the presenting complaint. It now became unclear how often blood had been observed. The history was further confused by the fact that mother reported that the boy wore dark underpants, which made it difficult to identify any staining on them. It was agreed with the mother that the general practitioner would be contacted to discuss her own recent illness and to establish whether there might be an inherited bleeding tendency. Mother agreed to keep a careful record of the reported bleeding over the next month and to make sure that observations were not obscured by the type of clothing worn. An interview one month later was agreed with time to review the problem fully.

Comment

Many incongruities in this clinical story merit exploration: discrepancies in the parental complaints (haematuria is, on the whole, a very worrying sign for parents and it would be very unusual if this did not lead to prompt reconsultation), surprising lacunae in the history ('forgetting' a history of bleeding tendency in herself when this was the supposed concern in her son), and a clinical account which does not fit with common disease patterns (it would be most unusual and clinically improbable for visible haematuria to occur on every single day for a number of years).

Rather than embarking on further investigations it was important to try to assess the current facts about the boy, who had no blood in his urine at clinic and no abnormality on cystoscopy. The only investigation required was a telephone call to the general practitioner to establish the existence or otherwise of a bleeding tendency in the mother, and to discuss with him or her the nature of mother's recent ill-health, plus an understanding of the consultations for the boy in primary care over the last few years.

Thus the hypotheses at this point included:

1. There may be a bleeding tendency in the family.
2. The boy may have haematuria, but it does not conform to any common disease and investigations have already taken place.
3. There is something wrong with the mother's account, which contains many internal inconsistencies. In the absence of any evidence that the mother has significant disabilities or some form of dementing process, she must be assumed to be 'embroidering the truth', but the reasons are not obvious.

At the subsequent appointment, the mother reported that no more bleeding had occurred and suggested, again in contradiction to her previous history, that there had been no bleeding for several months. The GP's records had not confirmed a bleeding tendency.

Hypotheses one and two are then unlikely and hypothesis three must be assumed to be accurate. At this stage, the question was raised: how harmful were these fabrications? The boy had already been harmed by a cystoscopy that was possibly unnecessary, but some time had passed and no significant increase in fabrications had occurred. Thus it was deemed best to bear this in mind rather than to act upon it. The protocol for managing abnormal consultation behaviour when the threshold of harm has not been reached was employed (see Chapter 9). Unless there is other evidence of problems with parenting (not explored here), such a case can often be managed by containment of consultations and investigations and limitation of the number of clinicians involved. However, increasing the awareness and vigilance of the GP and other health professionals (e.g. community paediatrician, school nurse) is essential too.

Dawning of 'private concerns in the mind'

This title implies that a clinician is crossing an important threshold of concern about the child. He or she has an awareness of discrepancies that cannot be explained away or dispersed by any of the more or less benign explanations or management strategies described so far. Either there is an undiscovered illness or there is something else very wrong with the situation and it is not being contained by firm resistance to unnecessary health care (sometimes, but rarely, both are true). In other words, the time to dichotomize has arrived because the clinician is worried that the child is either suffering harm because doctors are missing an illness, or because someone is pretending or making him ill. In this section these two hypotheses are explored, together with a summary of some of the most worrying kinds of incongruity in consultations – ones that should alert clinicians to less benign aspects of parental behaviour. Even so, it should be remembered that many have explanations that are not harmful to children.

Concerns might arise at any stage of the assessment of a clinical problem. They might slowly develop as more and more circumstantial evidence of fabrication emerges over months or years and 'benign' explanations become implausible, or they might suddenly become an urgent possibility because of an episode which cannot be explained except by illness induction. These concerns will vary considerably depending on the harm that the clinician thinks has occurred or is at risk of occurring.

This critical threshold is a matter of individual professional judgement. As private concerns in the mind move towards the preliminary consultation with a colleague, a systematic, dispassionate, objective review of all the data is essential. If the system of assessing clinical problems set out in this chapter has been followed, a careful and detailed evaluation of the clinical problem will have collected most of the relevant information, but systematically summarizing all the information is crucial.

Informing parents about concerns

How should parents be informed of concerns? Up to this point, parents should be treated in a normal way with regular discussions. In tertiary practice one is frequently faced with difficult diagnoses, uncertain clinical courses, unpredictable outcomes. It is normal practice to discuss the dilemmas with parents in such a way that they can have understanding of the situation, participate in clinical decisions and help their child. There is no need to share all one's thoughts with them. It is appropriate to tell parents if you do not know the explanation for the findings and what steps are being taken to establish these. At an early stage possible factitious illness abuse can and should be handled in the same way.

Hypothesis one: doctors are missing an illness

We do not deal here with the child who is already in hospital when the need for the investigation of severe illness induction is recognized, such as when smothering is suspected. This is dealt with in the next chapter.

Throughout this chapter the consideration of an overlooked or undiscovered intrinsic illness is raised. If must be raised again here, as one of the possibilities. It is difficult to describe precisely how the appraisal of this differs when the clinician is also seriously concerned about extrinsic causes. Of course, to those clinicians implicated in the damage to children in early reported cases and in an American system with no primary care as a filter for referrals, extenuating circumstances (ignorance of the way doctors are used to serve parental needs) can be granted. Even with the benefit of hindsight, some of these scenarios remain difficult to understand. Guandolo (1985) reported a five year old with no intrinsic pathology who had '250 office visits' including consultations with an otolaryngologist, orthopaedic surgeon, nutritionist and three neurologists. The mother would also frequently inform the paediatric office that a physician neighbour or emergency room had diagnosed and treated a specific problem.

The number of consultations that may be attained by a child with a serious handicapping disorder (spina bifida with multiple anomalies, perhaps, or severe congenital heart disease) may, of course, reach 250 or more by the age of five, but here there is no difficulty establishing the diagnosis. Main, Douglas and Tamanika (1986) reported a case where, over a period of seven years, a mother consulted about her child's health over 300 times. The main complaints were of abdominal pains and difficulty breathing, but there seemed to be a constant state of ill-health and crisis. Other examples of ill-health that were 'diagnosed' by the mother included heart trouble, kidney failure, ulcers, loss of vision, loss of hearing, bone problems, depression, refusal to eat, glandular problems, asthma, agoraphobia, curvature of the spine, a collapsed lung, 'nerves' and gastric reflux. It is difficult to imagine, in the absence of a clear pathology, what child condition could explain these and the confusing mixture of pseudo-medical, pseudo-psychological and fanciful symptoms. They appear to give clear evidence of maternal pathology. It is therefore frankly incredible that this paper continues '...over fifty investigative procedures have been performed'.

Perhaps the results of Lacey *et al.*'s (1993) case series of ten MSBP abuse identifications in a five year period should be considered here too. These children, aged from five and a half months upwards, had between two and eighteen admissions and up to ten formal assessments by paediatric subspecialists, most with normal results, before the 'dawning of awareness'.

These examples are quoted in an attempt to remind paediatricians of their great power to abuse. They are accompanied by the suggestion that the question of an undiscovered illness be reviewed and discussed with expert and sympathetic colleagues in a well-planned meeting where all information, including that from the repeated corroboration sequence mentioned below, is available. The recommendation is then that it is the key clinician, not the patient, who requires colleagues' advice; it is the key clinician who must formulate the case in all its complexity. It is essential that responsibility for intervention is not dispersed between many consultants and specialists.

Hypothesis two: factitious illness by proxy, either by invented symptoms or induced illness

Further evaluation of unresolved clinical problems will give rise to numerous incongruities. As these are explored and innocent explanations are excluded, the possibility of more dangerous incongruities including factitious illness increases. The list discussed below includes the commonly cited incongruities. Some are probably more specific for factitious illness than others. Examples are given of most of these issues: some have been selected to illustrate 'benign' explanations and others more 'dangerous' explanations; some may not cross the threshold of harm.

More worrying incongruities that might contribute to private concerns in the mind

Parental consultation behaviour meriting serious concern

• Erroneous information.

> One mother, to emphasize the severity of her child's vomiting, reported that the child had vomited faeces, even describing the smell. She claimed that the event had been observed by a GP and suggested he should be phoned. She was probably encouraged because her other implausible and dramatic stories had been accepted without corroboration by paediatricians. This failure of corroboration had been partly because the reported witnesses had not been contactable. Thus it was not possible to trace the emergency doctor who had asked the mother to ensure that the hospital doctors were aware that he had never seen such a distended abdomen: 'it looked as if the child was nine months pregnant'. Neither the GP who was said to have observed the copious haemoptysis, nor the laboratory who, it was reported, had analysed the sputum, had a record of this. The story of faeculent vomiting was completely fabricated.

Verbal communication between doctors through the patient/parent unfortunately seems to be commonplace. This certainly presents an opportunity to perpetrate factitious illness. In the above vignette, this led to the elaboration of a complex story that had no factual base. Manipulation of communication can lead to further referrals and investigations which are not clinically indicated. Never accept at face value the helpful suggestion that 'to save you time doctor X asked me to say…'.

Falsification of letters is a marker of clear deception, as is tampering with charts during admission (discussed in the next chapter).

Incomplete or false information about previous medical contacts. This describes something beyond what poor memory, rushing through a history or anxiety will justify. Lorber (1980) provides the following example.

'Further enquiries into the family history were made. Although no mention was made of this, it was discovered that the mother had been married previously and that two children by that marriage were in care. The general practitioner with whom the family were supposedly registered in the south of England, before moving to Derbyshire, had no record of the family. Previous addresses provided by the mother, in different cities, were found to be false and the general practitioner with whom she claimed to be registered currently, had no knowledge of either the mother or the child. A London hospital had 'lost' records of her admissions to them in 1974 and 1977, but an admission in 1976 … was confirmed. She had claimed to be a state registered nurse, but enquiries with the General Nursing Council showed that she had not so qualified. The hospital where she was said to have trained had no record of her.'

Major and unexplained incongruity between the clinical story and the clinical assessment

This scenario can involve a well child but a striking clinical story, including complex and changing histories. It often includes a changing clinical story with a clinically improbable and aetiologically implausible element. Thus the incongruity may be in the content of the clinical story, or the process by which this revealed and often includes elements of both of these.

> A girl of six was reviewed in the out-patients with reported haematuria. The story of persistent, very heavy macroscopic haematuria and clots in the urine was very convincing. Because of this, and a report of extreme lethargy, the possibility of serious renal disease arose and the child was admitted for immediate investigations. A full family history was taken in out-patients and checked on admission with specific reference to a family history of renal disease and of haematuria. No previous family illnesses of note were reported.
>
> On admission, basic renal function and ultrasound were normal and no haematuria had recurred. It was assumed that the girl had a self-limiting problem such as acute haemorrhagic cystitis and no further problems were expected. This was discussed fully with the parents.
>
> On review in the clinic one month later mother reported seeing blood in her daughter's urine every day and she reported that the child's lethargy had become even worse. On talking about the family, the mother reported she had discovered that two aunts had had serious problems with their kidneys, one with cancer and the other with renal failure. Eventually, permission was obtained to obtain these notes and one family member had had a mild orthopaedic problem and the other had had cystoscopy on one occasion 10 years previously but with no subsequent problems.
>
> Although the mother continued to report haematuria in out-patients the child remained well and attended school full-time and no other symptoms developed.

As there were no other suggestions of exaggerated illness or other evidence of parental difficulty and no triggers in this family, the possibility remains that this was simply a misunderstanding on the mother's behalf – but in no way could her account and the professional view be reconciled. The solution was to discount her reports because the child was well and objective information was available, but close monitoring by community professionals was recommended.

Incongruity between the seriousness of the story and the actions of the parents

An example of this would be avoidance of review when the child is 'unwell' but reports of symptoms then being used to justify new treatment. In circumstances where parents report symptoms that are intermittent but may be serious, it is a basic tenet of good medical practice to arrange for a child to be reviewed when clinically unwell. The parents should be asked to do this, while the professional needs to ensure that they can get up to the hospital when appropriate (e.g. transport and child care need to be available). The family need to know who will be available and the different ways to contact the hospital at different times of day and night and that the accepting clinician has instructions as to what clinical assessments are to be performed. If, despite these arrangements, the child is not presented for assessment when unwell, then the parents are behaving in a way which is incongruent with their complaint. Avoidance of review in these circumstances justifies frank discussion with parents, and a sceptical approach to reports of symptoms with a high threshold for investigations. The following vignette illustrates an incongruous failure to present a child who is unwell.

> A six year old boy has been followed for six months in the outpatients department. He was reported to have numerous problems including haematuria, episodes of going yellow, extreme lethargy, and marked abdominal extension. The mother was provided with a letter introducing her to the hospital and telling her how important it was to bring him in when unwell. On review one month later the mother was extremely concerned about his condition and said he had been unrousable for 48 hours. When asked why she had not brought him in she said she had not been specifically told to bring him in if he was unrousable, and it occurred at the weekend and she thought the consultant would not be available. Arrangements for emergency review were again explained. At the next outpatient visit she reported severe vomiting but claimed the boy had begged to be allowed to go to his friend's birthday party rather than visit the hospital.

The implausibility of treatment failure

Whilst complete success in treatment is rare, so is total failure. Like any other 'litmus test' this is not infallible, as the following vignette illustrates.

The vignette includes features that were difficult to explain. The failure of so many treatments meant a clear need to dichotomize had arrived: either there was an overlooked pathology or something else was maintaining the illness. There were repeated infections with no obvious cause and persistence of infections despite antibiotics being used to which the organisms were sensitive, even when these antibiotics were given intravenously. No doubt in an out-patient setting the most common explanation for this situation would be parents not giving antibiotics. The story in this vignette raised suspicions of induced illness but critical review of the radiology identified an overlooked pathology.

This explanation was not the only possibility. There are numerous reports in the literature of recurrent infections of intravenous lines, soft tissue infections, osteomyelitis and joint infections in which failure to respond to treatment was due to the parent interfering with the treatment. (Kohl, 1978; Liston, 1983; Sefarian, 1997).

> The three year old son of a paediatric nurse had six urinary tract infections over four months. On three occasions there had been positive urine cultures. Infections persisted despite being treated with appropriate antibiotics intravenously. Because of the persistence of infection despite adequate treatment with appropriate antibiotics the possibility of induced infections was considered. Review of the radiology revealed overlooked renal abnormality (occult non-functioning duplex element to the kidney). This was removed surgically. Before surgery the patient was treated with appropriate antibiotics which sterilized the urine, despite which the non-funtioning element of the kidney was still full of organisms sensitive to antibiotics previosly administered.

Constant welcoming of intrusive treatments for problems of, at worst, moderate severity

This applies especially to problems in which parent–child relationships are highly significant causes, including resistant and unexplained vomiting, starving, fatigue, wetting and soiling. After careful initial physical assessment has excluded likely organic causes, all such children merit assessment by skilled mental health specialists (in liaison with the paediatrician), and the persistence of such problems and avoidance of mental health inputs must not be viewed uncritically (see Chapter 9). This should take place before rare intrinsic causes are postulated or invented: the failure of basic relationships concerned with feeding and excretion are much more likely than a new or rare disease, but such an explanation is also likely to be unwelcome to the parent.

Symptoms or signs that begin only in the presence of one parent

This observation can carry very different weight depending on the symptom: great weight if the concern is of apnoea or seizures, but much less weight for less acute complaints. It can only be established with patient, sensitive, detailed history taking, although information from other witnesses may help. It must always be remembered that the child often spends more time with one parent than another and one parent, particularly the mother, is often much more alert to possible illness in a child than the other. Once again, carefully recorded notes about who reported what and who was present, will gradually allow the picture to be built up, whilst other hypotheses are able to be explored simultaneously.

Where factitious illness has resulted in major illness

Also to be considered here is the possibility that the factitious illness has resulted, both by virtue of the actions of the parents and those of the medical investigations, in major illness. There are numerous examples of this in the literature and some are quoted elsewhere in this book (Kosmach *et al.*, 1996; McClung, 1988; Porter *et al.*, 1994; Santangelo *et al.*, 1989; Sullivan *et al.*, 1991).

There is no doubt that major chronic illness (for example, chronic renal failure) and factitious illness can co-exist. This is, perhaps, not surprising because a burdensome child who disappoints their parents is likely both to prove very stressful and to bring out attachment relationship difficulties. This will also mean that the disjunction between a well child and a striking story of ill-health will not apply.

Testing the two hypotheses

Further corroboration of the story and review of family history including siblings

In the previous section on 'the unresolved clinical problem', a precise approach to observations of the child's illness and a review of the GP's view, and of letters from other clinicians about the child and probably the mother, was advised. These matters may need to be revisited at this stage: first, by reviewing the history with the parents, second, by seeking independent professional witnesses about what the parents report, and third, by scrutinizing notes from other establishments for this child, relevant siblings and perhaps a parent, if he or she agrees. A clear answer must be gained about what illness the child has had, and what is uncertain.

This requires adequate time, patience and no prejudice (believing everything the parent says and nothing the parent says). It is critically important to establish exactly who is supposed to have seen what, when and where. Establish a level of detail that can be checked. In a situation of fabrication there is almost invariably an element of uncertainty and lack of clarity. Follow up meticulously every clue offered in the history and make a clear record. The interview must not be curtailed. Concentrate on identifying and agreeing elements of the history which are open to corroboration from other sources, personal or documentary. The history must include the past medical history of the child, siblings and other family members. In the context of factitious illness, often stories about illness in neighbours and acquaintances will be volunteered. Two approaches may be useful:

- Encourage the parents to give a complete list of presenting complaints. This is often very extensive.
- Establish a chronology of the illnesses in the family and where they were treated, gaining permission to contact all institutions and witnesses if this has not been discussed earlier.

Seeking independent corroboration of the history and observation from professional witnesses

Talking to the child

Of course, even preschool children can feign some symptoms as a 'learnt' behaviour that can be encouraged by a parent. The child's view of the history may, however, show clear conflict with the parent's account or may even disclose abusive activities. A two and a half year old boy alerted authorities to problems when he complained to his mother's friend that his thigh was sore because 'Mommy gave me shots' (Boros, 1992). A four and a half year old boy reported that 'Johny forced the hose into my mouth and made me drink' (Mortimer, 1980). An adult survivor's story of her experience of MSBP abuse starting at the age of two years and continuing for eight years demonstrates that she was aware of the abuse from the age of two to three years (Bryk, 1998). Abuse such as suffocation may be 'played out' by the child whilst on the ward with a play worker, for example, and whilst of little value in a legal context, this is very helpful to alert the clinician to possibilities.

Discussing symptoms and observations with other professionals

The family doctor is an invaluable source of information (not all of it written in the notes), although some family doctors have little awareness of and are unwilling to consider the possibility of factitious illness. There may be problems gaining consent to discuss illness in other members of the family without the consent of the parent. The clinician may be able to explain to the GP that, where child abuse is considered possible, their duty to the child ranks higher than their duty of confidentiality to the child's parents, i.e. the child's interests are paramount. Or it may be necessary to wait for legal protection of this step (see Chapter 12) if the parent or GP is unhappy (see Chapter 11).

Other independent witnesses

Nurses, health visitors and other health professionals, day care/nursery school personnel, teachers and other family members are generally easily accessible. Fabricators will often 'volunteer' witnesses. These should always be contacted and asked to provide a simple, precise description of what was observed. Failure of corroboration of the story by reliable witnesses is very concerning. The reverse situation is more difficult to interpret:

- Factitious and non-factitious illness can co-exist, so that the witnesses may be truly observing pathology which the perpetrator then exaggerates.
- Witnesses, particularly those in the family, might have been deceived, be protecting the perpetrator or be denying the situation.
- Perpetrators of MSBP abuse mislead even the most experienced doctors and hence it is probable that they can persuade less clinically experienced individuals and, even more so, family members and non-professional witnesses. This also needs to be borne in mind when the medical notes are being reviewed.

Review of medical records

The possible sources should be identified by discussion with the parents, other family members, the family doctor and any referring paediatrician. A systematic review of all relevant notes is then necessary. It may be of particular value to examine the primary care records or to talk with relevant professionals who will be able to clarify the status of the observations (reported or observed) and will often share concerns which they have not written in the notes. They may show clear inconsistencies with the hospital records or may show problems hitherto unidentified. Siblings' records may need similar review. In several recent cases, these have clarified longitudinal patterns of parental behaviour in a stark and uncompromising way.

It is important to obtain the original records including nursing notes, not just the letters, and photocopies of the notes often include only medical notes. It is particularly important to check on the evidence for each new reported symptom – these are often accepted uncritically and gain enormous credibility as they are copied from one medical entry in the notes to the next.

Organizing the information

Organizing the substantial amount of information in cases where MSBP abuse is seriously considered is a daunting task. One generally recommended approach is given below.

1. Develop a detailed chronology of the medical care.
2. Develop a list of presenting features which documents the number of symptoms that have been reported and their development over time. New features tend to be added to the history, are not checked and become incorporated into the story and drive further investigation and referral. The evidence for each new symptom needs to be checked.
3. This template can be then be used to:
   (a) Review the differential diagnoses explored.
   (b) Consider whether there are alternative diagnoses that should be considered after a discussion with a colleague.

It is important to emphasize that this clinical process is aimed at understanding any complex/unresolved problem and not at proving factitious illness. If the reason for the underlying clinical problem *is* factitious illness, then during this process incongruities will persist and often more will emerge.

After the review process

The possibilities after this further review process are as follows:

1. A diagnosis is established and/or the consultation behaviour is explained. *Beware a rare diagnosis* – Meadow (1985) has made the point that many cases of MSBP abuse have been labelled as rare diagnoses (porphyria etc.) when MSBP abuse would be a more common explanation of the clinical phenomenology. Always ask someone with experience of the rare disease whether

or not the clinical picture is consistent with it. Published reports are a help but first hand experience is best.

2. Continuing uncertainty. The uncertainty lies on a continuum from a suspected as yet undefined, perhaps new, pathology, through to a bizarre illness with many features in the consultation behaviour that are suggestive of MSBP abuse. But, more commonly, the situation lies somewhere in between. In these circumstances, the extent of the harm to the child must be a factor in future decision making. It may be possible to continue the existing management of the child whilst maintaining vigilance. Uncertainty should always be respected and creating a plan of what would resolve this, in any of the possible directions, may help in the development of a clear plan to gain further evidence, either of health or disease. Chapter 9, 'Dealing with uncertainty', explores a number of these situations and suggests ways to resolve uncertainty.

3. Probable evidence of fabrication is established. At this stage the paediatricians should describe as accurately and as objectively as possible the observed situation on the basis of the history, examination and appropriate investigations (e.g. factitious epilepsy or parental exaggeration of asthma) rather than diagnosing 'factitious illness' (Fisher and Mitchell, 1995). At this point the clinician will wish to contact social services and discuss how to proceed with a strategy meeting. This point marks the bridge from Stage 1 to Stage 2: awareness and identification (or refutation) of possible factitious illness.

Integrating existing knowledge and collating facts

Concerns about possible harm to the child (child abuse) should not be managed alone by the paediatrician caring for the child. As a minimum, such concerns should be discussed with a independent colleague, often the designated doctor for child protection, and certainly one with experience in this field. There may be value in having a *meeting of health professionals* (community and hospital based general, specialist, child psychiatry) with or without social workers present. This should be strictly confidential, minutes taken and decisions made on the appropriateness of further medical investigations, or alternatively a formal referral to social services. They might decide to call a 'multi-agency strategy meeting' (without parents) to establish the need for a more detailed child protection investigation or for the use of more forensic diagnostic techniques (toxicology, covert video surveillance etc.). Chapter 10 further describes the process.

These meetings offer an opportunity to plan and to check historical, medical, social and family details, some of which may have been verified already. The result of this may be an increasing level of concern because of conflicting/inconsistent reports. Such details must be maintained confidentially at this stage to avoid alerting parents to the concerns and hence losing the opportunity to obtain additional information which might help to secure child protection proceedings. A strategy or professional meeting is a more formal process. After such a professional or strategy meeting talking to parents should be carefully planned. Both the meeting itself and the conversation with parents are discussed in Chapter 11.

If parents break off contact at this point, there may be sufficient concern to approach social services and to hold a strategy meeting or professionals' meeting in any case. This may be a great help to the GP who is likely to be faced with requests to initiate further referrals and who will be assisted by a full discussion of medical and child protection/harm and risk issues.

Professional barriers to identification of MSBP abuse

The commonest reason for not identifying this form of abuse is the professional's failure to consider the possibility of fabricated illness. Reasons that contribute to the delay in considering this form of abuse include the following:

- There is a lack of awareness of the range of behaviours.
- Concentration on 'making a diagnosis' rather than appraising all presentations and the whole of the child's health in a broad and holistic fashion. Faced with a difficult clinical problem there is much personal prestige invested in making a rare diagnosis, especially if other colleagues have already been consulted.
- Minor abnormalities on investigation are unquestioningly accepted as explaining a substantial level of fabricated illness presentation, rather than being evaluated critically.
- There is a tendency to consider this form of abuse as a 'diagnosis' of exclusion or last resort. It should be considered early in the assessment of any repeated or unusual presentation. Early consideration will enhance the careful collection of historical details, close documentation of signs and prospective verification and cross-checking of health records. More thought will be given to the decision to request further investigations and their interpretation and to initiation of trials of treatments.
- Failure to take even the most rudimentary steps to corroborate the story given by the parents. It is time consuming to pursue the information required to establish the history of medical contact and background in such families.
- Many children in whom illness is exaggerated or fabricated also have intrinsic illness. It is more difficult to identify fabrication in the context of an existing well documented illness.
- There is a professional (and legal) risk in deciding to stop investigations.
- This form of abuse questions our beliefs about parenting and the doctor–patient relationship and is, therefore, emotionally challenging. It is only human to try to avoid thinking about such difficult ideas, especially with parents with whom one has already apparently developed a trusting professional relationship.

Conclusions

This chapter has attempted to find a clinical approach that will allow the early identification of factitious illness because it adopts a broad view of the clinical process.

The focus has moved from a routine consultation, through the unresolved clinical problem, to the dawning of 'private concerns in the mind' about factitious illness. At this point, the situation may remain uncertain and various approaches to this are discussed in Chapter 9. Alternatively, concern will be sufficient to justify a strategy meeting with social services. This meeting may decide that the evidence is clear-cut and that it is appropriate to proceed to an initial child protection case conference (see Chapter 11). More often, further information will need to be collected in the investigation phase, using the methods discussed in Chapter 4.

The chapter started by emphasizing the centrality of history taking. There is, perhaps, a danger that the structure we have used is taken to suggest, that as concerns about possible factitious illness increase, the standard of history taking changes from a cursory routine to a much more alert, meticulous and detailed approach. Nothing could be further from the truth. Inevitably, as a clinical presentation fails to clarify itself following initial efforts, particularly if there is a possibility of factitious illness, the history taking process becomes more complex and the need for precision and corroboration increases. But a good enough doctor taking a good enough initial history, with sufficient attention to both detail and context, sets the firm foundation, the base on which hypotheses rest from the beginning. At that first consultation there may be a 'good enough fit' between the presented complaints, the history, the child's physical state and the parent's level of concern. Exploring the reasons for subsequent discrepancies depends on the quality of information at the outset, if MSBP abuse is to be identified and contained.

References

Baumer, J.H., David, T.J., Valentine, S.J. *et al.* (1981) Many parents think their child is dying when having a first febrile convulsion. *Developmental Medicine and Child Neurology*, **23**, 462.

Bools, C.N., Neale, B.A. and Meadow, S.R. (1992) Co-morbidity associated with fabricated illness (Munchausen syndrome by proxy). *Archives of Disease in Childhood*, **67**, 77–79.

Bools, C., Neale, B. and Meadow, R. (1994) Munchausen syndrome by proxy: a study of psychopathology. *Child Abuse and Neglect*, **18**, 773–788.

Boros, S. J. Brubaker, L. C. (1992) Munchausen syndrome by proxy: use accounts (1992). FBI Law Enforcement Bulletin, **61**, 16–20.

Bryk, M. and Siegel, P.T. (1997) My mother caused my illness: the story of a survivor of Munchausen by proxy syndrome. *Pediatrics*, **100**, 1–7.

Cooper, P.J. and Murray, L. (1998) Postnatal depression. *British Medical Journal*, **316**, 1884–1886.

Donald, T. and Jureidini, J. (1996) Munchausen syndrome by proxy: Child abuse in the medical system. *Archives of Pediatric and Adolescent Medicine*, **150**, 753–758.

Eminson, D.M. and Postlethwaite, R.J. (1992) Factitious illness: recognition and management. *Archives of Disease in Childhood*, **67**, 1510–1516.

Fisher, G.C. and Mitchell, I. (1995) Is Munchausen syndrome by proxy really a syndrome? *Archives of Disease in Childhood*, **72**, 530–534.

Garralda, M.E. and Bailey, D. (1987) Psychosomatic aspects of children's consultations in primary care. *European Archives of Psychiatry and Neurological Sciences*, **236**, 319–322.

Goldbloom, R.B. (1992) Family interviewing and history-taking. In *Pediatric Clinical Skills*, pp. 1–16. Churchill Livingstone.

Gray, J. and Bentovim, A. (1996) Illness induction syndrome: Paper 1. A series of 41 children from 37 families identified at the Great Ormond Street Hospital for Children NHS Trust. *Child Abuse and Neglect*, **20** (8), 655–673.

Green, M. (1998) The pediatric psychosocial diagnostic interview. In *Pediatric Diagnosis: Interpretation of Symptoms and Signs in Children and Adolescents*, 6th Edn (Green, M., ed.), pp. 471–482. W.B. Saunders.

Guandolo, V.L. (1985) Munchausen syndrome by proxy: an outpatient challenge. *Pediatrics*, **75**, 526–530.

Kohl, S., Pickering, L.K. and Dupree, E. (1978) Child abuse presenting as immunodeficiency disease. *Journal of Pediatrics*, **93**, 466–468.

Kosmach, B., Tarbell, S., Reyes, J. *et al.* (1996) Munchausen by proxy syndrome in a small bowel transplant recipient. *Transplantation Proceedings*, **28**, 2790–2791.

Lacey, S.R., Cooper, C., Runyan, D.K. *et al.* (1993) Munchausen syndrome by proxy: patterns of presentation to pediatric surgeons. *Journal of Pediatric Surgery*, **28**, 827–832.

Liston, T.E., Levine, P.L. and Anderson, C. (1983) Polymicrobial bacteremia due to Polle syndrome: the child abuse variant of Munchausen by proxy. *Pediatrics*, **72**, 211–213.

Lorber, J., Reckless, J.P.D. and Watson, J.B.G. (1980) Non-accidental poisoning, the elusive diagnosis. *Archives of Disease in Childhood*, **55**, 643–646.

McClung, H.T., Murray, R., Braden, N.J. *et al.* (1988) Intentional Ipecac poisoning in children. *American Journal of Diseases in Children*, **142**, 637–639.

McClure, R.J., David, P.M., Meadow, S.R. *et al.* (1996) Epidemiology of Munchausen syndrome by proxy. *Archives of Disease in Childhood*, **75**, 57–61.

Main, D.J., Douglas, J.E. and Tamanika, H.M. (1986) Munchausen's syndrome by proxy. *Medical Journal of Australia*, **145**, 300–301.

Meadow, R. (1977) Munchausen syndrome by proxy – the hinterland of child abuse. *Lancet*, **ii**, 343–345.

Meadow, R. (1985) Management of Munchausen syndrome by proxy. *Archives of Disease in Childhood*, **60**, 385–393.

Meadow, R. (1999) Unnatural sudden infant death. *Archives of Disease in Childhood*, **80**, 7–14.

Mortimer, J.G. (1980) Acute water intoxication as another unusual manifestation of child abuse. *Archives of Diseases in Childhood*, **59**, 166–167.

Oski, F.A. (1994) The diagnostic process. In *Principles and Practice of Paediatrics*, 2nd Edn (Oski *et al.*, eds), pp 51–53. J.P. Lippincott Co.

Porter, G.E., Heistch, G.M. and Miller, M.D. (1994) Munchausen syndrome by proxy: unusual manifestations and disturbing sequelae. *Child Abuse and Neglect*, **9**, 789–794

Santangelo, W.C., Richey, J.E., Rivera, L. *et al.* (1989) Chronic Ipecac ingestion. *Annals of Internal Medicine*, 1031–1032.

Sefarian, E.G. (1997) Polymicrobial bacteremia: a presentation of Munchausen syndrome by proxy. *Clinical Pediatrics*, **36**, 419–422.

Sullivan, C.A., Francis, G.L., Bain, M.W. *et al.* (1991) Munchausen syndrome by proxy. *Clinical Paediatrics*, **30**, 112–116.

Walker, L.S., Garber, J. and Greene, J.W. (1993) Psychosocial correlates of recurrent childhood pain: a comparison of pediatric patients with recurrent abdominal pain, organic illness and psychiatric disorders. *Journal of Abnormal Psychology*, **102,** 248–258.

Waring, W.W. (1992). The persistent parent. *American Journal of Disease in Childhood*, **146**, 753–756.

Wolkind, S. (1985) Mothers' depression and their children's attendance at medical facilities. *Journal of Psychosomatic Research*, **29**, 579–582.

Yudkin, S. (1961) Six children with coughs: The second diagnosis. *Lancet*, **ii**, 561–563.

4

Confirming factitious illness

Martin Samuels and Robert J. Postlethwaite

Introduction

The previous chapter developed a clinical method which integrated consideration of MSBP abuse into the assessment of any difficult clinical problem. The method leads from the out-patient appointment (even communication before the appointment) through to significant concerns about the possibility of factitious illness. Depending on the clinical circumstances the next task will be to confirm abuse. The level of confirmation required for a clinician simply to stop investigations will differ from that required for child care proceedings, and this will again differ from that required for criminal proceedings. Discussions with colleagues and strategy meetings often clarify what level of confirmation is appropriate and how best to obtain this. For any case in which child care proceedings or criminal proceedings are likely, the most direct and incontrovertible evidence of abuse that can be obtained without risk to the child should be sought.

The methods discussed in this chapter assume that concerns have been sufficient to justify a strategy meeting and it has been agreed during the strategy phase (see Chapter 11) that the information is sufficient and serious enough to warrant a child abuse investigation. In planning the investigation phase, consideration is given as to which of the methods described below maximizes the chances of acquiring suitable forensic evidence.

Confirmation of factitious illness

This could be summarized under the headings document, admit, independent observation (and further documentation), video and analyse. Before discussing these methods it is important to remember that there are circumstances in which direct proof of MSBP abuse is not possible. One obvious circumstance is fabricated stories. In many fabricated stories there will be symptoms reported with associated signs which could be confirmed by independent observers, professional or non-professional (for example, swollen abdomen, convulsions, the child going yellow etc.). Entirely subjective symptoms, however, which do not have related clinical signs, such as those in the first vignette in Chapter 2, page 27 ('not being with it', 'having a banging in his head', pain, frequency of micturition and tiredness), cannot be directly confirmed.

It is often difficult to judge what harm has been suffered and what further harm is likely to occur. It is even more difficult to achieve a level of proof that will persuade social services departments to take action, and yet more difficult still to achieve a level of proof that would stand cross-examination in a court of law. In these circumstances, the evidence required to persuade social services to take action will depend on meticulous documenting of all the improbabilities and implausibilities.

Another much rarer circumstance in which direct proof of fabrication is difficult, if not impossible, is induced illness that occurs infrequently and takes a different form on each occasion. Again in these circumstances the proof of factitious illness will depend on meticulous documentation of all improbabilities and implausibilities.

In general this chapter assumes that the strategy meeting has occurred and the optimum way of proving (or disproving) fabrication has been agreed. Admission to hospital does not easily fit into the scheme of things. Concerns about the possibility of factitious illness might arise during an admission to assess a puzzling clinical problem or, conversely, the admission might be planned at a strategy meeting to confirm factitious illness. The first situation is much commoner than the second, with the need for a strategy meeting becoming apparent during an admission. In this situation the precision of observations and record keeping needs to increase as concern increases (see the section dealing with nursing observations later in this chapter).

In Chapter 3 it was stressed that, when parents report symptoms that are intermittent but may be serious, it is a basic tenet of good medical practice to arrange for a child to be reviewed when clinically unwell. This is often best achieved by a short admission to hospital. Similarly, in the situation where there is a story of persistent symptoms that seem clinically improbable, a short admission often clarifies the situation. Such admissions allow for verification of symptoms and parents are often helped by simple explanations.

In the second vignette in Chapter 6, page 146 on admission to define the nature of the child's reported episodes of loss of consciousness, by virtue of routine, high standard nursing observation, a high suspicion of factitious illness was rapidly established.

In the first vignette in Chapter 6, page 145 the patient was admitted because of serious private concerns in the mind of the professional. The story of loss of consciousness was clinically improbable on at least two accounts, namely the type and frequency of seizure disorder, which was normally associated with developmental delay in a developmentally normal child, and frequent seizures not observed by the father. Before admission, in such circumstances, concerns must be shared with members of the nursing staff as discussed below and in Chapter 14.

Admission to hospital

If an admission is planned to prove factitious illness, there would need to be a likelihood that episodes would occur in hospital because of their frequency and agreement that, if this was not the case, this proved beyond reasonable doubt that the story was either factitious or due to induced illness. It must always be remembered that the more persistent parent who is inducing illness can do this in hospital, so that whereas cessation of symptoms in hospital is highly suggestive of factitious illness, continuing symptoms in hospital does not exclude factitious illness. This is further discussed in the context of covert video surveillance later in this chapter.

In addition to episodes not occurring in hospital (or being reported by parents but not observed by staff), on occasions records are tampered with.

A fourteen year old, previously healthy boy, was admitted with generalized swelling. Investigations showed him to have acute renal failure with nephrotic syndrome. He was commenced on dialysis and fluid restriction but still remained grossly oedematous. His father was of limited intelligence and his mother suffered from severe obsessive compulsive disorder. Attempts to explain fluid balance to the family were repeatedly unsuccessful and they seemed unable to grasp the simple concepts concerning it.

A two year old girl with nephrotic syndrome was admitted with intractable swelling. She required intravenous albumin and the IV drips needed frequent re-siting. On more than one occasion, the cannula was said by the mother to have fallen out within a few minutes of having been reviewed by the nurses. Mother claimed to have been advised by various members of staff that a central line should be sited but the staff denied any such discussions and some of the claimed discussions were said to have occurred when the staff concerned were not in the hospital. Despite a good urine output that should have ensured the child lost weight steadily, the weight increased day by day. The consultant discussed with the mother the fact that the child taking more fluid than the fluid balance chart recorded was the only possible explanation but she made no comment. After this, the mother asked if any messages from the consultant could be passed through the nurses, as she was upset at meeting the consultant. There had been numerous other concerns about the situation and other children in the family. The child was mobile and would have been difficult to confine to a room. Additionally, covert video surveillance would not be able to measure how much fluid the child was given by the mother. With the agreement of social services it was decided that exclusion of the mother was the only option. The child rapidly lost weight.

An eight year old girl was reviewed in the out-patient clinic. She had been attending doctors since the age of two years when she had had a Shigella infection and mother had been convinced since then that she had had chronic diarrhoea and recurrent pyrexias. There was extreme anxiety about possible short stature that antedated this illness, but the child continued to grow along the tenth percentile for height and weight. At each out-patient review the mother raised anxiety about the child's health and poor growth and reported persistent diarrhoea and recurrent temperatures occurring at least three times a week. The child was otherwise well, attending school full-time and showed no evidence of any effects from mother's concern about the illness.

With time, the child became more involved in the illness story and, when reviewed in the out-patients at the age of eight years, had various joint symptoms that were clearly not organically based. Mother was encouraged to keep a record of the temperature and diarrhoea over two weeks, which showed diarrhoea occurring six times a day and a temperature of more than 38°C on at least five days a week. After this the child was admitted, and there was no diarrhoea and no pyrexias documented by independent observation by the nurses over a four day admission. This was discussed with the mother who said the absence of diarrhoea was attributed to the fact that she had given a single dose of kaolin before admission because the diarrhoea had been so severe. Subsequent to this interview the temperature chart disappeared and reappeared some twelve hours later with new values inserted on it.

Clearly in all three of these vignettes, the charts were inaccurate but the likelihood of significant factitious illness is different in each case. In the first vignette, there was a combination of problems with a difficult period of adjustment to a very much more restricted lifestyle and diet, complicated by cognitive limitations and serious illness in the mother. It was difficult for the mother and child to grasp the fundamentals of fluid balance. This is clearly not factitious illness. In the second scenario, there might have been similar benign explanations for the inaccurate fluid balance, but the mother was considerably more articulate and had some nursing background. Her action in not wishing to see the doctor subsequently suggested that she had understood the points that were being made about the discrepancies in the fluid balance charts. The other suggestions, that the mother was perhaps interfering with treatment (IV drips requiring frequent re-siting) and wanted to escalate the treatment (requesting the insertion of central lines), and other concerns about other children in the family, led to the conclusion that, although charts had not been deliberately tampered with, the manipulation of fluid balance was considerably more deliberate than in the first case and the possibility of factitious illness was much greater. In the third vignette, there was deliberate tampering with the charts together with other clearly fabricated symptomatology. This clearly indicates pathological behaviour by parents which is highly suggestive of factitious illness.

Though, as discussed above, hospital admission is useful in the pre-strategy phase of management, there are problems in planning admission to definitively prove factitious illness. Tampering with charts, which is much more specific for fabricated illness, cannot be planned for. Additionally, there is always the risk of illness induction continuing in hospital. For these reasons it is usual to employ some other method of proof at the investigation stage.

Close nursing observation

Good nursing practice often alerts the team to the possibility of factitious illness in situations where it had not previously been considered. In the present context, however, close nursing observation means a conscious decision to increase the surveillance of a mother and child specifically because there are concerns about factitious illness (often induced illness). Historically this has been achieved by nursing the patient on a one to one basis or transferring the child to a unit in which one to one nursing is usual (for example an intensive care unit). Even with such close observation, on occasion crucial episodes have been identified serendipitously, the nurse returning to the room to find, for example, that the IV line had been disconnected (Kohl, Pickering and Dupree, 1978), or that there was saliva in the central venous line (Rosenberg, 1987). Additionally acute life threatening events have occurred when, inadvertently, the mother has been allowed to bath the baby (Berger, 1979) or the observer has been called away to deal with a cardio-respiratory arrest (Porter, 1994). This emphasizes that even close observation cannot prevent all abuse and may fail to collect crucial evidence.

As concerns increase and when any professional has private concerns in the mind, a much greater level of precision of record keeping by nurses is necessary. Unless these private concerns are shared confidentially between senior nursing and medical staff, this increased level of precision will not be achieved. Any paediatric ward in which nurses and doctors work as a team and have a respect for confidentiality should be able to achieve this quality of care and recording whilst maintaining the confidentiality. The sharing of concern elicits the nurses' support in collecting the information. This would usually mean that the routine nursing records are kept with even more care than normal, paying particular attention to whose observations are recorded (nurse's or parent's), the behaviour of the parent, circumstances 'around' observations, who was present and any consequences of an observation. Senior nursing staff will often assume personal supervision of such cases.

This crucial record may have two results, in that hypotheses about the source of the ill-health may turn out to be apparently unfounded or the suspicions could be confirmed and often increased, in which case a strategy meeting or case conference will be necessary depending on the level of suspicion or risk.

There are a number of considerations if it is decided at the strategy meeting that one to one nursing is the appropriate way to try and establish fabrication.

- There is the practical consideration of the demands on nursing resources, which may have a knock-on effect in the care of other children on the ward. This argument holds even more strongly for an ICU admission.
- Is close nursing observation to prevent abuse? If so, it places a heavy responsibility on the nurse and, whenever the nurse leaves the mother's side or turns her back on the mother, the mother will always have an opportunity to harm the child. Berger (1979) and Porter (1994) provide graphic examples.
- Is it policing to produce evidence? If so, this is a high risk strategy if there is significant concern about induced illness. Clearly this aim and the one set out above are incompatible – you cannot simultaneously prevent abuse and collect evidence.
- The 'detective' conspiratorial role conflicts with the nurse's normal open, confiding role with parents and child, and can cause considerable psychological stress for nurses (see Chapter 14).
- Even if the aim of close nursing observation has been clarified (investigation of symptoms, proving abuse, preventing harm?) and the nurses are willing to accept the responsibility, there is a remaining problem of how such close observation can be put into place and maintained? With the changes in relationships between professionals and parents set out in Chapter 2, it is highly unlikely that the parents would accept such close nursing observation either on the ward or on ICU without specific explanation. What happens if they reject this close nursing observation? Such discussions might alert abusive parents to the professionals' concern before crucial information has been collected.

For all these reasons, if there is an alternative way of obtaining direct proof of factitious illness at the strategy phase or beyond, then it is almost always a better course rather than using close nursing observation. If close nursing observation is the only way of collecting crucial information, then a detailed strategy needs to be worked out with the nursing staff about how the monitoring is to be presented to the family and what to do if: (1) abuse is observed or (2) mother disagrees or becomes suspicious. The level of concern must be high and social services need to be involved in planning the strategy. The nurses MUST be involved in the decision and willing to accept the responsibility.

Close nursing observations have sometimes been accompanied by searches of the mother's personal belongings or accommodation. 'In the light of all this evidence, a locker search was made' (Lorber, 1980). Meadow (1985) advocated this approach. Such approaches may have been acceptable in the past but these methods of confirmation may rightly be criticized as an infringement of civil liberty. The role of the doctor is to collect appropriate samples to identify the causation of a child's symptoms and signs. 'Detective work' is a role that should be left to the police. There are reports of other parents suspecting abuse, or finding medication in the mother's belongings. Medication has also been discovered by chance by nurses. McClung (1988) provides examples of both these events. Such fortuitous findings should be gratefully accepted and must be followed up.

Exclusion of parents

Historically this has been a useful means of confirming factitious illness. Meadow considered this an ideal diagnostic test (Meadow, 1985). He suggested that this should be possible if it only required the mother to leave the ward for a short time, up to a weekend, but acknowledged that it would be difficult for longer periods. However, nowadays, the parents are unlikely to leave the ward even for a weekend without a clear reason and, if the reason is explained, they are unlikely to agree. There is the added difficulty as to whether access is given to other family members and friends. As with close nursing observation, this approach has largely been superseded by direct proof of fabrication such as covert video surveillance. At all stages up to the strategy phase it is highly unlikely, and probably inappropriate, for social services to support any legal action to exclude the parents. It is also essential, if this course of action is being considered, that there is agreement beforehand between social services and the medical team that the planned exclusion will provide highly probable evidence of fabrication. It needs to be remembered that such evidence will be challenged by experts in child care proceedings and even more so in court proceedings.

Forensic analysis of specimens

Specimens relevant to the suspected factitious illness should be retained for forensic examination. There are numerous and extensive tests available through the local pathology service, police forensic service and other specialists. It will often be possible to identify abnormal constituents of a specimen provided there are some clues as to what is being sought. Conversely, on occasions routine analysis of artefacts in what seems to be intrinsic illness may alert the unsuspecting clinician to the possibility of factitious illness. The authors have seen rice particles, vegetable matter, putty, rust and plastic balls presented as renal stones, gravel allegedly passed per rectum, water presented as vomitus and saliva as mucus in the stools. Lyall reported a case of adding egg white to the urine (Lyall, Stirling and Crofton, 1992). A similar case is reported by Tojo (1990) but in this case was thought to be self induced, and administration of frusemide has been described to produce a biochemical picture identical to Barrter's syndrome (D'Avanzo, 1995).

Where there is a possibility of poisoning, it is important to have good liaison with the laboratory and to understand the limitations of the tests. The pharmacokinetics of the possible toxin(s) must be taken into account. A negative screen may be because the drug is excreted rapidly, the wrong specimen has been obtained (e.g. blood as opposed to urine), the timing of the collection of the specimen was wrong, or the specific test used cannot detect the toxin. Thus a negative toxicology screen does not exclude poisoning. The more specific the information given to the laboratory, the better the advice that can be given about the appropriateness of sampling and the greater the likelihood of identifying any poison (Henretig, 1995). The pharmatocokinetics of anti-epileptic drugs are discussed in Chapter 6.

It is important to remind people that the mere identification of an artefact in a sample does not prove factitious illness nor does it demonstrate risk of further harm. Some of the artefacts presented in the urine could have been accidental and, on occasion, credulous parents have maintained biologically implausible explanations of how this has occurred when there is clearly no other evidence whatsoever of a factitious illness in the index child or any other children in the family. In other children the urinary artefacts occurred in the context of other fabrications and a high risk of recurrence and the possibility of severe harm.

In handling a specimen in the context of Munchausen syndrome by proxy it is important to take account of chain of evidence procedures. These procedures (also known as chain of custody procedures) ensure that the results of any laboratory investigation can be reliably traced back to the patient. The procedures must be adopted in any case where there is a possibility of court proceedings, so that the results of analysis of the specimen cannot be challenged. Ideally the requirement means that a separate set of samples should be taken and analysed by a forensic laboratory while specimens used for routine patient care can be handled using normal practice. Chain of evidence involves carefully witnessed steps, documented with signatures, involving patient identification, specimen collection, and transport to and receipt by the laboratory. In the laboratory, details of specimen, storage and analysis must be recorded. Finally, a secure procedure for issuing reports must be used.

Samples for forensic analysis by the police should be transferred to a police officer who will document his part in the chain of evidence.

This whole procedure is onerous and chain of evidence procedures can be facilitated by the use of clearly drafted local standard operating procedures and forms (Dufour, 1996). These instructions should be available in accident and emergency departments, admissions units and relevant wards. Child protection training should include an awareness in the importance of chain of evidence procedures for relevant professions.

The possibility of MSBP abuse is often not considered until after specimens have been taken and sent to the laboratory, and sometimes even after it is too late to take the appropriate samples (e.g. urine for drugs). It is better to take samples under chain of evidence arrangements, which later prove not to be required, than to attempt the impossible task of trying to establish the chain in retrospect.

Overt video recordings

Video recordings provide an invaluable method for observing events or behaviours that health professionals would not usually see, but which may help in the management of a reported clinical problem. For example, they may help in the diagnosis of abnormal movements, colour changes or breathing abnormalities. For infrequent and less serious events that are unlikely to be witnessed during a hospital admission, home video recordings can be used. In situations of fabricated history, events may not be recorded for a variety of reasons (e.g. interference or breakdown of equipment), or fabricated events may be observed on tape. This also applies to physiological recordings taken at home (Poets et al., 1993).

Covert video surveillance

Uses of covert video surveillance

For more serious events, such as attempted suffocation, overt recordings will not show abnormal behaviour (Rosen, Frost and Glaze, 1986) as the parent will aim to keep this behaviour concealed. It is in this situation that covert video surveillance has been used to diagnose potentially life-threatening assaults (attempted suffocation) or other severe MSBP abuse (Rosen, Frost and Glaze, 1986; Southall et al., 1987; Epstein et al., 1987). This line of approach would be considered in infants and young children who suffer recurrent events involving cyanosis, apnoea, loss of consciousness, fits, sudden onset stridor, aspiration pneumonia, pulmonary oedema or pneumothorax, and where no other readily identified medical condition can be found. Failure to consider and make this diagnosis can result in major morbidity or death (Southall et al., 1997). Other pointers to this diagnosis include blood in the nose or mouth, petechiae, bruising or other skin markings on the head or face.

Covert surveillance has also been used to diagnose poisoning (Epstein et al., 1987), where it can identify the perpetrator, and the method and nature of poisoning, particularly where the poisons cannot be measured in body specimens (e.g. bleach). Covert surveillance may also identify emotional abuse, although it has not been used as the principle evidence in this situation (Southall et al., 1997).

Identification of abuse as the cause of fits or respiratory arrests is not straightforward, because clinical abnormalities are usually not found between episodes. The clinical picture can be further complicated by positive investigations performed between episodes. For example, the finding of gastro-oesophageal reflux on a radionuclide milk scan or oesophageal pH study does not necessarily implicate these as explaining the cause of the events. Multi-channel physiological recordings at home and in hospital have been used to 'capture' further events (Samuels et al., 1993), and the pathophysiology during episodes of imposed upper airway obstruction has been described as characteristic, although not necessarily diagnostic (Samuels et al., 1992). The findings include markedly increased breathing and body movements, initial tachycardia followed by bradycardia, marked motion artefacts or loss of signal, and severe hypoxaemia. The electroencephalogram shows attenuation and flattening of cerebral electrical activity within sixty to ninety seconds, and the subsequent consequences of a cerebral hypoxic episode include slow waves and the development of epilepsy (Stephenson, 1990). Simultaneous multi-channel respiratory and neurophysiological recordings may help to identify whether epileptic discharges are primary or secondary phenomena in such an event (Hewertson et al., 1994).

The suspicion that hypoxaemic episodes may be the result of attempted suffocation by a parent is sufficient to warrant constant supervision of the child and referral to social services. It must be made clear that conclusive evidence is not available, but may need to be sought, and before social services undertake further investigations, they should consider convening a confidential, inter-agency strategy meeting at which health professionals, social services, police and other professionals involved with the family may share information. As previously discussed in this chapter, this may lessen or heighten concern, but if suspicion still exists and the family is alerted at this stage, there may be no further opportunity to establish the facts. This is because trust with the family will be lost through 'unproven' allegations. Failure to establish the fabrication may mean that the child can only be discharged home to remain at possible risk from further hypoxaemic episodes or other less apparent abuse (e.g. emotional abuse). Confrontation of the parent with suspicions of this nature has been followed by parents discharging the child and the child being returned to hospital subsequently either brain damaged or dead (Mitchell *et al.*, 1993). Furthermore, confrontation is likely to be followed by denial and the end of any therapeutic relationship with any agency.

Covert video recording of a subsequent event may prove a definitive identification of intentional suffocation. Such recordings obviously require a parent to attempt suffocation of their child in hospital. The likelihood of this can be difficult to predict, but may be more likely if episodes are frequent, have previously occurred in hospital and/or there are strong pressures on the parent to 'prove' illness in their child. Since the early 1980s, various authors have reported covert recordings as an aid to diagnosis in poisoning, attempted suffocation and emotional abuse (Rosen, Frost and Glaze, 1986; Southall *et al.*, 1987; Epstein *et al.*, 1987) and there are probably many other unreported uses. Such recordings are both legal (Williams and Bevan, 1988) and morally and ethically acceptable (Shabde and Craft, 1998; Shinebourne, 1996). The Royal College of Paediatrics and Child Health has accepted their use in appropriately selected cases (BPA, 1994) as have Area Child Protection Committees and the Department of Health in the UK. A fuller exploration of the ethical issues, as well as guidelines for the use of covert video surveillance, have been published (Southall and Samuels, 1996; various authors, 1996).

Planning covert video surveillance

Prior to undertaking covert video recordings, all issues that relate to child protection matters in an individual case should undergo full, multi-disciplinary discussion in a strategy meeting, convened by social services and run as recommended in Department of Health Guidelines for good practice (DOH, 1995). It is important to stress that this meeting and any preceding discussions must be entirely confidential – alerting parents to suspicions at this stage without adequate information may prevent adequate investigation by any agency and thereby fail to protect a child if abuse is occurring. This approach appears contrary to the ethos of working together with parents, but it is notoriously difficult to work in true partnership with parents who deceive.

Confidential professional consultation, as occurs in a strategy meeting, allows decisions to be made as to whether there is adequate information to proceed to case conference, emergency protection or interim care orders. Alternatively, professionals may agree that gathering of further information is required, and this may include the use of covert video surveillance. This would be used principally to establish the causation of events, to help distinguish between natural and unnatural mechanisms and, if the latter, to allow child protection procedures to proceed. Without this information, it can be difficult for clinicians to either feel certain enough or convince social services that action is required. The severity of this abuse necessitates an assertive approach to clarification. The allegation of attempted suffocation is serious and would certainly warrant separation of the parent from the child. It is therefore important that the court is given the best information upon which to make a decision as to whether this has occurred and thereby ensure protection of the child. The court is unlikely to find that suffocation has occurred based on the suspicions of health professionals. This particularly applies when parents are able to call other medical experts in their defence. Family court judges will usually require a higher level of evidence for serious allegations and covert video recordings have been accepted in both civil and criminal proceedings (Southall *et al.*, 1997).

Carrying out covert video surveillance

Covert video recordings are undertaken in an ordinary hospital cubicle with two to four cameras hidden in the ceiling or walls of the cubicle. These ensure that the whole area of the cubicle can be viewed at all times. In an adjacent office or room, video monitors and recorders permit continual observation of the well-being of the child and allow the onset of any abusive behaviour to be documented and stopped. The observers have been police officers, children's nurses or mental health nurses, and ideally would involve some combination of these professionals. This is usually limited by local resources, although it should be stressed that the short duration required for manning video surveillance may involve much less time and money than contested court proceedings.

The abusive behaviour that is expected is discussed in advance with the observers of the video monitors. When potential harm to the child is witnessed, the observers will alert ward nursing staff to intervene in the cubicle. This should take no longer than twenty to thirty seconds from the onset of the episode to ensure that no serious harm occurs to the child. At the same time, intervention should not be so early so that inadequate documentation is achieved. In court, medical experts that are instructed by the parent's solicitor may offer alternative explanations for minor, short-lived events that may represent the onset of attempted suffocation. These include activities such as playing peek-a-boo, cuddling the child to the breast and clearing the infant's airway. When surveillance is used, it is important that there is a full briefing for the observers and all ward staff who may be involved in intervention. There should also be safeguards in case of breakdown of any technical aspect of the video recording (Southall and Samuels, 1996).

In one report of thirty-nine cases of children undergoing covert surveillance, child abuse was witnessed in thirty-three cases after a median duration of recording of twenty-nine hours (range fifteen minutes to fifteen days) (Southall *et al.*, 1997). An important observation was the fact that the mother (or father in one case and grandmother in another) usually performed abusive acts in a calm and calculated manner; for example, ensuring the ward corridor was clear before positioning the child appropriately on the bed or cot. In one case, a mother concealed a roll of domestic plastic film (used to occlude her child's airway) in the cubicle locker. In another case, the mother used bottle sterilizing solution and a syringe (both commonly found in a hospital cubicle) to inject sodium hypochlorite solution down the nasogastric tube of a child with severe failure to thrive. Thus the behaviour appeared to be premeditated and the perpetrator appeared to have control over the impulse to harm the child.

A common observation on covert recordings is the change in nature of the relationship between mother and child when the cubicle door is closed and no third party is present. Some mothers have extremely low levels of interaction with their child, in others the interaction is predominantly negative, and in some interactions are near normal. Overt observations would not detect this and could therefore mislead professionals into a false assumption that the parenting seems 'fine'.

In cases where covert surveillance has confirmed suspicions of child abuse, including attempted suffocation, usual child protection procedures have been followed. The police usually interview the parent immediately after the police and social services have reviewed the videotape. An emergency or police protection order is obtained, a case conference convened and the child is cared for by members of the family or foster carers, ensuring that the abusing parent has no unsupervised contact with the child. Rehabilitation of child to parent is an uncommon outcome for this severity of illness induction (see Chapter 13).

Although not the aim of covert video recordings, the substantive nature of the evidence has meant that criminal convictions have followed in cases where abuse has been detected. An advantage of this is the fact that successful criminal conviction means that such Category 1 offenders' names are held on a national register that can be checked if the parent or family moves around the country. In cases where only civil proceedings are held, the child's name is held on the Child Protection Register only for the area in which the child is normally resident.

Criticisms of covert video surveillance

There have been several criticisms of the use of surveillance (editorial, 1994; Morley, 1995; Evans, 1995). The most important of these is that the use of covert video recordings allows continued contact between parent and child with a risk of further harm to the child. However, although separation of parent and child may be achieved in the short term based on suspicions of harm, the absence of evidence from surveillance may mean that the child will ultimately be returned to the parent with a much longer term risk of harm, either physical or emotional. Adequate guidelines for the use of covert surveillance should ensure that the risk of harm is minimized. Ultimately, for this severity of symptom, the end result (guaranteeing the child's protection and safety) may justify the means (Shinebourne, 1996).

Surveillance has also been criticized on the basis that there are no adequate control data for the normal patterns of behaviour of parents with their child in a hospital cubicle (Morley, 1998). Obtaining such data would probably be ethically unjustifiable. As most hospital wards have cubicles and parents value the privacy that this gives them in hospital, children are very frequently managed in nursing cubicles with parents present. Thus, it is highly unlikely that the adverse behaviour observed on covert video surveillance is a consequence of the child being nursed in a cubicle, as has been suggested. Cases undergoing surveillance have presented with recurrent cyanotic episodes or life-threatening events and the video recordings mostly show quite clear evidence of abuse. This is evident from the successful conviction of all cases where criminal proceedings have followed.

A further criticism of covert video surveillance has been that it does not affect outcome, in that those cases where covert surveillance has proved negative have also been followed by child protection procedures (Morley, 1998). This is supported by Davis *et al.* who state that most cases of identified suffocation were achieved without the use of covert video recordings (Davis *et al.*, 1998). In these cases, it is probable that there was either other evidence of significant harm, or the parents who had abused their child may not have contested such allegations. It is often our experience that, in cases where covert video surveillance has not been undertaken or has proved negative and where suffocation was suspected, the child has returned to the care of the parent after temporary separation. Although this may not be subsequently followed by any further cyanotic episodes, it is likely that a disordered relationship still exists between parent and child that may have adverse long term effects for the child. Overt surveillance has been suggested as more appropriate for the diagnosis of recurrent cyanotic episodes. It may certainly be useful for diagnosing naturally occurring events, but would fail to diagnose either a physical assault or the disordered relationship.

Paediatricians and nurses may be concerned that covert video surveillance involves a betrayal of trust between them and the parent. This is a specific example of the general problem of being expected to assume a detective role, and this issue has been discussed previously in the present chapter and is further discussed in Chapter 14. However, if the child's recurrent collapses or cyanotic episodes are, in fact, due to repeated attempted suffocation, the parent is already deceiving health professionals and has obtained inappropriate hospital admission and investigations for their child. The cause must be confirmed and covert surveillance is a quick and effective means for doing this. It is possible to opt for a period of separation of parent from child and to then establish that no further episodes occur. However, medical experts have argued in court that such episodes may have stopped because apnoea frequently resolves with age. Critics of covert surveillance have also argued that the videotapes may be over-interpreted. However, such tapes are viewed by members of social services, lawyers and ultimately a judge dealing with the child protection issue, and the last person in this list, in particular, will make his own findings of the facts.

Covert video surveillance has been shown to be of value in ensuring a definitive identification of the cause of attacks. It has also improved our understanding of one form of child abuse and shown the behaviour of parents perpetrating various forms of abuse. The form of abuse described here does not arise as a result of some sudden loss of temper or in an attempt to quieten a crying and struggling infant – it occurs as a result of controlled and premeditated behaviours undertaken by a parent, with the result that health professionals are deceived into believing the child is unwell. Covert video surveillance is a technique that should be available in all regions of the country, but the decision to implement its use should be according to agreed local guidelines, so that it is not used inappropriately or where other means for diagnosis are available (Shabde and Craft, 1998).

Conclusions

Some MSBP abuse, primarily that emanating from invented histories, may be stopped by ceasing unnecessary investigation and referrals. But, in induced illness, forensic analysis of specimens and covert video surveillance provide the most direct evidence for MSBP abuse, and the possibility of obtaining this level of proof is the aim of the strategy and investigation phase. With invented stories this level of proof is not possible, and if child protection proceedings are initiated it can be difficult to obtain a level of proof that is convincing in court.

References

Berger, D. (1979) Child abuse simulating 'near-miss' sudden infant death syndrome. *Pediatrics*, **95**, 554–556.

British Paediatric Association Report of a Working Party (1994) *Evaluation of suspected imposed upper airway obstruction*. BPA.

D'Avanzo, M., Santinelli, R., Tolome, C. *et al.* (1995) Concealed administration of frusemide simulating Barrters syndrome in a 4.5 year-old child. *Pediatric Nephrology*, **9**, 749–750.

Davis, P., McClure, R.J., Rolfe, K. *et al.* (1998) Procedures, placement, and risks of further abuse after Munchausen syndrome by proxy, non-accidental poisoning, and non-accidental suffocation. *Archives of Disease in Childhood*, **78**, 217–221.

Department of Health and Social Services Inspectorate (1995) *The Challenge of Partnership in Child Protection: Practice Guide*. Planning the enquiries and investigations, para. 5.13.

Dufour, D.R. (1996) Sources and control of preanalytical variations. In *Clinical Chemistry; Theory, Analysis and Correlation* (Kaplan, L.A. and Pesci, A.Y., eds), pp. 73–74. Mosby, St Louis.

Editorial (1994) Spying on mothers. *Lancet*, **343**, 1373–1374, and replies from Morgan, B., Feldman, M.D., Johnson, P., Morley, C. and David, T. (1994) **344**, 132–133.

Epstein, M.A., Markowitz, R.L., Gallo, D.M. *et al.* (1987) Munchausen syndrome by proxy: considerations in diagnosis and confirmation by video surveillance. *Pediatrics*, **80**, 220–224.

Evans, D. (1995) The investigation of life-threatening child abuse and Munchausen syndrome by proxy. *Journal of Medical Ethics*, **21**, 9–13.

Henretig, F. (1995) The deliberately poisoned child. In *Munchausen Syndrome by proxy* (Levin, A.V. and Sheridan, M.S. eds), pp. 143–160. Lexington Books.

Hewertson, J., Poets, C.F., Samuels, M.P. *et al.* (1994) Epileptic seizure-induced hypoxaemia in infants with apparent life-threatening events. *Pediatrics*, **94** 148–156.

Kohl, S., Pickering, L.K. and Dupree, E. (1978) Child abuse presenting as immunodeficiency syndrome. *Journal of Pediatrics*, **93**, 466–468.

Lorber, J., Reckless, J.P.D. and Watson, J.B.U. (1980) Non-accidental poisoning: the elusive diagnosis. *Archives of Disease in Childhood*, **55**, 643–646.

Lyall, E.G.H., Stirling, H.F. and Crofton, P.M. (1992) Albuminuric growth failure. A case of Munchausen syndrome by proxy. *Acta Pediatrica*, **81**, 373–376.

McClung, H.T., Murray, R., Braden, N.J. *et al.* (1988) Intentional Ipecac poisoning in children. *American Journal of Diseases in Children*, **142**, 637–639.

Meadow, R. (1985) Management of Munchausen syndrome by proxy. *Archives of Disease in Childhood*, **60**, 385–393.

Mitchell, I., Brummitt, J., DeForest, J. and Fisher, G. (1993) Apnea and factitious illness (Munchausen syndrome) by proxy. *Pediatrics*, **92**, 810–814.

Morley, C.J. (1995) Practical concerns about the diagnosis of Munchausen syndrome by proxy. *Archives of Disease in Childhood*, **72**, 528–538.

Morley, C. (1998) Concerns about using and interpreting covert video surveillance. *British Medical Journal*, **316**,1603–1605.

Poets, C.F., Samuels, M.P., Noyes, J.P. *et al.* (1993) Home event recordings of oxygenation, breathing movements, and heart rate and rhythm in infants with recurrent life-threatening events. *Journal of Pediatrics*, **123**, 693–701.

Porter, G.E., Heitsch, G.M. and Miller, M.D. (1994) Munchausen syndrome by proxy: unusual manifestations and disturbing sequelae. *Child Abuse and Neglect*, **18**, 789–794.

Rosen, C.L., Frost, J.D. and Glaze, D.G. (1986) Child abuse and recurrent infant apnea. *Journal of Pediatrics*, **109**, 1065–1067.

Rosenberg, D.A. (1987) Web of deceit: a literature review of Munchausen syndrome by proxy. *Child Abuse and Neglect*, **11**, 547–563.

Samuels, M.P., McClaughlin, W., Jacobson, R.R. *et al.* (1992) Fourteen cases of imposed upper airway obstruction. *Archives of Disease in Childhood*, **67**, 162–170.

Samuels, M.P., Poets, C.F., Noyes, J.P. *et al.* (1993) Diagnosis and management after life-threatening events in infants and young children who received cardiopulmonary resuscitation. *British Medical Journal*, **306**, 489–492.

Shabde, N. and Craft, A.W. (1998) Covert video surveillance is acceptable – but only with a rigorous protocol. *British Medical Journal*, **316**, 1603–1605.

Shinebourne, E.A. (1996) Covert video surveillance and the principle of double effect: a response to criticism. *Journal of Medical Ethics*, **22**, 26–31.

Southall, D.P., Stebbens, V.A., Rees, S.V. *et al.* (1987) Apnoeic episodes induced by smothering: two cases identified by covert video surveillance. *British Medical Journal*, **294**, 1637–1641.

Southall, D.P. and Samuels, M.P. (1996) Guidelines for the multi-agency management of patients suspected or at risk of suffering from life-threatening abuse resulting in cyanotic/apnoeic episodes. *Journal of Medical Ethics*, **22**, 16–21.

Southall, D.P., Plunkett, M.C.B., Banks, M.W., Falkov, A.F. and Samuels, M.P. (1997) Covert video recordings of life-threatening child abuse: lessons for child protection. *Pediatrics*, **100**, 735–760.

Stephenson, J. (1990) Specific syncopes and anoxic seizure types. In *Fits and Faints* (Stephenson, J., ed.), pp. 59–82. Heinemann.

Tojo, A., Nanba, S., Kimura *et al.* (1990) factitious proteinuria in a young girl. *Clinical Nephrology*, **33**, 299–302.

Williams, C. and Bevan, V.T. (1988) The secret observation of children in hospital. *Lancet*, **i**, 780–778.

5

Hospital presentations: general considerations

Robert J. Postlethwaite, Martin Samuels and Eileen Baildam

Introduction

This book has focused on developing a critical, broad-based clinical method which will facilitate earlier recognition of MSBP abuse by a more thoughtful approach to all consultations. The presentations most commonly reported in MSBP abuse include, in order of frequency, poisoning, vomiting, seizures, diarrhoea, apnoea, fevers, unconsciousness, lethargy, dehydration and haematemesis. If all presentations of bleeding from generalized bleeding tendency to isolated bleeding, such as haematoma are grouped together bleeding in general is another very common presentation. All of these presentations are non-specific and many are very common in childhood – for example, all children experience a fever at some time. This reinforces the need to build awareness of MSBP abuse into all consultations rather than only considering it in unusual cases, thought to be possibly rare diseases.

Cases have been reported from virtually all branches of surgery, particularly general surgery (Lacey *et al.*, 1993) and otorhinolaryngology. For example, reports from otorhinolaryngology include bleeding from the ears (White, Voter and Perry 1985; Grace and Grace, 1987; Pickford, Buchanan and McLaughlan, 1988), chronic otitis externa (Obiako, 1997; Zohar *et al.*, 1987) and perforated tympanic membranes (Porter, Heitsch and Miller, 1994) and simulated CSF otorrhoea (Grace, Kalinkiewicz and Drake-Lee, 1984). There is a similar list of factitious nasal and oral presentations (Grace and Grace, 1987). Thus all surgeons who operate on children must remember the possibility of MSBP abuse.

There is increasing recognition of links between factitious illness in pregnancy, obstetric complications and MSBP abuse (Jureidini, 1993), which means that neonatal paediatricians and obstetricians also need to be aware of this form of abuse.

This chapter discusses the relationship between subspecialization in paediatrics and MSBP abuse. It will then discuss MSBP abuse in a variety of specific circumstances.

MSBP abuse and paediatric subspecialization

Donald comments that 'Severe abuse is more likely to occur when there is a medical system that is specialized, investigation orientated, fascinated by rare conditions, often ignorant of abusive behaviours' (Donald and Jureidini, 1996). Subspecialization in paediatrics is inevitable and for children with uncommon, often life-threatening conditions, subspecialization has led to dramatic improvements in outcomes, for example, the dramatic improvement in the survival of children with malignant conditions. What are the tendencies in subspecialization that could lead to the undesirable outcomes Donald fears?

Subspecialization inevitably entails a narrowing of the medical view so that the subspecialist is fully conversant with the rapidly expanding knowledge in his particular field. The subspecialist deals with rare problems, usually in a tertiary children's facility. Such an environment is far removed from the commonplace awareness of childhood abuse in all its forms to which general paediatricians and, even more so, community paediatricians are exposed in day to day practice.

In some health care systems, such as the National Health Service in the UK, referrals to subspecialties are filtered through general practitioners and, subsequently, general paediatricians. These practitioners, particularly the paediatricians as noted above, are experts in child abuse and often identify cases of MSBP abuse before referral to a subspecialist. This will further reduce the specialist paediatrician's exposure to all forms of abuse. Additionally, it probably means that the traditional implied bargain (that parents bring children who are sick and tell the truth about them and that doctors bring expertise and technology and like to do their best for the children – see Chapter 2) may hold more true in tertiary paediatrics than it does in community and general paediatrics.

Specialist paediatricians have highly developed expertise and access to technology. As these are the tools of their trade they are predisposed to put trust in them, and they have a predilection for using their expertise and technology to do their best for the children by seeking a medical solution to any difficult clinical problem.

Many referrals to subspecialists result from dogged parental demands that may or may not be justified (Waring, 1992). All specialist paediatricians will have personal experience of cases where such persistence was more than justified, with the child's previous treatment being sub-optimal or completely inadequate, or a major intrinsic problem having been overlooked. Again, this will reinforce the specialist paediatrician's predisposition to use his expertise and technology to resolve problems by ensuring that no intrinsic disease has been overlooked.

All this is further reinforced by the pressures towards not missing a diagnosis or perhaps making a rare diagnosis. Reputations are built on this and are equally well eroded if the specialist gets it wrong. In some health care systems there are financial advantages in pursuing more and more investigation and missing a diagnosis might have a negative financial impact.

There is a stigma attached to psychological causes of illness and, conversely, high status accorded to physical causes of illness.

Can these dangers be avoided?

The narrow medical view that a subspecialist necessarily adopts can be used to advantage. It means that within this narrow field the subspecialist is very familiar with clinical presentations and has a highly developed ability for pattern recognition. These skills should enable the subspecialist to spot incongruities that are not readily apparent to a generalist. For example, in the vignette on page 95 of Chapter 3, the incongruent pattern of the haematuria was immediately apparent to the specialist because of his familiarity with the range of presentations of haematuria and his confidence that the likelihood of serious intrinsic illness was very low. The generalist understandably did not have the same detailed knowledge of the patterns of haematuria nor confidence about the diagnostic possibilities. Stated more generally, the subspecialist should compare each presentation with all the similar presentations, so he will acquire a library of clinical pictures that should allow identification of incongruities which the generalist does not have the experience to identify. Provided the subspecialist further realizes that illness behaviour is an equally likely and equally valuable explanation as some unusual pathology for an atypical presentation, the narrow view of the specialist becomes an aid rather than a hindrance to the identification of factitious illness.

There is increasing recognition of the importance of psychosocial factors in the outcomes of illness, quality of life and response to treatment. For example, the importance of non-adherence as a multi-dimensional problem that seriously limits the treatment of many conditions has increasingly been recognized. Because of the importance of psychosocial factors in chronic illness in children, many subspecialists, both medical and surgical, now work within multi-disciplinary teams. This should provide an opportunity to remember that abnormal illness behaviour might be an important factor in an unusual persistence within the context of a chronic illness. These teams also usually include professionals with a child mental health background who should be able to help to maintain awareness of the wider dimensions of illness in childhood. These liaison practitioners (psychiatrist, psychologist) are better placed to suggest the possibility of factitious illness both by virtue of their training and because they are outside the team caring most immediately with the chronic illness.

Thus, at worst, subspecialist practice can degenerate into the stereotype that Donald set out, particularly if the system of health care offers financial rewards for increased investigation. On the other hand, good tertiary paediatric (both medical and surgical) practice, particularly when supported by a psychosocial team, is well placed to identify patients with factitious illness within their service.

Specific clinical situations

Intensive care

Intensivists, whose focus is on life-saving and technical approaches to management, increasingly lead the care of critically ill children. It is particularly in the intensive and high dependency care units that there needs to be a high index of suspicion. Patients with the most severe illness induction will present to such units. Intensivists whose background training is in a speciality other than paediatrics may be less aware of this form of abuse than paediatricians. Furthermore, in the intensive care setting with acute life-threatening presentation, the perspective that comes from a careful evaluation of previous contacts with medical services is often unavailable. Any acute life-threatening event in a child, therefore, which does not have an obvious and proven explanation, should have a factitious cause included in the differential diagnosis. Toxicology should be performed, taking into account the clinical signs and medication to which the family has access. There should be a low threshold for the performance of skeletal surveys, ophthalmic examination, toxicology screens and cerebral imaging. Such investigations are even more important if the child is dying or has died.

The importance of MSBP abuse for surgeons

In discussions about 'the bargain' in health care in Chapter 2, it was pointed out that certain subspecialties were particularly vulnerable to manipulation of this bargain because of their reliance on the history as opposed to the findings on clinical examination. This, with possible exceptions such as urology, does not apply to much of general surgery. In urgent and non-urgent surgical practice, physical signs are frequently present (a hernia, an undescended testis, an abdominal mass, signs of acute appendicitis etc.). Thus, for much of paediatric surgical practice, the traditional bargain holds. Surgeons often have to make a decision urgently on the basis of physical findings, which inevitably means relatively less attention is paid to other aspects of the consultation. This is partly the reason why paediatric surgeons rarely invoke child protection measures; they are often dealing with much simpler relationships with less complex clinical stories. Thus the specialist surgeon is even more remote from everyday contact with child abuse than the specialist paediatrician.

An additional but separate issue is that the specialist surgeon, in common with some other paediatric subspecialists, sometimes appropriately works within a narrow technical framework. If he works regularly with a gastroenterology team or an oncology team there will be general agreement about, for example, when central venous lines should be inserted and, when requested to do so, the surgeon will probably concern himself with whether the indications for a central line are in agreement with usual protocols and with the medical fitness of the patient. He would not be expected to review the overall problem. It is, however, important to be clear which consultant is doing this.

For all these reasons, when MSBP abuse presents to a surgeon, he/she will probably be less familiar with such abuse and have a clinical method which is orientated much more towards an assumption that there is an intrinsic physical cause for the child's symptoms.

Details of case reports illustrate, however, the frequency with which victims of MSBP abuse are subjected to surgery. The commonest procedures are central venous catheterization (often repeated), fundoplication and gastrostomy, even though most of the reports date from an era before the recent explosion in the use of gastrostomy feeding in numerous different circumstances. Much more radical surgery has often been performed. Surgical intervention may also be required for repeated injuries, the removal of foreign objects and to deal with unexpected bleeding or recurrent abscesses.

Lacey *et al.* (1993) reviewed all the cases of MSBP abuse identified in a surgical facility over five years and found the following:

- All ten patients referred to the institution subsequently recognized as having been subject to MSBP abuse had been referred to the surgeons at some stage in their clinical course.
- Nine out of ten underwent endoscopy of upper or lower gastrointestinal tract and/or bronchoscopy.
- Six of the ten had been operated on, with procedures including Nissen fundoplication (five), gastrostomy (three), and single instances of Broviac catheter placement, bronchial lavage, muscle biopsy, relief of small bowel obstruction, tonsillectomy and myringotomy.

This list does not adequately reflect the number of operations:

- Two of the children who had fundoplications required multiple dilatations because of changes in reported symptomatology and eventually the procedures were redone.
- In one of three children who had a central venous catheter placed for feeding, twelve revisions took place.

Lacey *et al.* concluded:

'It is important for paediatric surgeons to have an awareness of MSBP because children with this illness often require surgical evaluation. Though the illness induced in a child can be life threatening, paediatric surgeons may become the tools by which more serious illnesses are actually inflicted on the child. All ten of the cases in this institution were evaluated and treated by paediatric surgeons. Several children had major operations prior to the diagnosis of MSBP being established. It is hoped that by increasing surgeons' awareness of this entity and its patterns of presentation, the diagnosis might be arrived at earlier.'

This conclusion needs to be heavily endorsed and further systematic reviews from paediatric surgical services are required.

The following vignette graphically illustrates the extensive surgery that some of these children undergo.

A two and a half year old boy was referred with hydropneumothorax following several hours of bloody diarrhoea, coughing, retching and haematemesis. He had a history of frequent bouts of otitis media, intermittent bleeding from the ears and perforated eardrum of at least one year's duration.

The hydropneumothorax was shown to be due to a 2 cm perforation of the mid-oesophagus. No cause was identified for the oesophageal perforation. During this repair a gastro-jejunostomy tube was placed for feeding and the surgeon noted fresh blood in the peritoneal cavity and a fresh haematoma in the left paracolic gutter.

On hospital day five mother reported bloody oral secretions and loose teeth in her son. Two incisors were missing and one was so loose it had to be removed. A diagnosis of histiocytosis X was considered.

On hospital day ten, because of signs of bowel obstruction he returned to surgery. Generalized peritonitis and three perforations of the jejunum with the gastro-jejunostomy tube projecting through one were found. A retrograde intus-susception of the rectosigmoid colon, which appeared to be of at least several days duration, and a tear of the rectum were all found and received appropriate surgical treatment. Type IV Ehlers–Danlos syndrome was considered.

On hospital day twenty-nine, two episodes of acute respiratory distress occurred and the following day the abdomen was rigid. Surgical exploration revealed multiple abscesses, which were drained. Thereafter bloody drainage from the colostomy and the abdominal drain was noted but could not be explained by the surgeon.

On hospital day thirty-three, two episodes of brief apnoea occurred an hour apart. Review of these episodes revealed that mother was alone with the child at both times. At this point, MSBP was considered and constant sur-veillance by one to one nursing was ordered. When the nurse left the boy alone with his mother during another patient's cardiorespiratory arrest, mother reported that he had had a further brief apnoeic episode.

Further history was obtained at this point. The boy's two younger siblings had died. Both had been born with sepsis following premature rupture of foetal membranes at 22–24 weeks gestation. The first baby survived a stormy neonatal course but died a few weeks after discharge when he stopped breathing and could not be resuscitated by the mother at home. The second sibling died fifteen minutes after birth. A previous paediatrician who had cared for the index case reported periosteal elevation of both femora and tibia at three months of age and repeated claims by the mother that the boy had red urine, despite negative urinalysis. It was also suspected that the bilateral eardrum perforations had been traumatic.

The boy was taken into care and made a rapid and complete recovery.
(Porter, Heistch and Miller, 1994)

The authors of this report comment that oesophageal perforation in children is rare and usually has an obvious cause (endoscopy, inhaled foreign body etc.). Spontaneous oesophageal rupture can occur in adults (Boerhaave's syndrome) but, other than in adolescents with bulimia, only one case had been reported in a child. The authors also noted that oesophageal perforation with mediastinal and retropharyngeal abscesses secondary to trauma had been reported in physical abuse in children. Additionally, retrograde intussusception was identified as being very unusual in children – in one series only one out of 702 children with intussusception had this type. The eventual hypothesis for the causation of illness in this child was that the mother had inserted a foreign body into the rectum and the subsequent vomiting and retching had produced Boerhaave's syndrome. Alternatively, direct trauma by a foreign object to the oesophagus was a possibility. Many other features in the case were also only explicable on the basis of fabrication (Porter, Heistch and Miller, 1994).

This case is quoted at length to emphasize that even the most dramatic surgical presentations may have a factitious aetiology. The identification of two extremely rare conditions in a child should have prompted the consideration of factitious illness. Alternative rare physical diagnoses (histiocytosis X, Ehlers–Danlos syndrome type IV) were considered before MSBP abuse. If the identification of a rare presentation had prompted a review of the history, multiple other events would have been identified that pointed to factitious illness.

The final pathway of the patient with chronic intestinal pseudo-obstruction described by Kosmach et al. (1996) was repeated major surgery (small bowel and stomach transplant). It is difficult to tell from the details in the report at what point the factitious aetiology of this major illness could have been identified. It again reminds us that even the most major, apparently intrinsic illness can be the result of persistent fabrication and/or illness induction. This patient must have been cared for by numerous medical and surgical teams but it was the transplant team who finally identified the abuse. The observations that prompted the consideration of factitious illness were the facts that the mother seemed unable to de-escalate the amount of care she gave to the child and that she tampered with the notes, removing a psychology consultation from the notes. It would seem highly probable that an attempt to independently corroborate this child's symptoms much earlier would have interrupted this catalogue of abuse many years previously.

What precautions could surgeons take to try to minimize the chance of overlooking major factitious illness?

- In situations which are considerably more complex than the usual surgical transaction, remember to fully review the history; in such patients, a full review of all the information including consideration of consultation behaviour must be undertaken.
- Whenever a clinical scenario or presentation is unusual – or, as Meadow (1985) puts it, you have 'never seen anything like it before' – you must remember that factitious illness is a possibility, and probably more likely than a rare presentation of intrinsic disease.
- Independent corroboration of symptoms should be mandatory before invasive surgical treatment, even if functional studies (cystometry/ GI motility, pH studies etc.) are abnormal (this is discussed further below).
- Where there is escalating treatment with an apparent requirement of increasing surgical intervention do not assume that the previous paediatric medical or surgical team have reviewed all the possibilities including the possibility of factitious illness.

- Simple enquiry about previous illness, problems in siblings, details of the pregnancy and parents own health problems will often be sufficient to alert one to the possibility of more complex illness including factitious illness, which would prompt a much more detailed review, perhaps by a colleague who works more regularly in the arena of child abuse.

Misleading findings on investigation

Unexplained vomiting

A previously healthy 10 month old developed otitis and bronchitis, which resolved with antibiotic treatment. Severe vomiting and diarrhoea then began (sic) but subsided on hospitalization. Three times over the next two months vomiting recurred at home, resolved with hospitalization, but recurred as discharge was anticipated. Numerous laboratory tests were normal: chest radiograph, upper gastrointestinal and small bowel follow through, computerized tomography of the head with contrast, and oesophageal duodenoscopy with biopsy of the oesophagus, stomach and duodenum. Oesophageal manometry and gastric emptying time were also all normal. An oesophageal pH probe study was mildly abnormal and a trial of Bethanecol was begun. The child received continuous nasogastric tube feeding and the vomiting lessened.

There were concerns about mother and child's interaction. Emetine (a metabolite of Ipecac) was detected in the urine and in vomitus. When told about this, the mother denied knowing what Ipecac was or administering it to her child. However, when she allowed examination of her suitcase, a bottle of Ipecac syrup was found in the pocket of her trousers.

(Colletti and Wasserman, 1989)

Gastro-oesophageal reflux investigations

In all eight children with apnoea, work-up for gastro-oesophageal reflux led to pH probes, upper gastrointestinal contrast studies and oesophageal biopsy were performed in all eight patients. pH probes were usually only marginally positive but the persistence of symptoms despite medical treatment led to Nissen fundoplication in four. Persistent or changing symptoms thereafter led to multiple dilatation and eventually procedures were redone in two children.

(Lacey et al., 1993)

Chronic administration of toxins may be expressed in tissues. Leaving aside manifestations such as cardiomyopathy and myopathy, chronic Ipecac administration has given rise to erythema of the oesophagus, stomach, duodenum and colon, colitis ranging from mild to haemorrhagic and pseudomelanosis (Johnson *et al.*, 1991). Other laxatives have been reported to produce similar erythema of the gastrointestinal mucosa and colitis (Ackerman, 1981). Caustic substances have been administered, producing erythema or ulceration of the oesophagus (Rubin, 1986). This should be self-evident but there are many cases reported in the literature where such trivial findings have been taken as confirmation of an intrinsic problem which has been assumed to explain massive symptomatology. The two vignettes above illustrate over-interpretation of pH studies. With the first of these scenarios, it is tempting to say that, when such a massive investigation is employed to investigate such a straightforward problem, it is almost inevitable that some borderline results will be produced, which will then be invested with totally inappropriate weight and significance. The history as reported already gives a strong hint of the factitious nature of this symptomatology, and the pattern of no vomiting in hospital and recurrence on discharge was highly suggestive of fabrication or illness induction. It is difficult to see what hypothesis had been formulated on the basis of the pH studies that could possibly explain the symptomatology in this case. Similar comments apply to the second of the vignettes. It is not possible to identify the details of individual cases in this report but it is again difficult to see what hypothesis has been tested to explain the illness. Questionably abnormal results on investigation led to invasive surgical treatment when there seems no possibility that these results could explain the whole problem.

Unnecessary intrusion

A boy with pseudo-pseudohypoparathyroidism attended a school for the handicapped and participated in extracurricular activities such as the Boy Scouts. His school attendance and involvement in social activities was consonant with the mild intellectual impairment that always occurs in this condition. At the age of fifteen years he developed difficulty in urinating (and eventually required daily catheterization), vomiting, abdominal pain, diarrhoea and faecal incontinence. A diagnosis of intestinal pseudo-obstruction was made. A feeding gastrostomy was placed with little benefit and six months later (at the age of seventeen years) home total parenteral nutrition was initiated. By the age of eighteen years the patient was bedridden and was receiving total parenteral nutrition. All his needs were attended to by his mother who remained by his side day and night. She administered all medications and performed bladder catheterizations three times daily. Emetine (a metabolite of Ipecac) was detected in stool, vomitus and serum. With a court order, the mother was limited to one hour of visiting daily. Within one week, the patient was out of bed and could urinate spontaneously. He rapidly returned to pre-illness activities. The total parenteral nutrition was discontinued, he was discharged to a foster mother and six months after separation from his mother he continued to be well.

(Santangelo et al., 1989)

In this case and the cases reported by Kosmach (1996) and Sullivan *et al.* (1991) (see Chapter 6), the presence of an apparent neuropathic bladder and severe intestinal failure was assumed to indicate intrinsic disease, whereas in all three cases it was in fact due to induced illness. In these cases the cystometry and gastrointestinal motility studies were normal. This is a surprise – given that there was such abnormality of gastrointestinal and bladder function, it would be expected that the motility studies would show abnormality. There are certainly other reports in the literature of cases in which similar degrees of illness have been supported by abnormal functional studies but eventually the illness has been shown to be entirely factitious (Baron, 1995).

It is beyond the scope of this text to review the evidence for the existence of conditions such as chronic intestinal pseudo-obstruction or neuropathic bladder (in the absence of a demonstrable neurological disease) but, as emphasized by these reports, there are serious dangers of over-interpretation of such functional studies. If chronic administration of toxins can cause such obvious macroscopic effects on tissues, it is even more likely to produce abnormalities in functional studies such as cystometry and GIT motility. Abnormalities in functional studies are simply that; they are not diseases and the findings need interpreting within the context of all other available information. The problems with such studies are:

- Normal data are not available and, as a result, there is a lack of consensus as to what constitutes 'normality' and about the changes in values that occur during normal development.
- Clearly such physiological studies can be influenced by acute or chronic emotional factors.
- Poisoned children or those whose parents report symptoms which do not exist might either have abnormalities on functional studies as a consequence of the poisons administered, have trivial findings over-investigated or have abnormal studies because of the emotionally abusive situation they are in.

Before embarking on invasive investigations and management of bladder or gastrointestinal symptoms on the sole basis of parental reports of symptoms and possible abnormalities in functional studies it should be mandatory to independently corroborate the clinical story. Interpret positive findings in the light of a coherent hypothesis about a truly likely disease not as proof of a diagnosis.

The following vignette illustrates how far more weight was attached to a non-specific test on cystometry, while the independent corroboration obtained by hospital admission and by the reports from professionals in the community were ignored. Again it is not clear what hypothesis has been tested. How could marginal abnormalities on cystometry cause wetting at home but not in hospital or in school?

A five year old boy was presented with a maternal report of polyuria, polydipsia, daytime and night-time wetting. The mother had consulted a number of doctors about wetting since the boy was one year old. Mother had a complex history of wetting herself that had caused her major social inconvenience. A urinary diversion because of a 'small bladder' had eventually been performed, leaving the mother with a permanent urine bag. Full evaluation including appropriate investigations was normal. Mother was not reassured by the normal investigations, nor was she convinced that this was a developmental delay, which with time and training would be corrected. The extraordinarily early age at which this mother had sought advice about wetting and her persisting anxieties were attributed to her own very handicapping experience of wetting.

The boy was followed in out-patients and mother's complaints about the social inconvenience became so extreme and so convincing that a short admission to hospital was agreed. In hospital the child had absolutely normal daytime and night-time control. This should not be over-interpreted because many children with wetting improve dramatically on admission to hospital. There were concerns about the situation, however, and it was felt that psychological assessment was appropriate. The mother readily agreed to this. No psychological problem was identified in the child.

Mother's own medical problem had never been entirely clear and with mother's permission her own consultant was contacted to check out some of the details in a summary letter that had been previously requested. When pressed about the pathology the consultant said that it was not clearly defined and, with regards to the urinary diversion, he said that it was not clear why this had been necessary but that the 'mother had seemed to want it'.

Combined paediatric and child psychiatric follow-up was maintained for two years in order to prevent unnecessary intervention and to try to assist with the disturbed relationship between the mother and child which, together with mother's own personality difficulties, underpinned the grossly abnormal consultation behaviour. Mother would demand an extensive rediscussion of the wetting at each review but would not follow any training regime. Her repeated requests for further investigations were resisted. Over the two years the boy became increasingly disturbed and admission to an in-patient child psychiatric unit was agreed to be indicated because of his severe disturbance. Mother refused this and soon afterwards stopped attending out-patients.

Soon after this she contacted the school medical service because the wetting was said to be disrupting the boy's school work. The teachers did not confirm any problem and the community paediatrician maintained the same approach as had been pursued in the hospital out-patients.

Some time later both the hospital and community paediatrician received copy letters indicating that a further consultation had been requested and invasive investigations were being considered. Despite the concerns of both the hospital and community paediatrician being conveyed to the new consultant involved in the boy's care, these invasive tests were performed. Bladder function showed a minor non-specific abnormality and this precipitated a cascade of treatments, culminating in a urinary diversion for the child. Subsequent repeat cystometry showed normal bladder function.

Pregnancy and Munchausen syndrome by proxy abuse

Jureidini (1993) reported that, in approximately 70 per cent of those cases of MSBP abuse where obstetric history was available, there had been delivery before thirty-seven weeks, ante-partum haemorrhage or emergency caesarean section. He concluded that, even allowing for bias in ascertainment, this almost certainly indicates a significantly higher level of obstetric complications than the normal population. Furthermore, Alexander, Smith and Stephenson (1990) reported that previous perinatal bereavement (still birth or sudden infant death) was more common in mothers who perpetrated serial MSBP abuse.

It has been suggested that obstetric complications can contribute to the genesis of abnormal parental illness behaviour through unresolved grief secondary to perinatal bereavement or through the production of a damaged child. Either of these factors may disrupt the mother/child relationship in the context of maternal depression and other risks factors which might subsequently be expressed through abnormally frequent consultations or presentations. Another, more sinister explanation may account for at least a part of this higher than expected level of obstetric complication, namely that feigned symptoms of self injurious behaviour in the mother during pregnancy may be a severe form of (somatizing) factitious disorder in the mother herself.

In the obstetric setting, fabricated illness is still considered rare and in the obstetric literature is still at a level of individual case reports (Goodlin, 1985; Edi-Osagie, Hopkins and Edi-Osagie, 1997). The reported cases include feigned contractions, induced ante-partum and post-partum bleeding, self-induced vomiting presenting as hyperemesis gravidarum, feigned trophoblastic disease and feigned seizures. However, there were less than forty-nine reported such cases in the world literature (Jureidini, 1993; Edi-Osagie, Hopkins and Edi-Osagie, 1997).

The first case report linking factitious illness in pregnancy to MSBP abuse is probably that of Pickford, Buchanan and McLaughlan (1988) but the information, however, is buried in a long (though very interesting) case report and is not the main message of the case report. The obstetric features are summarized in the following vignette, but not the many other factitious problems the mother had reported for herself.

The mother's gynaecological and obstetric history changes frequently, and varies from one to six miscarriages, a still birth, a fictitious child twelve months older than her son, a hysterectomy for failed abortion, up to seven curettages and approximately five ovarian cystectomies. She also reports having undergone a tubal ligation. Her obstetrician denies knowledge of any of the above conditions. She claimed repeatedly and falsely to be five to eight months pregnant.

During her pregnancy with her daughter, she was admitted to hospital five times with abdominal pain, which was described as 'feeling like a contraction'; she feigned rebound tenderness on abdominal examination and placed urine on perineal pads to simulate amniotic fluid from ruptured membranes. She later claimed that these hospital admissions were for hyperemesis gravidarum, although vomiting was never recorded. The mother had multiple hospital admissions when not pregnant (Pickford et al., 1988).

The first report that specifically related self-induced pre-term delivery to subsequent MSBP abuse was that of Goss and McDougall (1992). Again this is summarized in the following vignette.

A twenty-seven year old Caucasian woman had recurrent ante-partum haemorrhage from eighteen- to twenty-eight weeks gestation when, following premature rupture of foetal membranes, premature delivery occurred. This led to a prolonged stay in neonatal intensive care for the baby and subsequently bronchopulmonary dysplasia. As the child recovered from the effects of extreme prematurity, he became a victim of fabricated illness and recurrent smothering episodes.

In the court case following identification of the MSBP abuse, the mother admitted she had used a knitting needle to induce her delivery. Her justifications were: 'I was sick of being in hospital', 'the doctor said the baby would be premature anyway' and 'the hospital wanted the child to be born earlier'. She said she only used the knitting needle once and 'did not jab it around so as to maybe damage the cervix'. She claimed she did not tell anyone 'because no one asked'.

(Goss and McDougall, 1992)

Jurcidini (1993) reviewed the literature and reported six mothers known to him. These six mothers had a total of nineteen children, of whom fourteen were victims of MSBP abuse. There was a complex catalogue of pregnancy complications and factitious illness in the mother, plus pre-term delivery, neonatal deaths, sudden infant death and major factitious illness in these children. Additionally, there were still births, neonatal deaths and neonatal intensive care resulting from the pre-term deliveries. The rarity of a reported association between factitious disorder in pregnancy and subsequent MSBP abuse in a child does not imply that this association is uncommon. More reports will occur as awareness of factitious disorder in pregnancy increases and links with subsequent MSBP abuse are recognized. At present probably many cases go undetected as was previously the case for child abuse in general and subsequently for MSBP abuse. It is likely that the dialogue between obstetrician and paediatrician in this disorder is limited, as much of the further factitious illness in the child may occur years later and not necessarily be reported to the obstetrician.

Goss and McDougall (1992) called attention to the 'battered foetus syndrome', a term coined by Condon in 1987. Condon's report highlighted cases in which there had been an assault by the mother upon the unborn child and where this abuse had continued postnatally.

The presence of factitious symptoms during pregnancy should alert the paediatrician to the possibility of MSBP abuse arising later. There is a possibility, as happens with the management of infants abused in utero by exposure to drugs, that teams caring for the mother view the newborn infant at low risk of harm post delivery (apart from the symptoms of drug withdrawal). They may deal with this primarily as a maternal issue. Clearly it is essential if factitious symptoms are identified in pregnancy to have an assessment of risk to the infant, and in this the rights of the newborn infant for protection become of paramount concern. In this assessment there are issues of abuse against the foetus versus maternal self injurious behaviour. This may be viewed in some cases as the transition of self harming to an external focus of harm. This, combined with the poor prognosis of severe early MSBP abuse, makes it vital that institution of appropriate child protection procedures occurs early rather than waiting to see what occurs.

Jureidini concludes that 'both obstetric factitious disorder and MSBP abuse are dangerous conditions that can easily be missed'. There are important implications to this novel claim. This is an association that is entirely consistent, however, with an understanding of severe maternal psychopathology expressed through the use of the body. This can be worked out through factitious illness and other somatic complaints for oneself and for others considered a part of oneself. These mechanisms and associations are discussed further in Chapters 2 and 8. Prior identification of MSBP abuse or of any less severe form of abnormal illness behaviour for her children by a pregnant woman should suggest to the obstetrician an increased risk of obstetric factitious disorder. Conversely, the presence of any factitious symptoms during pregnancy should alert the paediatrician to the possibility of MSBP abuse.

Factitious child sexual abuse

Sexual abuse is an important problem which often presents difficulties in identification. Both true and false allegations of sexual abuse in the context of parental separation or divorce are not uncommon and they have been studied quite extensively (Jones and McGraw, 1987; Schuman, 1987; Thoennes and Tjaden, 1990). Meadow (1993) reported fourteen cases from seven families of false allegations of sexual abuse made by the mother. These accusations were made in the context of factitious illness, as either the children themselves had been victims of factitious illness or they had a sibling who had suffered from such abuse. In none of these families did the accusations occur in the context of parental separation, divorce or a custody dispute concerning the children. False allegations of sexual abuse in the context of mental health problems are discussed in Chapter 8.

The case in the following vignette was managed by a professionals' meeting (strategy meeting) to contain repeated presentations for examination and investigation. It was not felt that sexual abuse was occurring here but the possibility had to be borne in mind. This possibility had to be balanced by the fact that repeated

Two young sisters were repeatedly presented with reports of vaginal bleeding. Precocious periods were ruled out by normal uterine dimensions and normal FSH/LH levels. The management plan always included obtaining a sample of the blood on the pants for analysis. However, this was never forthcoming despite repeated complaints of persistent symptoms. Urinalysis at the time of so-called 'bleeding' was always normal. A single examination of the genitalia of the first child failed to reveal evidence of sexual abuse. The issue of whether or not to examine the second child was more difficult and the decision was made to defer examination of the genitalia until such time as evidence of bleeding was produced.

genital examinations of a child are in themselves abusive. The discrepancy between maternal complaints and absence of evidence of abuse was taken to indicate an invented history, i.e. a form of factitious illness.

Police surgeons are aware of cases of Munchausen syndrome itself where women present with repeated claims of rape. Some of these women have been severely abused previously or are limited in their ability to cope with their lives and appear to respond to the attention given them at the hospital, with a desire to repeat the contact with caring staff.

It is an observation in some cases that when the women have children they stop presenting themselves as having been raped, and the question must remain as to whether they then transfer their attention to their children and present them as possible cases of sexual abuse. These women have all the vocabulary necessary to describe suspected sexual abuse. There are no reports in the literature of such a direct link between claims of repeated rape in Munchausen syndrome patients and subsequent presentation of a child. However, most police surgeons and paediatricians dealing with child sexual abuse are aware of cases where spurious allegations of abuse towards the child are made. It is highly likely that the two are linked and there should be a level of awareness of this issue in the same way as for a link with obstetric factitious disorder.

Management

We recommend that the possibility of factitious sexual abuse is considered in confusing cases presenting with vaginal symptoms.

Remember that repeated genital examination is abusive. The aim should be to perform one examination in the presence of a police surgeon or specialist and then only to repeat the examination if there is a definite and corroborated indication of a new episode of sexual abuse. The only exception to this would be in conditions such as genital warts or lichen sclerosis et atrophicus where ongoing assessment of response to treatment is necessary.

Remember too that a diagnosis can be made using forensic evidence. For example, blood on the pants can be studied for blood group, to confirm that it is human blood, to define menstrual blood and for DNA analysis. This analysis is best arranged through the police surgeons. Samples can be saved but it is important to maintain chain of evidence procedures to avoid claims that the evidence has been tampered with (see Chapter 4).

Conclusions

It is clear that any attempt to approach the identification of MSBP abuse by describing specific disease patterns is doomed to failure. Any symptom or sign will at some time be fabricated or induced, though this is more likely with some than others. Identification of abuse depends on a highly skilled professional remembering the possibility, having a clinical method that takes account of this possibility and being willing to explore his concerns. This chapter has discussed the clinical method described in Chapter 3 in some specific circumstances where there are particular problems in identifying factitious illness. The next chapter illustrates application of the methods in one medical speciality (neurology) and subsequently the particular problems of community settings and child mental health settings are discussed.

References

Ackerman, N.B. and Strobel, C.T. (1981) Chronic diarrhoea in Munchausen's child gastroenterology. *Gastroenterolgy*, **81**, 1140–1142.

Alexander, R., Smith, W. and Stephenson R. (1990) Serial Munchausen syndrome by proxy. *Pediatrics*, **86**, 581–585.

Baron, H.I., Beck, D.C., Vargas, J.H. *et al.*, (1995) Overinterpretation of gastroduodenal motility studies: Two cases involving Munchausen syndrome by proxy. *Journal of Pediatrics*, **126**, 397–400.

Colletti, R.B. and Wasserman, R.C. (1989) Recurrent infantile vomiting due to intentional Ipecac poisoning. *Journal of Pediatric Gastroenterology and Nutrition*, **8**, 394–396.

Condon, J.T. (1987) The battered fetus syndrome: preliminary data on the incidence of the urge to physically abuse the unborn child. *Journal of Nerve and Mental Disease*, **175**, 722–725.

Donald, T. and Jureidini, J. (1996) Munchausen syndrome by proxy: child abuse in the medical system. *Archives of Pediatric and Adolescent Medicine*, **10**, 753–758.

Edi-Osagie, E.C.O., Hopkins, R.E. and Edi-Osagie, N. (1997) Munchausen syndrome in obstetrics and gynaecology. *Obstetrical and Gynecology Survey*, **53**, 45–49.

Goodlin, R.C. (1985) Pregnant women with Munchausen syndrome. *American Journal of Obstetrics and Gynecology*, **153**, 207–210.

Goss, P.W. and McDougall, P.N. (1992) Munchausen syndrome by proxy – a cause of preterm delivery. *Medical Journal of Australia*, **157**, 814–817.

Grace, A. and Grace, S. (1987) Child abuse within the ear, nose and throat. *Journal of Otolaryngology*, **16**, 108–111.

Grace, A., Kalinkiewicz, M. and Drake-Lee, A.B. (1984) Covert manifestations of child abuse. *British Medical Journal*, **289**, 1041–1042.

Johnson, J.E., Carpenter, B.L.M., Benton, J. *et al.* (1991) Hemorrhagic colitis and pseudomelanosis coli in Ipecac ingestion by proxy. *Journal of Pediatric Gastroenterology and Nutrition*, **12**, 501–506.

Jones, D. and McGraw, J.M. (1987) Reliable and fictitious accounts of sexual abuse of children. *Journal of Interpersonal Violence*, **2**, 27–45.

Jureidini, J. (1993) Obstetric factitious disorder and Munchausen syndrome by proxy. *Journal of Nervous and Mental Disease*, **181**, 135–137.

Kosmach, B. Tarbell, S. Reyes, J. *et al.* (1996) Munchausen by proxy syndrome in a small bowel transplant recipient. *Transplantation Proceedings*, **28**, 2790–2791.

Lacey, S.R., Cooper ,C., Runyan, D.K. *et al.* (1993) Munchausen syndrome by proxy: patterns of presentation to pediatric surgeons. *Journal of Pediatric Surgery*, **28**, 827–832.

Meadow, R. (1977) Munchausen syndrome by proxy: the hinterland of child abuse. *Lancet*, **ii**, 343–345.

Meadow, R. (1985) Management of Munchausen syndrome by proxy. *Archives of Disease in Childhood*, **60**, 385–393.

Meadow, R. (1993) False allegations of sexual abuse and Munchausen syndrome by proxy. *Archives of Disease in Childhood*, **68**, 444–447.

Obiako, M.N. (1987) Eardrum perforation as evidence of child abuse. *Child Abuse and Neglect*, **11**, 149–151.

Pickford, E., Buchanan, N. and McLaughlan, S. (1988) Munchausen syndrome by proxy: a family anthology. *Medical Journal of Australia*, **148**, 646–650.

Porter, G.E., Heistch, G.M. and Miller, M.D. (1994) Munchausen syndrome by proxy: unusual manifestations and disturbing sequelae. *Child Abuse and Neglect*, **18**, 789–794.

Rubin, L.G., Angelides, A., Davidson, M. *et al.* (1986) Recurrent sepsis and gastrointestinal ulceration due to child abuse. *Archives of Disease in Childhood*, **61**, 903–905.

Santangelo, W.C., Richey, J.E., Rivera, L. *et al.* (1989) Chronic Ipecac ingestion. *Annals of Internal Medicine*, **110**, 1031–1032.

Schuman, D.C. (1987) Psychodynamics of exaggerated accusations: positive feedback in family systems. *Psychiatry Annals*, **17**, 242–247.

Sullivan, C. A., Francis, G.L., Bain, M.W. *et al.* (1991) Munchausen syndrome by proxy: 1990. A portent for problems? *Clinical Paediatrics*, **30**, 112–116.

Thoennes, N. and Tjaden, P.G. (1990) The extent, nature and validity of sexual abuse allegations in custody/visitation disputes. *Child Abuse and Neglect*, **14**, 151–163.

Waring, W.W. (1992) The persistent parent. *American Journal of Diseases in Children*, **146**, 753–756.

White, S.T., Voter, K. and Perry, J. (1985) Surreptitious warfarin ingestion. *Child Abuse and Neglect*, **9**, 349–352.

Zohar, Y., Avidan, G., Shvili, Y. *et al.* (1987) Otolaryngologic cases of Munchausen's syndrome. *Laryngoscope*, **97**, 201–203.

6

Neurological presentations

Richard Newton

Introduction

Up to a third of consultations in general paediatric practice will involve central
nervous system symptoms. Episodes of loss of consciousness are particularly
common where the diagnostic possibilities include epilepsy or more commonly
syncope. Bouts of apnoea in young infants are also frequently seen (Southall *et
al.*, 1987). Children with these conditions are usually healthy and symptom-free
between episodes and carry no interictal signs. Few people will go through life
without having witnessed someone lose consciousness and the vividness of what
is seen is usually carried by that person for the rest of their life. Given that this
accurate detail is commonplace, and that confirmatory evidence may well be
lacking between bouts, it is understandable how epilepsy, syncope and apnoea are
commonly presentations of MSBP abuse.

Where epilepsy is confirmed, long term anti-epileptic drug therapy is often
given. This offers new opportunities for parents, who may withhold the medication to induce seizures, give too much to induce intermittent coma or simply fabricate the story of the evolution of the seizure disorder. These possibilities are
probably even more likely if epilepsy has not been independently confirmed and
inadvertently anti-epileptic drugs have been prescribed for factitious epilepsy.

The birth of a disabled child necessarily leads to the need for readjustment on
the part of all family members. At times this process is incomplete and for the
psychologically vulnerable an undue dependence on the hospital services may
emerge. Again this is an area rich in possibilities for fabricated symptoms involving epilepsy or gastrointestinal symptoms.

The case histories presented in this chapter will illustrate how, at times, complicity is present in other family members and perhaps in the child themselves,
especially where there are learning difficulties and undue immaturity. At times,
unwitting support may come from a sympathetic relative, themselves alarmed
and concerned and wanting to do 'the best for the child'. With all these possibilities in mind, it is very important to draw up an investigation plan carefully.
Doctors must remember that, not only may investigations undermine reassurance
in the innocent setting of a benign condition and prolong the unhappiness of a
young person with illness behaviour, but they may also consolidate a behaviour
pattern of contrived malice in the setting of the Munchausen syndrome by proxy.

Episodic loss of consciousness: epileptic and non-epileptic seizures and the scope for fabrication

Neurologists themselves still argue about whether epilepsy should be a clinical or neurophysiological diagnosis. The present author prefers the latter and, given modern electroencephalographic techniques and the availability of standard, sleep, peripatetic and video EEG recordings, this is usually possible. Measurement of prolactin may also be useful (French, 1995). This principle should not become an obsession, however, and at times it is reasonable to act on what seems far more likely than not. Diagnosis is frequently difficult. Young people presenting with syncope often convulse due to transient brain hypoxia. Epilepsy is a huge 'pantechnicon' word that fills people's minds. Once the diagnostic label is applied it is very difficult to take it away. Medical records bear evidence of this and trainees still commonly but deplorably write 'known epileptic', and each follow-up visit carries an entry involving 'two fits' or 'three fits'. Once the initial diagnostic assumption has been made, it is common for the detail of the history to be lacking at follow-up consultations and, in the context of MSBP abuse in particular, this allows the consolidation of the behavioural pattern of all concerned, professional as well as non-professional! The following case scenarios are illustrative of some of these points.

A ten month old girl with normal development was presented by her mother with a description of a four month history consistent with myoclonic and astatic seizures. These were said to appear in clusters two or three times on a daily basis. An EEG was normal. Treatment with Valproate and Nitrazepam by the general paediatric service had brought no improvement. At presentation the author's attention was caught by the incongruent facts of frequent seizures of this type, which often in infancy are associated with developmental delay, the girl's obvious good developmental progress and the EEG which, when repeated, was normal. The telling question then became, 'Has your husband ever seen these episodes?', to which a negative reply was given. Given the seizure frequency, the statistical chance of this possibility was very small. Further observation in hospital established a pattern of seizures never being seen when nurses were present, only when the mother (an ex-nurse in her mid twenties) was alone with the child. The MSBP abuse was confirmed when these findings were discussed with the child's mother. She explained how she had fabricated the story. Appropriate advice and help were supplied through the child psychology and social services and the child remained with her mother and has remained well.

A young, single, unsupported Afro-Caribbean woman presented her eight month old child with loss of consciousness. She was a bright little girl with normal development and no interictal signs. The episodes sounded like white breath holding syncope or reflex anoxic seizures. The story given was that the little girl would become very pale, inaccessible, lose tone and fall to the floor. There were no apparent triggers. At times convulsive movement would be reported. An ECG and EEG were normal. Assessment in hospital was arranged. During admission it was evident that the bouts only ever occurred when the mother was alone with the child in her cubicle. Nurses would be called to a pale and hypotonic child who, on one occasion, was seen to be convulsing: a quick recovery would usually follow. As the diagnosis became clear, a much longer episode occurred involving prolonged cardiac arrest. The child developed hypoxic ischaemic encephalopathy and survived with severe motor and intellectual impairment. Her mother later admitted that she had induced the bouts by compressing the child's mouth and nose.

Jones *et al.* (1986) similarly described a twenty-three month old with induced apnoea, some episodes of which required mouth to mouth resuscitation. There had been two previous hospitalizations in other hospitals. The child was placed in foster care and the mother had psychiatric treatment. Pickford, Buchanan and McLaughlan (1988) described a young infant with repeated cyanotic episodes and the child was described as 'not breathing, stiff, floppy, cyanosed and in asystole'. The diagnosis of 'near miss' sudden infant death syndrome was considered. The pattern of uncorroborated frequent episodes then emerged but it was many months later, following a long train of events involving an additional hospital and a multiplicity of symptoms, that a formulation of MSBP abuse was arrived at and appropriate intervention made.

The risk to young infants when apnoea is induced by asphyxiation or vagal nerve stimulation is made very evident by Alexander, Smith and Stevenson (1990). They described a thirty-three month old who had evidence of apnoea on every third Tuesday of the month, requiring cardiopulmonary resuscitation (an earlier sibling had also been affected). In all, thirteen of the eighteen children of the families in this series were involved in MSBP abuse. Four of these (31 per cent) died.

Valentine, Schexnayder and Jones (1997) reported on a fifteen month old little girl who presented to the accident and emergency department on several occasions and had two admissions. The parent reported episodes of ingestion, apnoea and seizures. She was admitted following several unusual episodes of syncope with convulsive movements, was diagnosed as having epilepsy and started on treatment. The day after discharge she was brought in dead, resuscitated but declared brain dead two days later. Post-mortem studies failed to establish a diagnosis. Approximately three months later her four month old sister was brought to the hospital with a similar story and a stool analysis was shown to contain

Lorazepam and Temazepam. The child's symptoms disappeared and the child was removed from her parent.

The key issue in identifying abuse in the children involved in the above vignettes was that frequent events were described yet never seen by others (failure of corroboration). In the first account, corroboration was not forthcoming from the father even though bouts were said to be very frequent, and then in both cases nurses were unable to define the presence of these episodes on the ward, unless the mother was with the child alone. The combination of normal investigations and other features in the 'story' was clinically improbable and this led to the search for independent corroboration.

A six year old girl with mild learning difficulties presented to the hospital on two or three occasions unconscious. The family background was complicated. Her parents too had learning difficulties, had poor coping strategies and lived in very disadvantaged conditions at home. They fell prey to a rather well-dressed, smooth-talking Australian couple who lavished the child with presents and then persuaded the child's natural parents that they would be able to give her a better life. They took the child into their home nearby. Social services were aware of the situation but did not intervene. The 'fostering' parents told how each of these episodes of loss of consciousness had been preceded by the little girl stopping, staring, falling and then exhibiting convulsive movement. EEG studies showed a non-specific dysrhythmic slow wave abnormality, present in about 6 per cent of the population, but this finding together with the story led to the clinical diagnosis of epilepsy and the child was started on carbamazepine.

When reviewed in the clinic her affect was obtunded and serum analysis showed the level of the parent drug, carbamazepine, to be 72 fmol/l (general guidance range 20–50 fmol/l). The dose was adjusted. However, on a subsequent occasion the girl was admitted in coma and again the carbamezepine level was found to be very high. The child was admitted to hospital. She was continued on her prescribed dose of carbamezepine and her serum level was seen to fall. This, together with her persistently normal EEG (in the face of three volumes of notes!) and the fact that no one had ever seen her have a seizure but her 'foster' mother, led to the understanding that this was MSBP abuse. Further evidence for this formulation was added when one morning her mother called the nurses into her cubicle on the ward and pointed out that the bed was wet, indicating that this must mean the child had had another seizure. The nurse involved, however, knew that she had taken the child from a dry bed and, in fact, had changed the sheet. The wet patch did not smell of urine.

Court proceedings were pursued to take the child into care. The 'foster' mother did not attend. Indeed she absconded and left the country. A directive was made to the Crown Prosecution Service for her to be arrested should she ever return.

This and other cases serve to emphasize how it may not only be natural parents who involve themselves in MSBP abuse. Foster parents or other 'caretakers' may also become involved.

In the above scenario involving poisoning, the same sort of background issues, involving failure of independent corroboration coupled with the prudent use of a laboratory test and knowledge of the pharmacokinetics of anti-epileptic drugs, secured an accurate formulation but only after substantial harm had occurred.

The measurement of serum anti-epileptic drug levels is rarely indicated in clinical practice. However, this is one scenario where it can be useful. Carbamazepine is a particularly illustrative drug in this respect, as the levels of the parent drug may fluctuate quite markedly in the course of a day, whereas the active metabolite, the epoxide, stays at a fairly constant level in serum if the drug is being taken regularly. This allows quite sophisticated interpretation of data (Tomlin, McKinlay and Smith, 1986). A number of similar cases have been reported in the literature (Deonna et al., 1985).

When MSBP abuse is suspected it is essential that, prior to admission of the child, the nursing team is fully appraised. This allows accurate observation of infant and child behaviour and, in our third case scenario, the wet sheet offered corroborative evidence that the history was fabricated. Video-telemetry now offers new opportunities to corroborate parents' accounts of 'funny dos' in their children. Many units also have the facility for covert video surveillance, which may be particularly indicated where it is felt that the seizures are being induced in hospital. (Further discussion of the issues surrounding covert video surveillance is presented in Chapter 4.)

Where older children are involved, corroborative evidence should be sought from the child him or herself. It was lack of corroborative evidence that led to the correct formulation in the eleven year old described by Roth (1990) presenting with a fabricated story of recurrent headache and the seven year old presenting with seizures described by Alexander, Smith and Stevenson (1990). MacDonald (1989) described how a mother presented her twelve year old boy with a multiplicity of symptoms, which she believed to represent myalgic encephalomyelitis. He was unable to corroborate this story when interviewed alone. The mother herself, in fact, was demonstrated to have hypothyroidism yet she was convinced that she too had ME.

Poisoning and consequent neurological presentations

The previous vignette reminds us that perpetrators of MSBP abuse may induce illness by poisoning with prescribed drugs. Of course children may not only be poisoned by drugs that have been prescribed for them. Poisoned children may present with a number of different neurological symptoms and signs: intermittent lethargy, coma, ataxia and muscle weakness have all been described. Lorber (1978) described intermittent coma in a two year old poisoned with ultra-short-acting barbiturates. Livingston (1987) described a three year old with intermittent vomiting, ataxia and lethargy whose symptoms were always worse when mother visited. There had been multiple hospital admissions and ultimately phenobarbitone was identified as the cause. Jones *et al*. (1986) described intermittent dipheniramine poisoning in a three year old.

Again MSBP abuse was identified because, in the context of normal investigations, it was noted that the child was well except when symptoms appeared during the mother's visits. The importance of carrying out a toxicology screen in this context is evident.

The confusing clinical picture that poisoning may create is exemplified by the eight month old little boy described by McClung *et al*. (1988). Here, intermittent hypotonia was ascribed to muscle weakness before the correct diagnosis of intermittent ipecachuana poisoning was made.

Disability: dependency and unresolved grief

A child with severe learning difficulties and proven epilepsy had had numerous investigations but no underlying cause had been found. The seizure types described were of atypical absences and frequent tonic-clonic seizures. The presence of the seizures was noted independently by staff on the ward when the child was admitted for investigation and EEGs confirmed the presence of epilepsy. A number of epileptic drugs were used. However, no improvement was ever achieved. Over a two or three year period from the age of eight years onwards the girl was repeatedly admitted to the ward for periods of assessment. On the ward it was noted that the seizures, reported to be so very intrusive at home, were much less frequent. Additionally, they were reported to be more frequent at the times the mother visited. Measurement of anti-epileptic drug levels indicated a pattern of erratic drug administration.

Over this two or three year period the child's mother and father had separated. The mother involved behaved in an immature way and clearly was quite dependent on the support she received from ward staff. Collation of data led to the conclusion that she was manipulating the situation for her own needs. The situation was resolved with the removal of the child to foster parents for a period whilst the mother's psychological needs were addressed. Unresolved grief over the birth of her disabled daughter was identified as one underlying issue.

A three year girl with profound motor impairment in the form of a spastic quadriparesis and profound learning difficulties of undefined aetiology was admitted with persistent vomiting and weight loss. On the ward, the child was seen to take an adequate amount of food if due attention was paid to food consistency, and weight gain was observed. This had been the previous pattern seen at home. Vomiting continued to be reported in the mother's presence (often cleaned up and dealt with by her alone). On one occasion the nurses were called to apparent faecal vomiting which was incongruent with the good clinical condition of the child. A search of the room was made and faecal material mixed with saline was found in a jar in the wardrobe in the mother and child unit. The family background here again was of a relatively recent split in the marriage and unresolved grief.

Disabled children are particularly vulnerable to manipulation by their parents and the specific difficulties involved in identifying significant abuse in the presence of disability is discussed elsewhere (see Chapter 7).

The two vignettes above have factors in common which alerted our clinical service to the presence of MSBP abuse. In each case an unusual degree of infantilization of the disabled child by the mother was noted. Hospital admission and contact with the consultant involved was frequent in each case and unusual in the context of the level of support being offered to the family at home. The hospital admissions then became an important investigational tool and no corroboration emerged in relation to seizure frequency in the first child or vomiting in the second when the mother was absent. The prudent use of the measurement of anti-epileptic drugs in the first case and the emergence of a biologically implausible symptom (faecal vomiting) in the second case then led to the correct formulation. The nursing teams skilfully recorded symptom frequency, type and context, but both of these cases would lend themselves to evaluation by covert video surveillance.

Older children and complicity: la folie à deux ou trois

A child of three years presented with her mother who gave a history of staring followed by a convulsion and a reduced conscious level. On a number of occasions the measured serum anti-epileptic drug levels were high enough to explain the reduced conscious level. Mother was asked if there had been any other witnesses to the event and she confidently asserted that her own mother had seen some of these episodes. A phone call was made and the maternal grandmother confirmed the account. Further investigation including serial anti-epileptic drug measurement led to the identification of MSBP abuse. Court proceedings were brought within the terms of the Children Act and the grandmother retracted her account in Court and indicated that she had never actually seen an episode. Driven by her own belief that the illness was genuine and out of concern for her granddaughter she had been manipulated by her daughter into giving a false account and had felt compelled to corroborate her daughter's story.

A grandmother induced illness with the rather unwitting complicity of a four year old grandson who had specific learning difficulties. Grandmother owned a health food store and gave her grandson excessive amounts of vitamin A which he took to school and ate continuously. This led him to be ill with fever and irritability and widespread muscle aching. He sustained hepatic injury and his grandmother denied her own involvement until teachers gave a true account of events.

(Shaywitz, Siegel and Pearson, 1977)

Where illness is contrived, there may be an advantage for other parties involved. This may lead to apparent independent corroboration of the story because of complicity, as illustrated by the scenarios above.

A twelve year old in his first year in secondary school presented with a significant degree of difficulty with sequencing movement (a developmental dyspraxia) and his difficulties with balance and co-ordination were compounded by the presence of ligamentous joint laxity, a trait he had inherited from his father. His mother and father were estranged and his mother disabled. On follow-up a year later, after due assessment by the remedial therapists, the boy re-presented, stating that there had been significant deterioration in his motor performance and that for distances of more than twenty yards he needed the use of a wheelchair. There was no objective change in his physical signs and investigation was refused by the family, the mother being the dominant figure. The boy was no longer attending school and home tuition was arranged. The boy was very content to continue in the 'sick role' at home and his mother enjoyed his presence. The assertion on the part of the family was that the education authority was failing to meet the boy's needs at school. The medical practitioners involved, the local GP and community paediatrician, were unable to pursue the case under the terms of the Children Act. Despite representation to each of these on the part of the author, together with case conferences being held involving education and social services, it seems that the mother's dominant character has convinced all concerned that home tuition is the only appropriate educational setting for her son. The general practitioner's opinion is that 'the boy will come through in the end...'. Meanwhile, the boy's psychological, educational and social development continue to be disadvantaged by this predicament.

Unwitting complicity by virtue of subservience was also seen in the case described by Sullivan *et al.* (1991). An eight year old girl with some learning difficulties was unnecessarily receiving hyperalimentation through a central venous cannula, was subjected to intermittent catheterization and had become a wheel-chair user. Unwitting complicity was clearly also present on the part of her attend-ing surgeons. As commonly occurs with MSBP abuse, a different hospital was consulted over her care who, on carrying out a complete reassessment, realized what the true formulation of her presentation was. Within a few weeks the catheterization, hyperalimentation and the wheelchair were all abandoned and psychiatric assessment pursued. Unfortunately, the child protection team was unable to prevent the removal of the child from hospital at this point. The family transferred to another service where the hyperalimentation and bladder catheter-ization have been resumed. Complicity of the child (usually an adolescent) and the role of different professional views are discussed further in Chapter 9.

A ten year old girl presented with disabling and chronic pain around her abdomen and legs. This presentation was associated with a clear depressive illness. Her mother had a strong family history of cancer and had lost her own mother and older sister from the disease. Her father, with an analytical mind and scientific background, spent much time on the Internet. There was no loss of function but intermittent changes in colour in the affected legs were described though never corroborated by the professionals involved nor by thermography. The girl continues to miss time from school though the situa-tion is improving. The family retain the firm belief that this is a reflex sympa-thetic dystrophy, which at one level remains irrefutable. Rehabilitation is continuing with the help of the child psychiatry team.

The last two case scenarios are illustrative of the point that, where complicity is involved and continues in a family who encourage, maintain and support illness behaviour, the psychological and educational development of a child may be harmed, and the issues involved in MSBP and illness behaviour merge imper-ceptibly in neuro-psychiatric practice.

Conclusions

All these cases serve to re-emphasize the importance of not using a 'pantechni-con' term. It is important to keep an open mind in diagnosis and, at every con-sultation, details of history must be addressed and then re-addressed. Doctors should be like a policeman at the scene of an accident. Attention should be paid to every detail of the story that is told and evidence from as many independent witnesses as possible should be gathered. Doctors, like policemen, should be pre-pared to treat everything they are told, initially anyway, with disbelief if diag-nostic precision is to be maintained (believe everything the parent says and nothing the parent says).

It must be remembered that organic illness may present in unusual ways and diagnosis may be difficult. Porphyria may present with unexplained bouts of confusion or coma or seizures, though sins of commission may be made (Kappas *et al.*, 1995). Narcolepsy may present with bouts of sleepiness, disordered behaviour or unusual episodes of loss of tone (Allsopp and Zaiwalla, 1992). All these possibilities need to be kept in the back of the mind if diagnostic precision is to be maintained.

References

Alexander, R., Smith, W. and Stevenson, R. (1990) Serial Munchausen's syndrome by proxy. *Paediatrics*, **86**, 581–585.

Allsopp, M. R. and Zaiwalla, Z. (1992) Narcolepsy. *Archives of Disease in Childhood*, **67**, 302–306.

Deonna, T., Marcoz J.P., Meyer, H.U. *et al.* (1985) Factitious epilepsy: Munchausen syndrome by proxy. Another aspect of child abuse: recurrent coma in a four year old child caused by non-accidental poisoning. *Revue Medicale de la Suisse Romande*, **105**, 995–1002.

French, J. (1995) Pseudoseizures in the era of video electroencephalogram monitoring. *Current Opinion in Neurology*, **8**, 117–120.

Jones, J.G., Butler, H.L., Hamilton, B. *et al.* (1986) Munchausen syndrome by proxy. *Child Abuse and Neglect*, **10**, 33–40.

Kappas, A., Sassa, S., Galbraith, R.A. *et al.* (1995) The porphyrins. In *The Metabolic and Molecular Basis of Inherited Disease.* (Scriver, C.R. and Beaudet, A.L., eds). McGraw-Hill.

Livingston R. (1987) Maternal somatisation disorder and Munchausen syndrome by Proxy. *Psychosomatic*, **28**, 213–217.

Lorber J. (1978) Unexplained episodes of coma in a two year old. *Lancet*, **ii**, 472 and 680.

MacDonald, T.M. (1989) Myalgic encephalomyelitis by proxy. *British Medical Journal*, **299**, 1030.

McClung, H.J., Murray, R., Braden, N.G. *et al.* (1988) Intentional Ipecac poisoning in children. *American Journal of Diseases in Children*, **142**, 637–639.

Pickford, E., Buchanan, N. and McLaughlan, S. (1988) Munchausen syndrome by proxy: a family anthology. *Medical Journal of Australia*, **148**, 646–650.

Roth, D. (1990). How 'mild' is mild Munchausen syndrome by proxy? *Israeli Journal of Psychiatry and Related Sciences*, **27**, 160–167.

Shaywitz, B.A., Siegel, N.J. and Pearson, H. (1977) Megavitamins for minimal brain dysfunction, a potentially dangerous therapy. *Journal of the American Medical Association*, **238**, 1749–1750.

Southall, D.P., Stebbens, V.A., Rees, S.V. *et al.* (1987) Apnoeic episodes induced by smothering: two cases identified by covert video surveillance. *British Medical Journal*, **294**, 1637–1641.

Sullivan, C.A., Francis, G.L., Bain, M.W. and Hartz, J. (1991) Munchausen syndrome by proxy: 1990. A portent of problems? *Clinical Paediatrics*, **30**, 112–116.

Tomlin, P.I., McKinlay, I. and Smith, I. (1986) A study on carbamazepine levels, including estimation of 10,11-epoxycarbamazepine and free levels in plasma and saline. *Developmental Medicine and Childhood Neurology*, **28**, 713–718.

Valentine, J.L., Schexnayder, S. and Jones, J.G. (1997) Clinical and toxicological findings in two siblings and autopsy findings in one sibling with multiple hospital admissions resulting in death. *American Journal of Forensic Medicine and Pathology*, **18**, 276–281.

7

Presentation to community paediatricians

Hilary Smith

Introduction

Clinical paediatrics in a community setting in the UK involves a mixed workload. Community paediatricians, health visitors and school nurses between them provide the majority of the statutory services required of health authorities under the 1989 Children Act and the 1993 Education Act. Acute referral of children with potentially serious symptoms is unusual. Most children referred to a community paediatrician have developmental or behavioural difficulties, or chronic illness that affects school attendance or performance. Some referrals arise from routine pre-school child health surveillance or school health programmes, so it is health workers rather than parents themselves who have triggered a medical consultation (Rogers, 1993). There is also a requirement for each health authority area to identify a designated doctor (usually a consultant community paediatrician) and a designated senior nurse (who must have a health visiting qualification) to co-ordinate all health-related aspects of child protection work in the district, working across the boundaries of primary and secondary care and of individual trusts.

In order to consider presentations of factitious illness in a community setting, it is important to understand parents' behaviour when seeking health care for their children, and the circumstances in which this behaviour is abnormal.

The nature of community paediatric work means that severe acute illness induction is unlikely to present in a community paediatric setting. Nevertheless, within a given locality, there are likely to be children who are affected by induced or invented illness. Community paediatricians need to be alert to the consequences of factitious illness and be prepared to liaise with hospital colleagues in deciding whether the child is being harmed. However, in some circumstances, community staff may find themselves asked to provide continuing supervision of a child who has presented to hospital with unusual symptoms.

Patterns of seeking health care

Knowledge of the family's pattern of seeking health care, and of attendances at other hospitals, may assist in the recognition of fabricated signs, as the following case examples illustrate.

Case examples

A baby boy was enrolled on a CONI (care of next infant) programme from birth, because a sibling had died the previous year. The sibling had failed to thrive and had a number of hospital admissions because of diarrhoea and vomiting, and also episodes when he had stopped breathing. Subsequently, he developed a seizure disorder and showed acute developmental regression following an episode of status epilepticus. Extensive investigations involving five different consultants did not reveal a diagnosis. He was found dead in his cot at the age of seven months. The death was attributed to epilepsy. The mother had initiated legal action against the two hospitals who had provided the baby's care.

The new baby had eight hospital admissions in the first eleven months with apnoeic spells, possible seizures and a severe respiratory illness which was of extremely rapid onset and required intensive care. Throughout this time, the mother maintained at least weekly contact with the health visitor and was also a frequent attender at the GP's surgery and the local child health clinic. The baby made satisfactory developmental progress and thrived. Suspicions were aroused one weekend when the infant was brought to hospital for the seventh time following an apnoeic spell and was noted to have bruising around the neck. Mother reacted angrily to questions about the bruising. The infant was discharged but presented a few days later at another hospital with non-specific symptoms. Discussions between staff at the two hospitals and those working in the community led to a detailed review of both children's records. This concluded that there was a strong possibility that many of the hospital presentations of both children had been the result of imposed upper airway obstruction. Following referral to social services, the surviving child was placed in foster care, a care order obtained and the symptoms have not recurred.

Comment

It is recognized that a proportion of sudden unexpected deaths in infancy are not due to natural causes (Emery, 1993; Meadow, 1999). In addition, studies of families where fabricated illness has been identified show that the siblings of an index child are also at risk of death or fabricated illness (Alexander, Smith and Stevenson, 1990; Bools, Neale and Meadow, 1992). Community staff asked by hospital colleagues to implement a CONI programme following the unexpected death of an infant should be alert to the possibility of MSBP abuse, particularly if the next infant displays unusual symptoms. Good communication between hospital and community services is essential if the full extent of parental behaviour is to be recognized.

Most factitious illness presenting in a community setting poses no direct risk to the child's physical health. Parents present their child as being in need of services, and are grateful for the advice and support they receive, thereby flattering the physician. The main consequences to the child are the emotional effects of assuming a sick role and experiencing repeated investigations and serial referrals to other specialists, and the disruption of education by prolonged absence from school (Schreier, 1996). While current UK child protection procedures can be used effectively to protect children from parents who actively induce symptoms, it can be more difficult to manage invented illness, especially when the symptoms are difficult to verify.

Unexplained physical symptoms and unusual patterns of consultation and illness behaviour are common in the parents who present their children with factitious illness (Bools, Neale and Meadow, 1994). The next case illustrates how a mother with a variety of psychiatric problems, including hysterical conversion and other psychiatric phenomena, has persisted in making a wide range of allegations about her children. Many of the allegations have demanded a rapid response from paediatricians before serious illness could be excluded with confidence.

Mr and Mrs G have four children living with them, two sons aged 12 and 10 and twins of 9. Mrs G says she has epilepsy and takes anti-epileptic medication. She also exhibits a range of symptoms including loss of function of limbs, which has been extensively investigated by neurologists and rheumatologists without identification of organic disease. Exaggerated reporting of her children's symptoms started with the birth of the oldest child, when mother contacted the press to say that he had 'been born a drug addict' as a consequence of her anti-epileptic treatment. There had been no evidence of withdrawal symptoms in the baby and he had not required any special care in the neonatal period. The boy went on to have a number of admissions to different hospitals in his first two years. Presenting symptoms included difficulty breathing, blood in the stools and a convulsion. Staff were not always informed of the admissions elsewhere and the reported symptoms were not confirmed during his hospital stay. By the time he was four years old, he had also attended the out-patient clinics of six different hospital consultants in three different hospitals, and seen a community paediatrician, clinical psychologist, speech and language therapist and physiotherapist. Symptoms included abnormal gait (and a reported family history of muscular dystrophy), wheezing, developmental delay, rectal bleeding and short stature, and prompted a number of investigations. Three of the consultations with consultants were the result of GP referrals; the remainder arose after the mother presented her son to hospital or when consultants referred on to colleagues for further advice. The clinic letters refer to 'a multiplicity of problems, the severity of which always seems less marked after he has been assessed professionally than the history would suggest'. Subsequently, he had a number of episodes of stridor associated with acute laryngotracheobronchitis, one of which required intensive care. He was found to have a congenital subglottic stenosis. During middle childhood, the boy's school attendance worsened. Parents claimed that the absences were due to illness and attendance at hospital and therapy appointments. These reports reflected an exaggerated view of the implications of symptoms and treatment. For example, following surgery for undescended testes, he did not attend school until after the surgical follow-up appointment six weeks later. Most children undergoing this procedure return to normal activities within a week.

The parents became increasing dissatisfied with their son's school progress and insisted he attend a special school. The education authority's initial refusal led to the child's withdrawal from school for most of an academic year. Ultimately, he was placed in a special school some distance from home, where his attendance (and his attainments) remain poor. Further referrals to hospital have recently recurred after a four year gap and coincide with the development of cardiac disease in the father.

The second child showed unremarkable developmental progress in his pre-school years. He is a well-built child, in contrast to his older brother. He has always attended school regularly. He was first reported to have seizures at the age of fifteen months and was started on phenytoin. There were no independent descriptions of seizures and EEG recordings have always been normal. He is rarely brought to paediatric appointments for review of his medication, but any discussion of withdrawing treatment prompts further reports of seizures.

The third child is of small stature, like his eldest brother, and also has some mild learning difficulties. He has attended numerous clinics with persistent complaints about his growth, behaviour and educational attainments. In addition, there have been reports of excessive drinking, prompting investigation for diabetes insipidus, tonsillitis leading to tonsillectomy, and diarrhoea. His school attendance is poor and there is increasing pressure from his parents to move him to a special school. None of the symptoms that the mother reports are verified by objective observation outside the home. While school staff agree that he has some mild educational difficulties, they do not substantiate the reports of extreme aggression or oppositional behaviour. This child's twin sister has mild asthma and minimal contact with medical services.

The medical records of all three children contain numerous references to the mother's reports of 'bizarre and inconsistent' symptoms which are multiple and severe. The mother often emphasizes the importance of the symptoms she reports by claiming a family history of serious illness in that organ system. While the oldest child did have a subglottic stenosis, which would predispose him to airway obstruction with croup-like illnesses and clinical assessment of other symptoms has rarely identified abnormalities. At recent consultations, the mother has described extreme behavioural disturbance and aggression in the oldest and youngest boys, but as reports from school give no support to this, it seems likely that these behavioural symptoms are part of the mother's fabrication. Although these two boys have mild learning difficulties, they would normally be supported within a mainstream school. Intervention by the local department of child and adolescent psychiatry has not been able to alter the mother's intensely over-involved relationship with her sons or her views of her sons' ill-health and unmanageable behaviour.

Attempts to consolidate the children's medical supervision in general practice and the local community paediatric clinic are undermined by the family's ability to seek out new members of the practice who are unfamiliar with the family's pattern of consultation. When serious symptoms are reported, yet another hospital referral results. A general practitioner has also been persuaded to write condoning school absence on the basis of mother's reports of both symptoms and a lack of special educational provision in a mainstream school. The need for close liaison with GPs is emphasized by this case.

Current legislation is ineffective in ensuring school attendance in these circumstances. Social services have attempted assessment of the family but made little progress. There is insufficient evidence of harm to justify action under child protection procedures. The community paediatrician contributes to periodic strategy discussions to reiterate the lack of evidence of serious ill-health in the children. Fortunately, the children have been spared invasive investigation.

Comment

This family has been able to engineer multiple medical contacts for three of their four children. The presenting symptoms are often unusual, multiple and cannot be verified by examination or reports from independent sources. While complaining about having to attend so many medical appointments, mother clearly relishes the opportunity to repeat her own and her children's medical history and makes false assertions about serious illnesses diagnosed at other hospitals. The pattern of parental behaviour is characteristic of factitious illness (Taylor, 1991; Bools, Neale and Meadow, 1992; Eminson and Postlethwaite, 1992) and there are strong indications that these parents (particularly mother) gain much satisfaction from assuming a sick role by proxy.

It is difficult to quantify the harm caused to these children. The main consequence of the parents' behaviour in recent years has been the children's erratic school attendance. Some of the absence has been occasioned by genuine problems that have received an inappropriate response, such as prolonged absence from school after minor surgery, and withdrawal from school when demands for special provision are not met. In circumstances such as these, it is important to have agreed channels of communication between the various components of the health service and schools, so that explanations for absence can be verified.

It is more difficult to assess the emotional effects that the multiple medical referrals have on children. There is little evidence that any of the children are adopting a sick role themselves, and it is too early to know how far they will be able to assert their independence during adolescence.

When a child is presented to a GP with unverifiable but potentially serious symptoms, by a demanding and apparently desperate parent, it can be hard to avoid hospital referral. However, this approach satisfies the parent's needs rather than the child's. If the child's welfare is to be paramount, it is essential to obtain as much independent information as possible, including findings from physical examination, assessment of growth, and reports from others such as school staff or the school nurse about the presence of symptoms outside the home. Practitioners in both primary and secondary care need to recognize factitious illness if they are to manage or contain it. Assessment of harm is difficult, and the circumstances and effects on the child may need to be considered from a multi-agency perspective before agreeing a management strategy, even if the responsibility for management remains with clinicians.

An important question about factitious illness, and one that will only be resolved by more systematic longitudinal studies, concerns the circumstances in which fabrications may become more harmful. The next case illustrates how parental behaviour can change over time, and shift from clear fabricated illness behaviour into the 'not quite Munchausen syndrome by proxy' domain (Fisher and Mitchell, 1995).

A ten year old boy is the third of four siblings. As an infant, he was investigated for failure to thrive and had two jejunal biopsies. No diagnosis was reached, but for a time he was treated with a cows milk free diet. His paediatric care at that time was provided by five paediatricians in four different hospitals.

When he was three years old, he was admitted to hospital for hernia repair. Post-operatively, his mother made four separate reports to ward staff that the child was convulsing, but no abnormal movements were witnessed. The duty paediatrician who attended became suspicious that the mother's account was a fabrication. Mother responded by removing the child from hospital and writing to the paediatrician concerned to discharge the child from his care. Concurrently, the boy had also been referred to a paediatric surgeon with penile pain and a poor urinary stream, an ENT surgeon because of reports of nose bleeds and poor hearing, and an orthopaedic surgeon because of limb pain and worries about his gait. No pathology was identified at any of the consultations. Five years later, the boy was referred to a community paediatrician by the school nurse. He remained small and thin and had frequent school absences. At the time of referral he had not attended school for ten weeks. Mother reported that the boy suffered chronic diarrhoea with periodic exacerbations, when he became acutely unwell and 'too weak to climb upstairs'. When admitted to hospital, the boy appeared well and passed normal stools. Investigations did not show any evidence of chronic illness and a screen for laxative abuse was negative. For some months he attended the hospital school regularly, but on return to his local school, attendance lapsed. Mother claims he is unable to go to school because of diarrhoea but fails to attend paediatric appointments for further evaluation of the boy's symptoms. He has had two further admissions to different hospitals for dental treatment. On each occasion, treatment has been delayed while further information is sought to determine the anaesthetic implications of mother's reports of post-operative seizures.

The boy is now in his final year at primary school and his attendance rate is barely 30 per cent of possible sessions. School staff have often see him playing in the neighbourhood during school hours. Not surprisingly, his educational attainments are extremely poor. Mother continues to claim that school non-attendance is justified by the child's bowel symptoms. She has requested that he attends a special high school because he lacks the literacy skills to cope with the mainstream curriculum. Attempts to challenge her claims produce angry reactions and threats of litigation against the education authority. Strategy discussions with representatives from social services have concluded that there is insufficient evidence of harm to justify a child protection investigation on the grounds of suspected emotional abuse.

Comment

In early childhood, this boy's presentations to doctors showed many features of factitious illness, with multiple but unverifiable symptoms leading to investigation in a multiplicity of clinics and hospitals. This boy is now rarely presented to doctors, despite his allegedly chronic symptoms. Because he is out of contact with medical and educational services, it is impossible to ascertain his physical or mental health and therefore impossible to determine the extent of any harm. Before recommending any legal action, such as seeking a child assessment order or starting care proceedings, local authority representatives would have to be satisfied that the child was suffering emotional abuse. This is currently defined as an 'actual or likely severe adverse effect on the emotional and behavioural development of a child caused by persistent or severe emotional ill-treatment or rejection'. Non-school attendance on its own is not generally regarded as causing significant harm, despite the likely consequences of educational failure and social isolation.

Apart from keeping her son at home, this mother does not appear to restrict his activities or enforce dependency. Again, effective intervention is difficult because of uncertainty about what constitutes significant harm. School non-attendance and poor educational attainment occur in many families for reasons unrelated to illness behaviour, and this rarely falls within the scope of child protection procedures unless there is other evidence of neglect. This child does not appear to regard himself as chronically ill in terms of his own behaviour and social activities. He is no longer being taken to doctors and clinics or experiencing investigations. The mother appears to have shifted her need to consult away from doctors on to educational psychologists and the special needs services. It might be argued that repeated educational and psychological assessments and unnecessarily segregated education are a form of emotional abuse, but are they severe and persistent enough to constitute 'significant harm'?

The attitude of the parent towards medical agencies varies widely in these community presentations. Distinguishing between different motivations for the behaviour, as has been proposed (Meadow, 1995; Jones, 1996), is not always easy. Many parents who report factitious illness give the impression of being in need of advice and guidance about their children's health and show gratitude to the network of health professionals they draw in. Others develop a hostile relationship when their demands for acceptance of a particular diagnosis or treatment cannot be met (McKinlay, 1986; Taylor, 1991; Schreier, 1996).

The next case illustrates how it can be difficult to distinguish between factitious illness, parental over-anxiety and benefit seeking in a parent's consultation behaviour.

A boy is the second of three children living with a single mother. As a pre-school child, he showed delayed speech and language development and received therapy. Over time, it became clear that he had some mild learning difficulties with immature gross and fine motor co-ordination. He also developed asthma, and mother reported pains in his knees, ankles and elbows which restricted his activities. This prompted successive referrals to a paediatric rheumatologist, orthopaedic surgeon and paediatric neurologist. After careful assessment, the neurologist pronounced him 'fit for the army'. However, the mother continues to regard the child as disabled by his learning difficulties and physical symptoms. At each consultation, a new problem is presented for the doctor to solve. Mother was disappointed when the local educational authority turned down her request for formal assessment of the boy's special educational needs, and his progress meant that the school reduced his ranking in their special needs record. She has applied unsuccessfully for disability living allowance and orthopaedic footwear for him, on the grounds that he requires considerable assistance with self-care and mobility. These assertions are not supported by the independent observations of school staff. Mother has also contacted the local specialist social work team for disabled children and has been allocated a social worker.

Comment

This boy has mild learning disabilities and a degree of developmental dyspraxia. It is difficult to know whether his limb pains were exaggerated or entirely fabricated. The application for financial benefits has arisen relatively late and does not appear to have been the initial reason for the multiple consultations. The mother continues to show a disordered perception of her son's abilities. Paediatric management includes regular liaison with the school and social worker to provide an accurate interpretation of medical issues, and giving advice to the mother that provides reassurance about the boy's potential and promotes a greater degree of independence.

Conclusions

Fabricated reports of illness are not uncommon and need to be recognized and managed in a way that contains the reported symptoms and minimizes potential for multiple referrals and invasive investigations.

In a community setting, verbal fabrications predominate and often relate to long-standing symptoms. Many fabrications arise alongside genuine medical conditions or disabilities. Investigation is rarely urgent, and lack of immediate access to laboratory and other diagnostic facilities can protect the child from an over-zealous approach. When communication between hospitals and community services is effective, community paediatricians may be in a key position to collate all the information on hospital attendances and recognize the underlying psychopathology. They will also have local knowledge of recent events and available services, which might influence consultations.

In any medical consultation, it is important to consider not just the presenting problem, but the reasons for seeking an opinion at that particular time in that particular setting. Waring has developed an algorithm to identify circumstances where parental persistence and severity of illness are incongruent and may indicate falsification of symptoms (Waring, 1992). For community paediatric consultations, it is also important to consider who has initiated the referral and what outcomes are expected. Parents who have sought referral themselves and bring a long list of unusual symptoms for which they expect extensive investigations may well be consulting about factitious illness. When others have initiated the paediatric opinion, perhaps because of school non-attendance, fabricated symptoms may also be given as an explanation. However, a careful paediatric history will usually determine whether the symptoms have previously been brought to medical attention, or whether they are being used as a cover for other pathology such as school refusal or maternal over-dependence on the child. In older children, the reports of symptoms may originate from the child rather than the parent and indicate a somatization disorder.

For much of the fabricated illness seen in a community paediatric setting, definitive action is difficult. As a first step, it is important to collate all available medical information from both hospital and community records, and compare this with the past medical history given by the parent. Reports about the presence and impact of symptoms should also be obtained from the child's school or nursery and, if possible, from other family members who care for the child. If this information confirms abnormal consultation behaviour, the next step would usually be informal consultation with colleagues. Community paediatricians will usually be members of a local liaison network which includes GPs, nursing colleagues, head teachers, social workers and education welfare officers. Confidential discussion with one or more colleagues will help to clarify areas of concern, identify resources that may help, and consider thresholds for further action. It may also identify problems with parents' health and illness behaviour. When several different doctors and specialists are seeing the child, the community paediatrician will need to ensure that information is shared between all clinicians, especially if they are working in separate hospitals and keeping separate records. It is sometimes possible to negotiate the child's discharge from one or more out-patient clinics and for the community paediatrician to assume the role of lead clinician. This will consolidate the child's specialist follow-up in a local clinic and limit pressure for referrals elsewhere by agreeing to provide prompt appraisal of new symptoms as and when they arise. In addition, the community paediatrician will need to ensure that those in frequent contact with the child do not form a distorted view of the child's health, and to see that they encourage the child to attend school regularly and take part in normal activities. Regular paediatric follow-up is useful to judge the impact of new symptoms if they are reported and to try to increase parents' understanding of their behaviour and its effects on the child. Sometimes, referral to a child psychiatrist will be needed for more detailed assessments of the child's emotional state and family functioning.

For many families, this approach will contain the situation and allow normal childhood activities to continue. When symptoms escalate, the paediatrician will need to consider the consequences in terms of school attendance, reduction in social activities, imposition of treatment, and the child's perception of his or her symptoms. In this situation, a strategy meeting with social services will be helpful to consider the extent of any harm to the child. In making this assessment, it is important to consider all aspects of the child's life, including unnecessary investigations or hospital admission, loss of educational opportunities, loss of social contact with peers and signs of emotional distress such as adoption of a sick role.

Harm would be significant when there is a serious change in one or more areas such that the child is no longer taking part in normal activities in the home, local community and school. Although evidence for the long term psychological sequelae following MSBP abuse/fabricated illness is accumulating (Jones,1994; Bools, Neale and Meadow, 1993; Libow, 1995), this can be hard to quantify in the individual case and so it is difficult to initiate action on the basis that the child is likely to suffer harm if the situation continues.

Only a minority of community presentations of fabricated illness will result in formal referral to social services for a child protection investigation and case conference. Legal action to remove the child from the family would be a last resort for situations where a child is suffering significant harm and it has been impossible to negotiate any change in parental behaviour.

References

Alexander, R., Smith, W. and Stevenson, R. (1990) Serial Munchausen's syndrome by proxy. *Pediatrics*, **86**, 581–585.

Bools, C.N., Neale, B.A. and Meadow, S.R. (1992) Co-morbidity associated with fabricated illness (Munchausen syndrome by proxy). *Archives of Disease in Childhood*, **67**, 77–79.

Bools, C., Neale, B. and Meadow, S.R. (1993) Follow up of victims of fabricated illness (Munchausen syndrome by proxy). *Archives of Disease in Childhood*, **69**, 625–630.

Bools, C., Neale, B. and Meadow, S.R. (1994) Munchausen syndrome by proxy: a study of psychopathology. *Child Abuse and Neglect*, **18**, 773–788.

Emery, J.L. (1993) Child abuse, sudden infant death syndrome and unexpected infant death. *American Journal of Diseases in Children*, **147**, 1097–1099.

Eminson, D.M. and Postlethwaite, R.J. (1992) Factitious illness: recognition and management. *Archives of Disease in Childhood*, **67**, 1510–1516.

Fisher, G.C. and Mitchell, I. (1995) Is Munchausen syndrome by proxy really a syndrome? *Archives of Disease in Childhood*, **72**, 530–534.

Jones, D.P.H. (1994) Editorial: the syndrome of Munchausen by proxy. *Child Abuse and Neglect*, **18**, 769–771.

Jones, D.P.H. (1996) Commentary: Munchausen syndrome by proxy – is expansion justified? *Child Abuse and Neglect*, **20**, 983–984.

Libow, J.A. (1995) Munchausen by proxy victims in adulthood: a first look. *Child Abuse and Neglect*, **19**, 1131–1142.

McKinlay, I.A. (1986) Munchausen's syndrome by proxy. *British Medical Journal*, **293**, 1308.

Meadow, S.R. (1995) What is, and what is not, 'Munchausen syndrome by proxy'? *Archives of Disease in Childhood*, **72**, 534–538.

Meadow, S.R. (1999) Unnatural sudden infant death. *Archives of Disease in Childhood*, **80**, 7–14.

Rogers, M. (1993) The growing pains of community child health. *Archives of Disease in Childhood*, **68**, 140–143.

Schreier, H.A. and Libow, J.A. (1994) Munchausen by proxy syndrome: a modern pediatric challenge. *Journal of Pediatrics*, **125**, S110–115.

Schreier, H.A. (1996) Repeated false allegations of sexual abuse presenting to sheriffs: when is it Munchausen by proxy? *Child Abuse and Neglect*, **20**, 985–991.

Taylor, D.C. (1991) Outlandish factitious illness. In *Recent Advances in Paediatrics*, Vol. 10 (David, T.J., ed.), pp. 63–76. Churchill Livingstone.

Waring, W.W. (1992) The persistent parent. *American Journal of Diseases in Children*, **146**, 753–756.

8

Presentations in mental health

Jonathan Green

Introduction

The systematic description of factitious medical symptomatology by proxy is now over twenty years old (Meadow, 1977), but that of the factitious presentation of psychiatric symptoms by proxy has only very recently become the subject of clinical writing, debate and research. The literature is correspondingly small. Fisher, Mitchell and Murdoch (1993), in a single case report, describe a young boy presented by his mother as psychotic, who was found on psychiatric examination to be without any psychotic symptoms, although having fears of victimization, rejection, abandonment and poor self-image. Schreier (1997) published a review of a series of cases under the heading of 'Factitious presentation of psychiatric disorder'. However, he comments in the review that it is 'difficult to be certain that these cases involve the *motivation* that defines MBP'. These uncertainties about definition may at least partly explain why thinking in this area has taken longer to evolve than it has in cases of physical presentation. But why should such difficulties have arisen, especially when one might have thought that psychiatry would have been the natural home for discussion of MSBP abuse?

A number of features of psychiatric presentations may explain this:

1. Psychiatric diagnosis is often particularly dependent on the history. In these cases a significant distorting of the history is the rule.
2. Psychiatric symptomatology, particularly in younger children, can be strongly related to specific contexts or relationships. It is common for children to have symptoms at home which cannot be verified at school; this does not necessarily mean that the symptoms at home are being factitiously reported. Even independent verification from a spouse (as is often advocated; see Schreier, 1997) is not foolproof. Children commonly behave very differently with each parent, and differently with a parent when the spouse is present as against when the spouse is absent.
3. The phenomenology of mental illness can often be more difficult to ascertain than physical illness (particularly in younger children) and more prone to examiner bias and reporter error.

4. Psychiatric symptomatology can, on occasion, be actively produced by parental suggestion without this necessarily constituting a factitious phenomenon.

It is thus the interpersonal context of symptomatology in child psychiatry that can make it difficult (or inappropriate) to formulate a straightforward factitious illness label in relation to psychiatric symptoms. The bread and butter of child psychiatry is to be working with disturbed parent–child relationships and situations in which parental views of children's behaviour or development are highly charged and sometimes distorted. To bring all these phenomena within a notion of MSBP or factitious illness by proxy would be misleading as well as dangerously counter-productive, particularly when the notion is so highly pejorative to parents. To take one example, some factitious presentations may be associated with parental over-protection or anxiety in both physical and psychological domains, but it would be wrong to ascribe a categorical definition of MSBP abuse to all situations of parental over-concern or enmeshment.

Consequently, it will be important to establish clear conceptual definitions of MSBP abuse as a context in which to consider psychiatric presentations. The approach of the present author, reflected in this chapter, is to attempt to give a fairly 'narrow' viewpoint on the definition of MSBP abuse and to confine this in the main to clear-cut examples of psychiatric presentations where the child's symptoms can be determined as factitious. A key feature for definition and ascertainment is that resulting harm accrues for the child, and it is this which brings the syndrome into the ambit of child abuse. Additionally, it is suggested here that a characteristic feature of the syndrome is commonly that the 'care giver' shows what can be understood as an abnormality in health belief in relation to the child's symptoms. In psychiatric MSBP it is usually a psychological rather than physical injury that is done to the child, thus falling into the category of emotional rather than physical abuse.

Factitious allegations of sexual abuse

Factitious allegations in the context of parental conflict or custody disputes

Studies have suggested that false allegations of sexual abuse are particularly found in the context of custody battles and disputed care (Schreier, 1997; Kelly and Loader, 1997; Jones and McGraw, 1987). Allegations may simply be blatantly cynical attempts to defame a partner by fabricating abuse. In more complex cases, the parent may have developed diffuse or confused psychological boundaries (including the use of projective identification, which will be described further below) with the effect that her own experience of abuse at the hands of a spouse is transformed into a belief that their child has experienced the same. Such disruption of a sense of psychological boundaries is particularly likely in families organized around repeated major trauma and fear (Bentovim, 1992). For these reasons, clinicians will need to be particularly wary of allegations of sexual abuse when they are made within the context of disputed care or abusive spousal relationships. However, to be overly dismissive of such claims is equally wrong. Recent evidence suggests that much parent–child abuse is concurrent with parent–spouse abuse: the traumatized spouse may find the boundary between herself and her child's suffering blurred – but this does not exclude the possibility that both abuse of the spouse and child is occurring (Shipman, Rossman and West, 1999). Vignettes are presented below to illustrate the background factors (family and otherwise) associated with diverse presentations of neuropsychiatric disorders.

Presentations of child sexual abuse

A mother presented to social services and then to psychiatric services saying that both her young school-aged children had been sexually abused. The details were vague but the abuse seemed to have happened a little time before and had been perpetrated by a friend who was a visitor to the house. The mother, who was black, said that her children had been subjected to systematic institutional racial abuse and victimization. Because of this she said she had progressively restricted the children's activities outside the home and had withdrawn them from school; at presentation to psychiatric services they were essentially house-bound.

The mother was suspicious, querulous, and often hostile towards 'authorities' of all kinds, whom she accused of institutional racial discrimination. During different contacts, her mental state fluctuated between states of high arousal and disorganized, at times deluded, thinking; on other occasions she was more relaxed, collaborative and integrated. She recounted her own history of a disorganized, frightening upbringing with multiple care givers, a period of sexual abuse from her father from four until nine years, school failure and extreme emotional difficulty in adolescence. She had a history of drug use, including cocaine and marijuana and had had multiple liaisons with partners, one of whom she said had been physically abusive to her (this was the partner who she had accused of abusing her own children).

The children, a boy and a girl aged seven and five, presented with fluctuating anxious states of mind and disorganized attention and communication. They were anxious, somewhat frightened of their mother's moods, and confused about their situation. The older boy had a more organized view about the fact that he had received racial taunts at school; the younger girl did not talk about this. Neither gave any indication of having been subject to sexual abuse.

As the psychiatric team gathered in information from different agencies over a period of time, a complex pattern emerged which gave cause for increasing concern. They found evidence of repeated previous contacts with other agencies, including social services in different areas. These contacts had gone back over a number of years and had all taken a similar pattern.

The mother had presented her children as having been abused, had been querulous and inconsistent with the professionals, had been vague in her descriptions and resisted further investigation, and had broken off contact abruptly with the agency. As this pattern emerged it became clear that none of the agencies had known about the contacts with others and there had been no systematic overview of the case. The mother had had intermittent psychiatric care, primarily for symptoms of anxiety, and had been described as having an abnormal personality. She had not sustained treatment. The family was isolated within its own community and well known to local primary care agencies, who described mother as 'unusual'. The school described relatively conformist children who attended poorly and denied there had been episodes of racial harassment by peers or staff (both had been alleged by the mother). They did comment, however, on the mother's unpredictable and often bizarre behaviour and their concerns about the children. No objective evidence to suggest abuse of the children had been reported by any of the agencies.

A professionals' conference concluded that there was no reasonable doubt that the mother's allegations represented a factitious presentation of child sexual abuse. Mother was thought to be suffering from a personality disorder with both borderline and 'sensitive' elements. Her presentation of a proxy allegation of abuse was possibly a displaced form of seeking help in relation to her own distress, perhaps related to her own experience of abuse as a child. A risk assessment was undertaken regarding developmental harm to the children. The combination of their distorted social experience, their exposure to the mother's fluctuating and sometimes borderline psychotic mental state, and their progressive removal from school and other social contact, led to a view that significant developmental harm was occurring.

Careful and sustained attempts were made to engage the mother along these lines. The consensus formulation was put to her in the context of a number of interviews and she was offered community mental health support. Her response depended a good deal upon her mood but overall the frequency of her querulous rejecting responses increased and she broke off contact. The professionals decided that the child protection issues were of such concern that action needed to be taken. A care order was taken by social services and the case went to court. The mother showed energy and competency in mobilizing her case and saw an adult psychiatrist with special interest in transcultural issues. He was of the view that the difficulties described represented a transcultural misunderstanding on behalf of the child care professionals and that there were no grounds for proceeding with the care order. The case was dismissed by the court. The child mental health and social work agencies could do no more than alert other agencies to whom they assumed the family would be likely to present in the future. No more has been heard.

This kind of case is not common but has been experienced by the present author on other occasions taking a similar form. The parental personality difficulties make insight and alliances with professionals very difficult. The children's predicament is a cause of huge concern and a disagreement among professionals about the formulation can make successful child protection proceedings impossible. It is certainly possible to interpret such a case – as the mother's psychiatrist did in this instance – in terms of a conflict of health beliefs, with the mother's beliefs seen as culturally understandable and the professionals' views misconceived. The issue turns on whether the mother's health beliefs are seen as abnormal and culturally dissonant, and whether the children have suffered objective harm because of them. Psychiatry has considerable experience in forming judgements about the abnormality of beliefs within cultural contexts. There are, of course legitimate grounds for debate in particular cases, particularly perhaps involving transcultural issues, but methods for ascertaining the phenomenology of abnormal beliefs (delusions or 'over-valued ideas') are well described and provide a useful way of thinking about the issues involved. Similarly, there are practice guidelines deriving from the Children Act for establishing the presence of significant harm to a child. The application of both these judgements is suggested here, i.e. as to the abnormality (in a technical sense) of the beliefs held by the parent and the extent of harm accruing to the child, in that together these factors constitute useful criteria for ascertainment in such cases.

In their genesis, such cases may on occasions exemplify in extreme form phenomena typical of highly enmeshed parent–child relationships, including a blurring of the psychological boundaries between parent and child. An experience of this kind (common in its mild form) is the way in which the presence of a child at a particular developmental stage will evoke unresolved memories and reactions from an equivalent stage in a parent's own development. So ubiquitous is this phenomenon that it can be a useful 'rule' for clinicians, when presented with unusual symptoms in their child patients, to focus on events in the parents' own developmental histories at around the current age of the child. Association with traumatic childhood events in the adult is especially likely to result in this almost uncanny echoing of child and adult experience.

An hypothesis for the mechanism of some factitious presentations follows from this. The unresolved traumatic emotions triggered by age-specific developmental signals from the child can be unbearable for an adult to bring to consciousness. An easier option is the psychological mechanism described as 'projective identification' in which an uncontainable feeling is (as it were) 'placed' into another person and is then experienced as actually emanating from that other person. This mechanism can lead a parent to confuse their child with themselves as a child – to perceive their own experience as existing in their child and thus come to believe that it is the child who has experienced the trauma. In a further twist, their consequent actions 'on behalf of' their child can also have a complex 'proxy' origin. In presenting the child for care and for action around the 'abuse', the current parent may be acting out what they wish their own parent had done for them. However, such an action activates the anger and ambivalence they felt towards their own parents in the context of their abuse (perhaps for their inactivity in preventing it) and this can introduce ambivalence into their current parental behaviour. Such intense recapitulation of unresolved traumatic experience can account for the observation that parents in this situation are unpredictable and ambivalent – that, at one moment, they are pressing forward their children's distress and demanding immediate action and yet, at another time, they are angrily breaking off contact from services. Professionals and 'authorities' are commonly cast into the role of uncomprehending and uncaring adults and much unintegrated aggression from the parent's own previous experience can be displaced on to relationships with them. Schreier (1997) states that, in these cases, the mother's 'primary goal is pursuit of a perverse relationship with powerful transferential figures – doctors, nurses and others – that contains various degrees of aggression and dependency'. However, rather than seeing the dynamics of these cases as primarily an issue of a relationship with the professional, it is suggested here that the primary focus of the psychological disturbance lies within the relationship between the parent and child (both the actual child and the 'child-as-projected-parent'). It is the parent–child relationship that suffers most intensely and the professional is often cast in the role of helpless onlooker.

The parent in these circumstances may come to need the child to be symptomatic or 'ill' until some relief is found or until the traumatic memory is deactivated by time passing or the child growing past a critical developmental period. In anything more than mild form, this process can be extremely pathogenic for the child. People receiving a projected identification often come to feel, in an intense and inexplicable way, the emotion that is projected into them. Children thus feel these intense emotions, which have an adult complexity and are often linked to trauma, in a context in which their parent is unable to assuage their distress and is indeed themselves distressed. The child can become disorganized and truly symptomatic under these circumstances, thus further confusing the picture.

Such dynamics of enmeshment may be common to a number of different factitious presentations. When serious, they can represent a critical failure of parenting and a serious issue of child protection. They will not, however, be a useful or relevant explanation in all cases and other factors in parents are no doubt also relevant to the genesis of the abnormal beliefs noted in many cases. Personality variables such as rigidity and perfectionism may predispose to the formation of inflexible attitudes and make adaptation to abnormal development in a child more difficult, as will be illustrated in the next section. A number of mental health problems in the parent such as borderline or paranoid personality disorder, psychotic or depressive illness, and substance or alcohol abuse may all make the sufferer vulnerable to abnormal belief formation. None of these clinically based hypotheses which have been formed to account for the aetiology of the syndrome has been formally tested, although the study reported in the next section makes a start at doing so.

Factitious presentation of autism and other developmental disorders

There is one case report in the literature (Stevenson and Alexander, 1990) describing a case in which a mother insisted that her child suffered from cerebral palsy, hearing impairment, mental retardation and seizures against all evidence to the contrary. There has been no published report of the factitious presentation of autism, attention deficit disorder or other neuropsychiatric disorders. However, the increasing currency of these disorders in the public imagination (as the result of public education, television documentaries, the activities of parental support groups, and widespread detailed information on the Internet) is likely to mean that these presentations will become more common. Additionally, the specific nature of each of these developmental disorders facilitates them standing as an emblematic, within-child explanation for particular difficulties in relationships between parent and child. For instance autism, with its core characteristic of abnormal social relationships, can become a proxy description for situations in which the parent feels either a lack of relationship or a disturbed relationship with the child. Attention deficit disorder, with its characteristic of impulsive, uncontrollable behaviour, lends itself as a description of problems of parental control. Tourette syndrome, with its episodic nature and the often abusive content of its complex tics, lends itself as an explanation of aggressive, insulting and 'revolting' behaviour that seem to 'come over' a child 'for no reason'.

There are also a number of potential secondary gains in the diagnosis of any of these disorders in the context of a scarcity of educational provision and specialized resources. There can be difficulty in many areas of the UK in getting some specialized forms of educational support without having an appropriate diagnosis. A diagnosis can also be a reassuring explanation in a situation of uncertainty and distress, one that objectifies the problem in the child rather than in the relationship, and which provides a useful explanation to others. A diagnosis can be an entry ticket for a variety of other social supports such as lay groups organized around specific disorders or Internet discussion groups.

A seven year old boy was referred to the child psychiatric unit for evaluation and querying of a diagnosis of autism. The child had originally been seen by paediatricians in the same hospital following a tertiary referral from a district general hospital. By the time of arrival to the child psychiatry unit, the mother had consulted neurologists and a dietician and was in regular contact with a clinical psychologist who supported the diagnosis of autism.

The mother described her son as being like 'two totally different children'. Firstly there was a fun loving, interesting and lovable boy with whom she enjoyed spending time, and then, and increasingly frequently, there was the other 'evil' son. This evil son had a characteristic facial expression with swollen slit-like eyes, and a photograph was produced to support this. He was loud and abusive, showing aggressive and threatening behaviour, which the mother felt was triggered by stress, excitement and certain foods. He often engaged in bizarre behaviour: specific incidents included squashing a hamster to death, hanging by a finger from an upstairs window and 'chasing the cat through the cat flap'. Against this background of a 'Jekyll and Hyde' personality, the mother worried about his lack of social awareness; he was 'shunned' by other children and had no friends, preferring to be alone. After watching a television programme on autism and researching the subject herself, the mother was convinced that this was her son's problem. Professionals who had told her otherwise were not believed.

PJ was the product of Mrs J's first pregnancy. Whilst the pregnancy was a happy time in her life, the birth was a traumatic experience (nine induction attempts) and, as a neonate, PJ was placed under a UV light, which his mother found distressing. Mrs J felt that PJ was always sleeping as an infant, but between six months and one year he became 'hard work', being difficult to get off to sleep and 'taking no comfort in my arms'. He had early locomotor development, sitting at four months and climbing stairs at eight months. At the age of eleven months she reported that he climbed on to the roof of the house and up a tree. He could vocalize in single words ('Mum', 'Dad') at ten months, and spoke in short phrases soon after. By eighteen months, however, he still referred to himself as 'the boy', never 'me' or by his name.

Mrs J sensed something was wrong as early as nine months. At two years of age PJ was referred to a dietician because of his 'Jekyll and Hyde' personality, which Mrs J insisted was caused by an allergy to food colouring, and a restrictive diet was introduced. Playgroup staff, however, did not substantiate her claims regarding his behaviour. At three years of age PJ was referred to a clinical psychologist who found him to have advanced locomotor development and average intelligence, but who empathized with the mother and felt strongly that PJ had some inherent and as yet undiagnosed disorder.

PJ was the eldest of three children, with the other siblings reported as being entirely normal. Mrs J, a thirty-three year old woman, described an isolated childhood, frequently separated from her mother who was in and out of hospital with a variety of ailments. Mrs J herself had suffered numerous illnesses in childhood, including kidney and chest problems, and had recently been diagnosed as having hereditary angioneurotic angioedema. PJ's father, who had been sexually abused as a child and feared the same happening to his son, was 'drained' by PJ's problems and sought comfort in an extramarital affair. The marital difficulties were acknowledged by Mrs J who felt that she had 'no self-esteem' since her husband had worn her down.

Following an initial consultation, PJ was admitted as an in-patient for assessment. A physical examination, blood tests, drug screen, chromosome studies, EEG and CAT were all normal and a normal diet was reintroduced without any change in behaviour. No autistic behaviour was noted on the ward and a Children's Autistic Rating Scale was performed which confirmed clinical suspicions that PJ did not have autism. Play assessment revealed no inherent disorder but someone who was extremely possessive and defensive about his own space. PJ seemed to feel alone and cut off from his peers and family. The formulation reached was that, whilst PJ had features of emotional distress, the supposed inherent disorders were factitious in nature. The parents refused to accept this diagnosis and insisted that a label of autism should be used. This argument was supported by the clinical psychologist who had been in contact with the family for a number of years and was felt by the unit to be an important maintaining factor.

A retrospective case note study to investigate family factors associated with MSBP abuse presentation of neurodevelopmental problems

To further investigate such factitious presentations of neuropsychiatric disorder, a case note study was undertaken*.

Sample

In the author's referral clinic for pervasive developmental disorders, seven cases were identified over a number of years which satisfied criteria for MSBP abuse. They had the following features in common:

- The history presented by parents had some features typical of autism but often involved bizarre or unusual symptoms. One case presented a very similar picture but in relation to Tourette syndrome (TS).
- On clinical assessment the child did not fulfil any criteria for diagnosis of autism or autism spectrum disorder (or TS).
- Despite feedback to the parent or parents of the detailed evidence against the diagnosis (if necessary with follow-up appointments), and despite the fact that this lack of diagnosis of a severely debilitating and lifelong disorder would normally be a matter of unambiguous relief, the parents refused to accept the results of the assessment and persisted with their view that the child suffered from an autistic disorder.

For the study, five further cases were ascertained by advertising to colleagues in the area. One presented with Tourette syndrome rather than autism. The resulting twelve cases were studied against a comparison group of twenty-two clinic cases matched for age and sex and where there had been a true diagnosis of autism.

Method

A literature review identified a number of family factors described in association with physical presentations of MSBP abuse. The reports were of variable quality and some were unsystematic, but the factors thus identified were taken as a starting point:

1. Maternal history of psychiatric illness (Rosenberg, 1987; Eminson and Postlethwaite, 1992; Fisher, Mitchell and Murdoch, 1993), sexual, physical or emotional abuse (Eminson and Postlethwaite, 1992; Fisher, Mitchell and Murdoch, 1993; Meadow, 1982 and 1985), or abnormal illness behaviour (Eminson and Postlethwaite, 1992; Fisher, Mitchell and Murdoch, 1993; Meadow, 1985; Fisher and Mitchell, 1992).

---

*The author would like to acknowledge the contribution of Claire Appleby who, at the time of the study, was a medical student and undertook the data collection and initial writing up of this study.

2. Medical related occupation in mother (Bools, Neale and Meadow, 1994).
3. Presence of marital conflict (Samuels *et al.*, 1992; Palmer and Yoshimura, 1984; Griffith, 1988), or distant or unsupportive father (Bools, Neale and Meadow, 1994; Lasky and Erikson,1974).
4. Associated abuse (physical or sexual) of other members of the family (Rosenberg, 1987).
5. Persisting consulting behaviour, with multiple referrals made either by the parents directly or other professionals involved (Rosenberg, 1987; Rogers *et al.*, 1976).

Further to these, a number of extra factors were hypothesized to be of potential additional relevance in factitious psychiatric presentations:

• Reported family history of psychiatric disorder/developmental syndrome (either a diagnosed condition or suggestive behaviour such as 'odd' or eccentric, socially aloof family members).
• Maternal loss of parents before fifteen years.
• Significant life events occurring around the index pregnancy and neonatal period (e.g. bereavement, relationship breakdown, traumatic birth).
• Report of postnatal depression with the index child.
• Report of early relationship difficulties with the index child.
• Involvement in self-help groups reported by parent.
• Evidence of parental over-protection.

These factors were included in a case note ascertainment form using operationalized criteria. The case notes were rated independently from the clinical assessment, but internal evidence within the notes made it not always possible for the rater to remain blind to clinical status. In eleven cases, the mother was considered the main parent responsible for presenting the child and insisting on the diagnosis, and details of her history were therefore recorded for the purposes of the study. In the remaining case, the father had a dominant role and his history was used. Reported history of abuse (physical or sexual) was recorded for the index child or a sibling, irrespective of the abuser's relationship to the child. 'Parental over-protection' was coded if the case notes specifically mentioned this term or if they recorded behaviours of the kind described by Parker (1983), i.e. excessive contact with the parent always around, excessively anxious preoccupation with the child's supposed vulnerability, child being 'infantilized' or treated like a baby or inappropriate restriction of independent behaviour. Early relationship difficulties were recorded if the parent specifically reported sustained difficulties with attributions or feelings about the child in the first year. The number of professionals consulted about the presenting problems was recorded – relevant professionals included psychiatrists, paediatricians, psychologists and specialist therapists such as speech therapists. A 'self-help group' was defined as a syndrome-specific local or national association. Coding of maternal 'abnormal illness behaviour' was based on reference in the case notes to a parental diagnosis of Munchausen syndrome or somatization, or to reports of multiple illness throughout life for which no cause had been found.

Results

Children were group matched for age and sex. No significant difference between case and comparison groups was found for maternal age, social class or route of referral. Summary findings comparing the two groups are shown in Table 8.1 (because of the small numbers in the study, significance levels of < 0.01 are emphasized).

Eight children (66.7 per cent) from the study group had a significant medical history, of which three (25 per cent) were allergic to various foods. This compares with 9.1 per cent of children reporting allergies in the comparison group. Additionally, 41.7 per cent of cases had other medical problems including asthma and nocturnal enuresis, whilst 9.1 per cent of the comparison group reported other medical conditions. A history of abuse was noted in 27.3 per cent of cases of the factitious group. In two cases there was physical abuse of the index child. Sexual abuse of a sibling occurred in one case, although the perpetrator was a family friend rather than a family member. In contrast, no abuse was noted in the comparison group.

Of the mothers in the factitious group, 36.4 per cent were noted to have a history of abuse. In two cases this was physical; a further two suffered other forms of abuse which both described as emotional neglect. This was in contrast to 4.5 per cent in the comparison group. Parental loss was more common in the factitious group, with 27.3 per cent of mothers losing a parent before adulthood. Descriptions of the relationship with their partner in the factitious group were: abusive (36.4 per cent), unsupportive (18.2 per cent), involves an extramarital affair (9.1 per cent), good (9.1 per cent) and unspecified (27.3 per cent). Descriptions of the relationships with their partner in comparison cases were: abusive (0 per cent), unsupportive (13.6 per cent), extramarital affair (0 per cent), good (36.4 per cent) and unspecified (50 per cent). Depression was found to be the commonest psychiatric illness in mothers, being reported in 27.2 per cent of cases and 9.1 per cent of comparisons. Postnatal depression was coded separately: one-third of index mothers suffered from postnatal depression as against 4.5 per cent in the comparison group. Two-thirds of the factitious group described early relationship difficulties with their child. Such descriptions included: 'she was odd, I felt like she was rejecting me'; 'he was difficult to bond with'; 'I didn't take to him'. Only 18.2 per cent of mothers in the comparison group experienced similar problems, but when they did their descriptions were comparable.

Regarding abnormal illness behaviour in care givers, no cases of Munchausen syndrome or somatization were recorded in the case notes studied and inferences about the 'abnormality' of illness behaviour reported by parents must, of course, be conjectural. However, 40 per cent of parents in the factitious group (compared to none in the other group) reported an extensive medical history of often unexplained symptoms. For instance, in one case a history was given of Bell's palsy,

Table 8.1 Case note comparison of variables between factitious and non-facti-tious groups

Variable	Factitious group ($n = 12$)	Comparison group ($n = 22$)	Fisher exact (p value)
Child:			
Significant medical history			0.008
None	33.3	81.8	
Allergies	25.0	9.1	
Other	41.7	9.1	
Family history of related disorder			0.09
Sibling	–	9.1	
Father	9.1	9.1	
Extended family	36.4	4.5	
None	54.5	77.3	
Abuse in family			0.03
Index child	18.2	–	
Sibling	9.1	–	
None	72.7	100	
Mother:			
Psychiatric history			0.4
None	63.6	81.8	
Depression	27.3	9.1	
Anxiety	9.1	9.1	
History of abuse			0.03
None	63.6	95.5	
Physical	18.2	4.5	
Sexual	–	–	
Other	18.2	–	
Early parental loss			0.09
Yes	27.3	4.5	
No	72.7	95.5	
Adverse life events			0.06
None	25	59.1	
Traumatic birth	50	31.8	
Bereavement	8.3	–	
Relationship breakdown	16.7	4.5	
Move of house	–	4.5	
Postnatal depression			0.04
Yes	33.3	4.5	
No	66.7	95.5	

Variable	Factitious group (n = 12)	Comparison group (n = 22)	Fisher exact (p value)
Early relationship difficulties with child			0.008
Yes	66.7	18.2	
No	33.3	81.8	
Abnormal illness behaviour			0.03
None	66.7	95.5	
Munchausen syndrome	–	–	
Somatization disorder	–	–	
Multiple illnesses	33.3	4.5	
Recruitment of professionals			0.03
More than one	72.7	100	
More than five	27.3	–	
Self-help group involvement			0.001
Yes	81.8	18.2	
No	18.2	81.8	
Parental over-protection			0.001
Yes	63.6	–	
No	36.4	100	

arthritis, lifelong sporadic fainting attacks (for which no cause had been found) and numerous hospital admissions for asthma.

Case note examples of 'parental over-protection' were significantly more common in the factitious group. Examples included a six year old child not being allowed to play in the yard at school because they might get injured, preventing a child from running because of fears they would have a heart attack and putting a four year old, toilet-trained boy in nappies while at home.

Comments on the study

This is a small-scale study and a number of provisos need to be made about the design before evaluating the results. Firstly the sample is small (reflecting the relative rarity of the problem) and significance levels are open to the risk of chance associations. Secondly there is a potential ascertainment bias due to the fact that the factitious group was recruited from a number of clinical settings and the comparison group solely from the author's own clinic. However, all the clinics were in the same region and one was in the same health trust as the author's clinic. Two of the clinicians involved had trained with the author and similar diagnostic procedures were involved in each case. A potentially more serious bias may relate to the effect of repeated consultations. The families in the factitious group had had, on average, a significantly greater number of health care consultations and thus would arguably have discussed their histories more times than the true disorder group. This could lead to a possible ascertainment bias in the information obtained, particularly perhaps relating to parental background factors, based on repeating tellings of the story or more probing history taking on the part of clinicians. (Many clinicians assessing autism would not routinely go into a detailed history of parental psychological development unless they were concerned about other sources of the problem.) It is also possible that the parents in the factitious group amplify or divert attention to their own histories during the consultation, as part of insistent help seeking or due to the pressure of their own distress. The clinics involved took standardized histories, which may mitigate against this potential bias; however, numbers in the sample are too small to test for its presence in any definitive way.

With these provisos in mind, one can cautiously conclude that the data does provide preliminary evidence that factitious and true cases presenting with these developmental disorders differ systematically on a number of family factors. The factors involved show similarities with many of those described in the literature on MSBP abuse with physical presentation and support clinical hypotheses made prior to the study. Striking findings include the report of multiple illnesses, including allergies, during the child's development, as has already been discussed in association with factitious illness by proxy in the medical field (Meadow, 1982), early relationship difficulties with the child (the nature of true autistic development is that early problems are rarely found), and patterns of over-anxiety and over-protection that seem inappropriate and which again have also been described in physical MSBP abuse (Meadow, 1985). The involvement in self-help groups is often highly insistent and the use of their information and Internet resources generates a large knowledge-base about the disorder. Clinically during consultations this often manifests as a strange experience of talking as if in a medical seminar rather than about an actual child or family.

Factitious conversion disorder and somatization

A fourteen year old boy was presented with a 'total allergy syndrome'. He was said by his parents to be allergic to many aspects of his environment, including rain, cleaning fluids of all kinds, dust and foam fillings in furniture. The child's 'allergic response' was to have a temper, to swear and to kick his mother. The case occurred at a time when considerable media attention was being given to so-called 'total allergy syndrome' and treatments for it: the child's predicament was reported in local and national newspapers. The family had seen a large number of practitioners and had been dissatisfied with all the advice they had received until they consulted a homeopathic allergist who prescribed a remedy that needed to be taken under the tongue daily. This remedy cost the family a great deal of money but they persisted with it while pursuing a referral to the child psychiatry service.

The family was extremely unusual. Father had had a paranoid illness and presented with a deficit state. Mother was hostile to professionals and passionate in her beliefs regarding the causation of illness of various kinds. The child's 'allergic' episodes were witnessed in the clinic and videotaped. They were just as described by the family. The boy became agitated and flushed. His mother said 'that's it, he's about to have one'. He then got up and assaulted his mother and swore at her. During admission to hospital the boy showed no symptoms except in the family's presence. The homeopathic remedy was discontinued during the in-patient stay. The boy himself was socially immature but showed no abnormality of mental state. He believed in the syndrome that his family said he had.

Because the boy had been withdrawn from school and virtually confined to his house for over a year for fear of the danger of allergies, and because of the lack of any insight by the family into these difficulties, care proceedings were carefully considered. However, because of the boy's age and the fact that he showed no signs of distress or any wish to change his predicament, it was concluded that proceedings were unlikely to be successful.

A large amount of therapeutic work was undertaken with the family and the child in an attempt to shift these health beliefs. The boy himself as an in-patient was symptom-free for four months, during which time he made progress in education and social areas. The treatment, however, was not sustained after discharge and the family were lost to follow-up.

Although this is an extreme and potentially tragic case which at times verged on the farcical, it does echo, in the drastic psychosocial effects of the disorder, Meadows' description of chronic MSBP abuse (Meadow, 1977). Some of the background factors described in the previous section are present. An additional element in this case was the way in which the abnormal health belief held by the family did link in with cultural concerns (powerful in the media at the time this case presented) about the adverse effects of the environment and the efficacy of 'alternative therapies' compared to conventional medicine. This exacerbated the hostility that the family felt towards the doctors that they saw and acted to entrench their belief in their version of events. As with many cases, the family also had a 'clinician' who supported their view. The fact remained, however, that even within the context of this belief system, the nature of the presentation and its consequences were bizarre and abnormal.

Summary of the presented cases

The case note study and the other cases reported here offer preliminary evidence that similar psychopathological processes are at play behind diverse presentations of factitious illness by proxy. Specific public preoccupations at any time may exert a shaping or even precipitating effect on the nature of the symptoms presented; thus the form of presentations has successively involved sexual abuse, pervasive developmental disorder, allergy syndromes and other conditions 'of the day'. At the time of writing, many clinicians report parental interest in attention deficit disorder as a key concern, although autistic disorders remain strongly in the public mind.

The underlying vulnerabilities necessary to develop these presentation, however, are likely to lie elsewhere, and go to the heart of the psychopathology of MSBP abuse. Possible specific vulnerability factors in the family are identified in the case note study above. It has been hypothesized here that a mechanism for their action in some cases lies in the dynamic processes of parent-child enmeshment and projective identification leading to the formation of abnormal health beliefs. It is an open question at present as to what other mechanisms may be at play in these cases and whether the psychopathology differs significantly in psychiatric and medical presentations.

Management

Assessment

The first key of management is evaluation; not just of the presence or absence of psychopathology in the child but of the underlying family variables. In this wider family evaluation, it is now the present author's practice to make systematic enquiry into the variables identified above in the case note study. This needs to be done with tact and consideration since such enquiry enters into intimate matters that are far from the initial concerns regarding symptomatology in the child that led to the parents' consultation. The assessment can, however, gradually be made in the course of a number of interviews, picking up the leads suggested by the family in conversation regarding family life and their child, without it seeming like systematic enquiry or interrogation. Similarly sensitive enquiry needs to be made into possible secondary gains that may accrue from the symptomatology. As outlined in Chapter 4, and in common with all similarly complex presentations, scrutiny of other records is essential. Permission needs to be sought for the gathering of information from other records: from previous professional consultations, from schools, and from professionals attending to parents as well as the child.

As with other forms of fabricated illness, admission for the child or assessment away from the family can be extremely helpful in clarifying symptomatology and interactions away from the intense family culture. This must be distinguished from the admission process that is described in detail in Chapter 13, where it constitutes a part of the decision making 'judgement' and/or treatment phase. Admission as described here is a part of the first and second stages of such cases, i.e. part of routine management of a child with such complex difficulties where extensive independent observations need to be made. However, the experienced clinician will be familiar with the changeable nature of children's symptomatology in different environments and great caution needs to be exercised in drawing inferences too rapidly from the child's behavioural reactions to admission.

Different symptomatologies present different difficulties here. Thus, disorders such as pervasive developmental disorder, ADD or conversion disorders will, in the end, clearly present themselves independent of environment. Emotional disorders can be more changeable. Complex tic disorders are difficult to evaluate because of the considerable liability of tics to degree of arousal and environmental conditions. Psychotic thought disorder, particularly in young children, can also be difficult to evaluate and may need repeated careful study.

A routine part of in-patient work would often be home-based liaison by members of the in-patient team. During home visits in these conditions it can be extremely informative to observe children's context-specific behaviours and gain other incidental information. Thus, the child above presenting with total allergy syndrome lived in a home environment that was totally chaotic, unmaintained and home to scores of dogs. The environment that the parents had built at home seemed to reflect their unusual mental state. Visits home can elicit the information about sleeping arrangements or other aspects of behavioural management that the parents conceal or never think to discuss in clinic.

Treatment

Generating a working alliance

The first key to therapeutic management is the development of a personal professional relationship and then a task-related therapeutic alliance (Hougaard, 1994). This task-related alliance normally needs to base itself around a progressively shared understanding between professional and parent about the nature of the problem, leading on to a shared understanding about strategies to manage it. A useful first approach to this, in these cases, is to try to understand, in as complete and non-judgemental a way as possible, the complex nature of the health beliefs underlying the parents' perception of the problem. There needs to be an attitude of genuine and open-minded interest on the clinician's part (which should not need to be forced: people's health beliefs in all their social, cultural and psychological ramifications and in their developmental emergence are fascinating things). Such an attentive approach from the clinician will give the parents a sense of being heard empathetically and, for some of the less extreme cases, this attitude itself is enough to develop a clinical relationship in which the true origin of the concern (often parental anxiety or other traumatic unresolved experiences) can be acknowledged and attended to. If this happens, then the preoccupation with the child's symptoms can melt away naturally as increasing focus is able to be given to core personal difficulties.

In this process of listening to and constructing the family's health belief, it is often valuable to concentrate on the 'episodic' detail of events, specific symptoms and functional difficulties, rather than 'semantic' inferences or generalizations that attach themselves to diagnoses. Thus, the clinician and the family can come to an agreement about the nature of the specific symptoms and impairments without needing to dispute about what the overall 'diagnosis' is or what the impairments 'mean'. This shared description of the symptomatology and functional difficulties is most useful if it is not solely concentrated on the child but includes issues to do with the impact of the child on the family and general family functioning. Sometimes the focus of the family's health belief is on the diagnostic construct ('autism' or 'ADD'), while sometimes it is on specific symptoms. Either way, this powerful and rigid adherence to a concept usually represents a crystallization of numerous and diffuse sources of fear and distress. Taking the focus away from this over-determined belief into other areas of symptomatology or experience can help the clinician get behind the rigid nature of the belief and to understand the intense perceptual biases that inform descriptions of particular symptoms.

Influencing beliefs

Having elicited these parental observations the clinician can then, with appropriate timing, introduce their own observations (again at the level of particular symptoms). The aim here is to develop an area of shared observations and a shared language to talk about them. The clinician will be hoping to introduce observations that begin to implicitly frame symptoms in a way that serves the clinical purpose. For instance, observations can be introduced linked in with an interactional context. Clinician and parent can agree, say, on overactivity behaviour in the child but the clinician can introduce the concept of an overactivity that is contingent on certain interactions, contexts or feelings. Thus implicitly rather than explicitly the clinician conveys the view that these symptoms are context-based and interactional rather than intrinsic phenomena within the child.

If such a common language for shared observations can be established, the way is open for the next step. Here the clinician can gradually reframe the observations during discussion with the family, in a way which can (in successful cases) allow parents, often dramatically, to alter health beliefs. The following vignette illustrates this point.

A mother of a five year old child with a mild spastic diplegia produced by birth injury was convinced that he was autistic. She had held rigidly to this view and convinced a number of professionals of her case. The child's behaviour patterns on which she based her diagnostic inference were his social avoidance of her, his withdrawal, the blankness of his affect and his lack of progress in school. There was agreement on all these phenomena, which were readily apparent in the child. As the child's avoidance of both parents, but particularly his mother, was investigated further, questions were asked about this phenomenon in its interactional context, about what her feelings were when she saw this in him and about particular contexts in which he showed these reactions. Gradually it was possible to link his social aversion to her feelings of negativity, disgust and anger towards him. These feelings in turn gradually linked to her reaction to his father (a quiet, unresponsive man who the son resembled in some ways), and, most profoundly, to her reactions to his birth and developmental difficulties. That link, in turn, enabled the mother to experience the full force of her grief and frustration at her son's difficulties, her frustration in her marriage, and her desperation about the boy's future. In a sudden, emotionally charged transition in one session, she was able spontaneously to reframe and reinterpret for herself her intense experiences and locate them, not in the child's supposed autism, but in her own desperation. This allowed a further working through of her complex emotions around his birth and development, and her mood and obsessive preoccupation with her son lightened as she did so. In consequence, her displaced anger and preoccupation, which had been perceived by her son as hostility and rejection towards him, were replaced by greater warmth and acceptance. The boy's social aversion decreased and his 'autism' disappeared.

Therapeutic failure

In more difficult cases it is impossible to form even the beginning of a therapeutic alliance; or a point comes in the middle of the therapeutic work where the parents feel a threat to their belief system and dramatically withdraw. The professional is denigrated as another one of the 'enemy' and the cycle of breaking professional contact and further help seeking elsewhere follows. Clinical experience suggests that parents with a more disturbed basic personality structure and those with more abnormal and rigidly held beliefs are more likely to break off in this way. Alternatively (and often more insidiously), the point of reframing is never really tackled and the clinician can slip into a kind of collusion with the family's belief – a state which can be rationalized as 'case management' or 'keeping a watchful eye'. This can go on for years and the harm to the child never really be grasped.

In any event of therapeutic failure or drift the crucial step is to make a risk assessment of harm to the child with all relevant professionals, leading to a decision as to whether legal action needs to be taken (see Chapters 11 and 12). There must be an informing of the network of professionals who may come into contact with the family. Gaining sufficient evidence to pursue a case successfully is not always easy and often requires an accumulation of carefully documented evidence from many sources (see Chapters 1 and 11). As the case examples illustrate, it is substantially more difficult to convince other professionals and the courts of the emotional harm that results from psychiatric MSBP abuse compared to the more classical physical kind.

Conclusions

Evaluation of psychiatric presentations of fabricated illness by parents is particularly difficult. This is because it is normal in child mental health settings to work with disparate perceptions of a child's problems and because a child's behaviour and responses can vary widely in different contexts.

Leaving aside cases where there is clear malingering, secondary gain or cynical manipulation of symptomatology, the presentation of factitious psychiatric symptoms in children by parents is often helpfully construed as relating to abnormal health beliefs in the parents. This allows the general psychiatric understanding of abnormal beliefs (such as delusions or over-valued ideas) to be used in understanding and treatment of a case. The other cornerstone of the syndrome is that the harm is accruing to the child; in psychiatric presentations this harm is less likely to be actual physical damage but more likely to be psychological stress and restriction of normal development and experience.

The propensity to form such abnormal health beliefs may at times be associated with mental health or personality type, or with an intense unresolved affect or traumatic experience whose true nature is unable to be named by the adult. Evidence regarding the developmental origins and markers of this propensity are now fairly well described in the literature on physical presentations, and preliminary data presented in this chapter suggest that similar factors may apply to factitious presentation of psychiatric as well as non-psychiatric disorders. The particular nature taken by the unusual health belief and symptomatic presentation may well be influenced by contingent factors such as the social and cultural preoccupations of the day and the ways in which individual diagnostic presentations lend themselves to be used as proxies for particular parental feelings. The fact that the child is used as proxy usually relates to the details of a child's effect on an adult at a particular age and sometimes their capacity to stir age-specific memories in parents.

Two essential features of ascertainment are to develop a good understanding of the health beliefs underlying the factitious presentation and to assess the resulting harm to the child. The core of treatment is to draw the family into therapeutic work in which such beliefs can be reworked. As is the nature of belief, such transformations in therapy can seem cathartic or sudden. As Eminson and Postlethwaite (1992) have pointed out, professional health beliefs and their particularities have also to be taken into account here, and professionals will need insight into their own beliefs as well as flexibility and persistence to work well with these cases. The insidious effects and occasional tragic consequence of such factitious presentations are a measure of the power of beliefs to mould perceptions and influence others. Treatment often fails and then the priority is to conduct a risk assessment focused on the harm to the child and the need for protective action.

References

Bentovim, A. (1992) *Trauma Organised Systems. Physical and Sexual Abuse in Families*. Karnac Books.

Bools, C., Neal, B. and Meadow, R. (1994) Munchausen syndrome by proxy: A study of psychopathology. *Child Abuse and Neglect*, **18**, 773–788.

Eminson, D.M. and Postlethwaite, R.J. (1992) Factitious illness: recognition and management. *Archives of Disease in Childhood*, **67**, 1510–1516.

Fisher, G.C. and Mitchell, I. (1992) Munchausen's syndrome by proxy (factitious illness by proxy). *Current Opinion in Psychiatry*, **5**, 224–227.

Fisher, G.C., Mitchell, I. and Murdoch, D. (1993) Munchausen syndrome by proxy – the question of psychiatric illness in a child. *British Journal of Psychiatry*, **162**, 701–703.

Griffith, J.L. (1988) The family systems of Munchausen's syndrome by proxy. *Family Process*, **27**, 423–437.

Hougaard, E. (1994) The therapeutic alliance – a conceptual analysis. *Scandinavian Journal of Psychology*, **35**, 67–85.

Jones. D. and McGraw, J.M. (1987) Reliable and fictitious accounts of sexual abuse to children. *Journal of Interpersonal Violence*, **2**, 27–45.

Kelly, C. and Loader, P. (1997) Factitious disorder by proxy: the role of child mental health professionals. *Child Psychology and Psychiatry Review*, **2** (3), 116–124.

Lansky, S.B. and Erilson, H. (1974) Prevention of child murder. *Journal of the American Academy of Child Psychiatry*, **13**, 691–698.

Meadow, R. (1977) Munchausen syndrome by proxy – the hinterland of child abuse. *Lancet*, **ii**, 343–345.

Meadow, R. (1982) Munchausen syndrome by proxy. *Archives of Disease in Childhood*, **57**, 92–98.

Meadow, R. (1985) Management of Munchausen syndrome by proxy. *Archives of Disease in Childhood*, **60**, 385–393.

Palmer, A.J. and Yoshimura, G.J. (1984) Munchausen syndrome by proxy. *Journal of the American Academy of Child Psychiatry*, **23**, 503–508.

Parker G. (1983) *Parental Overprotection: A Risk Factor in Psychosexual Development*. Grune and Stratton.

Rogers, D., Tripp, J., Bentovim, A. *et al.* (1976) Non-accidental poisoning: an extended syndrome of child abuse. *British Medical Journal*, **1**, 793–796.

Rosenberg, D. (1987) Web of deceit. A literature review of Munchausen syndrome by proxy. *Child Abuse and Neglect*, **11**, 547–563.

Samuels, M.P., McClaughlin, W., Jacobson, *et al.* (1992) Fourteen cases of imposed upper airways obstruction. *Archives of Disease in Childhood*, **67**, 162–170.

Schreier, H.A. (1997) Factitious presentation of psychiatric disorder: when is it Munchausen by proxy. *Child Psychology and Psychiatry Review*, **2** (3), 108–115.

Shipman, K.L., Rossman, B.B.R. and West, J.C. (1999) Co-occurrence of spousal violence and child abuse: conceptual implications. *Child Maltreatment*, **4**, 93–102.

Stevenson, R. and Alexander, R. (1990) Munchausen syndrome by proxy presenting as a developmental disability. *Developmental Behavioural Paediatrics*, **11** (5), 262–264.

9

Dealing with uncertainty

Eileen Baildam and Mary Eminson

Introduction

Identifying MSBP abuse may be straightforward in cases where a single, severe, dangerous and undisputed event has occurred to a dependent child. In this situation, the issue then is to achieve the most objective proof possible without further risk to the child. However, the majority of cases do not fall into this category and there can be a very real problem confirming abuse beyond reasonable doubt. In Chapters 3 and 4, a clinical method has been described to aid recognition and clarification of factitious illness and to help in identifying fabrications. In many cases there is as yet insufficient evidence to confidently identify abuse, or the nature of the risk (if any) to the child may be unclear. These cases present to all doctors dealing with children.

In this chapter we consider some difficult clinical circumstances in which uncertainty arises. This can be uncertainty about whether harm is occurring to the child as a result of parental actions relating to the child's health, uncertainty about whether there is a risk of future harm or uncertainty about the boundaries between abuse and other medical and treatment dilemmas.

Many of these situations would not usually be discussed in the context of factitious illness. We do so in the belief that none of these situations is black and white, and that all of them may, on occasion, shade imperceptibly into the category of abuse of children within the health care setting, which falls within the boundary of this book. Skills in analysing such situations and in finding ways to deal with them, and promoting children's health and protecting them from abuse, may all be assisted by contemplating the many situations in which abuse may occur in a medical setting.

In this chapter, we review examples of those circumstances where doctors may be uncertain as to whether parental pursuit of health care or the parental stance in relation to their child's illness is a harmful one. Included are a range of situations in which the child's professional attendants do not find that they can achieve agreement with parents about the management of the child's ill-health, at a time when this difference of opinion seems important in terms of the outcome for the child. Some of these situations have already been touched on in Chapter 3. The method suggested there was an analysis of abnormal illness behaviour by parents for children. The first part of this chapter restates some of the principal issues of that chapter and then discusses particular situations in greater depth. Risk assessment forms the second part of the chapter. The third section gives guidelines for the management of a number of such difficult situations, including an outline of management of those cases in which clinicians judge that significant abnormal illness behaviour and factitious illness exists, but where it is below the critical threshold for harm and hence MSBP abuse.

General issues increasing uncertainty

Some general issues that add to the uncertainty of work with factitious illness cases are outlined below.

A spectrum, not a category of behaviour

There is clearly a spectrum of abnormal parental behaviour towards children's health, from severe life-threatening concealed abuse through to minor exaggeration by the parent (Eminson and Postlethwaite, 1992). Although individual anecdotes provide exceptions, there is little concrete evidence to suggest that there is a progression from one end of the spectrum to the other in individual cases. There are difficulties, therefore, in making rules to manage the different ends of the spectrum from definite identification of abuse to minor suspicion. The point at which child protection procedures should be involved does vary from case to case.

Unfamiliar areas of history taking

A second issue emphasized in many parts of this book is the importance of establishing the correct facts of the case by using multiple sources of information in order to corroborate the history given by the parent with information from other sources. This includes information about the parents' own medical and psychiatric history. However, this in itself makes the enquiry more difficult, for this is the point at which paediatricians may move out of their normal lines of enquiry and where it becomes less comfortable to proceed, even if confidentiality is not an issue. In the psychiatric history-taking process such enquiry is more expected and if psychiatric colleagues are involved at this point, then they may be able to help with this information gathering. However, it is not uncommon for psychiatric involvement to be refused by the parent(s) at this stage. It may be the paediatrician who asks for the help in gathering information and weighing it up when gathered.

Lack of normal mutual trust between parent and doctor

A third consideration is the different climate that surrounds the doctor–parent relationship in these cases. The painstaking collecting of evidence and clarification of the exact causes of concern are similar to those processes needed for many complicated clinical cases. However, there is a fundamental flaw in these cases which must be remembered. The art of history taking towards a diagnosis stands on the assumption of mutual trust inherent in the normal doctor–patient relationship. It may take a long time for the fabricated nature of the history to dawn. This is particularly so with a very trusting or inexperienced doctor who has become engaged in the doctor–patient dyad with a diminished ability to stand outside the consultation process in order to analyse it. There is a need in medical consultations, as in psychiatric consultations, to remember that the reported history is a vehicle for many possible hidden agendas and that it requires care before the history is accepted as a factual account. This was summarized in Chapter 3 as 'believe everything the patient says and nothing the patient says'. Taylor (1992) described how uncomfortable this might feel: 'We might fear for our thought processes in each and every diagnostic encounter. Evil would leer out of any consultation where the aetiology was unclear'. Making the change to taking this stance towards parents may be uncomfortable for paediatricians and therefore difficult to undertake with confidence, thus making histories more difficult to appraise.

Lack of uniformity in judgement and management

The decision about how to proceed as a clinician in complex situations with risk of harm is further complicated by the variations in management of cases from area to area and from team to team. In other words, even groups of professionals make inconsistent judgements of harm. Thus, there was a situation where one local authority awarded a care order on three siblings where there had been very frequent attendance at the GP's surgeries with multiple referrals to hospital but without any definite evidence of fabricated illness. The risk stated by the local authority was that the girls would grow up 'medicalizing' all their emotional problems and that this *per se* constituted emotional abuse. At the other extreme, another case was reopened to consider whether or not there was any danger to a six month old baby currently in the care of its mother who had already been convicted of the murder by suffocation of a previous infant.

Cultural issues

There may be some specific problems in deciphering the MSBP abuse puzzle in different ethnic and cultural groups, including those groups with firm and unfamiliar views but who are members of the majority culture – Jehovah's Witnesses for example. In families from a different culture, the clinical method outlined in Chapter 3 may be almost impossible to follow. Sometimes there is an active exclusion of outsiders to a community which makes accurate risk assessment difficult. Independent corroboration of symptoms or current or historical events may be impossible to find. In these situations it may be difficult to know what value is placed on health-related issues and therefore judgements about 'persistence' and 'incongruence' are uncertain. Also difficult to appraise is the success with which the clinician has communicated what he intended if there is a lack of shared language. There may be specific disease anxieties that generate excessive seeking of medical advice until the patient feels fully reassured. It may be difficult to decide what is outside the norm when one does not really understand the norm in the first place. There may also be a lack of access to various cultural constructs regarding illness.

It is important to recognise benign causes of high anxiety about health and to understand why the anxiety is there. For example, there are families where several medical opinions may be requested before the parents are finally reassured. There are areas of the world with very high infant mortalities where minor symptoms such as a cough or fever may herald a serious illness or death. If the family have had experiences that sensitize them to illness then this must be understood and subtracted from the frame before judgements about over-investigation or treatment can be made. Clarification of the anxieties and the underlying beliefs is essential but may be especially difficult if an interpreter is necessary. Reading body language cues is unreliable in a cultural context different from one's own. However, the UN Convention on the Rights of the Child is clear that all children have the same rights whatever the culture. It may be important to remind doctors of this if they are struggling to assess a difficult situation and gather evidence of harm or otherwise. To sum up the aspect of cultural differences, all the elements of abnormal illness behaviour (e.g. sympton perception, illness beliefs, consultation patterns and illness behaviour) and 'invalidity' patterns are subjective judgements of deviance from normal values which are culture bound. Both access to and influence upon these beliefs and behaviours are very difficult from the standpoint of another culture.

Confusion of the responsibility

Tensions may exist between the rights, responsibilities and needs of the parents and the child. Social workers with limited training in child protection and adult mental health specialists may feel that the parent is the main client or over-value the notion of 'working in partnership with parents' and forget that the needs of the child are paramount. For example, with drug abusing parents the drug team needs to be fully aware of the child's needs and that this may require that confidentiality issues to a parent are over-ridden. If legal proceedings are not undertaken, the child will not have the benefit of a guardian *ad litem* and solicitor to consider their interests exclusively (see Chapters 11 and 12).

Extra difficulty when the parent has mental health problems: Mental Health Act or Children Act?

When a parent has a psychiatric disorder causing risk of harm to the child, tension and confusion may arise about the appropriate legal action and about responsibility. Curiously this uncertainty may be greater in these cases than in circumstances where parental mental health is apparently intact. This is probably because it seems evident that the mentally ill parent 'doesn't mean to harm the child': she or he is 'mad', not obviously 'bad' as in other MSBP abuse cases. Residual sympathy with the involved parent prevents recognition that the harm is the same as in other cases, as is the need for decisive action. Even if the Mental Health Act (1983) cannot be invoked for the parent, a judgement about the harm and risk to the child must be made in order to decide whether taking child protection procedures is the right path to follow. An example of this difficulty is included in a later vignette (see p. 199), which also illustrates the special difficulties of adolescent patients caught up in factitious illness.

Clinical circumstances where uncertainty arises

There are a number of 'grey areas' in clinical practice which increase uncertainty about current harm, risk of future harm and the way to proceed. These include areas where a confident identification of factitious illness is more elusive, and where a clear management plan may prove difficult to institute. We now discuss some of these areas.

The disabled child

There are specific difficulties in assessing presentations in the presence of disability and chronic organic illness. This is particularly so for children with severe learning difficulties and in the presence of multiple physical problems. In these circumstances it can be hard to differentiate organic illness from functional presentations due to genuine psychological difficulties and, in turn, factitious illness. A community perspective on these difficulties is also outlined in Chapter 7. The following vignette is complex and disturbing because it describes late recognition of obstetric factitious illness and lack of awareness of risk. It is included because delayed and partial recognition of MSBP abuse and uncertainty about future harm are all issues which will present increasingly to clinicians as our medical system becomes more technological and as more parents are drawn in to demonstrate their difficulties in this area. Hopefully, as recognition of MSBP abuse increases, such late presentations will become more unusual.

A baby was severely disabled following a premature delivery caused by the mother simulating repeated factitious ante-partum haemorrhages at twenty-five weeks. The adult psychiatrist's assessment at the time was that the future risks to the baby were small and that child protection procedures were not necessary as it was a desire to end the pregnancy rather than to destroy the baby that lay at the root of the problem. The baby suffered brain damage, hydrocephalus and epilepsy as a result of the pre-term birth. He also had feeding difficulties, gastro-oesophageal reflux and failure to thrive.

It was initially very difficult to separate out the organic physical complaints from the mother's search for ever-increasing medical involvement by exaggeration of symptoms. The baby's situation may also have been made worse by unnecessary administration of anticonvulsants and sedatives. The baby underwent many operations, some of which were clearly necessary, e.g. insertion of a shunt for hydrocephalus. In retrospect, some other operations were only carried out in response to unsubstantiated parental complaints and were probably unnecessary.

Comment

The problems in this case included an over-optimistic initial risk assessment which proved to be inaccurate and which lacked later follow-up and revision. This emphasizes the importance of expert assessment of parents who fabricate illness by those with a knowledge of the range and seriousness of obstetric factitious presentations (which are discussed further in Chapter 5). The mother's ability to communicate convincingly and to rationalize her actions obscured her very serious unresolved problems.

In the legal process the child's disability became a confusing issue. Protection and care are of equal importance within a disabled child's rights. The case was complicated by spurious legal arguments about the actual timing of the child protection procedures in relation to the event causing the harm. The defence argued that because legal procedures were instituted two years after the main event causing damage, that child protection procedures were in contravention of the Children Act (1989). There were arguments that it was the child's prematurity that caused his brain damage, and that the mother had not set out to damage him but to end the discomfort of her pregnancy.

It was also stated that because the child was brain damaged already there was less risk of further damage from maternal over-sedation as there was less brain left to damage. In other words, because there was less capacity for learning it was too late to protect his development and therefore too late to act to prevent significant harm; in essence the defence argued that a risk of a little further damage was insignificant as there was less left to hurt. The issue of the child's life expectancy (which was initially stated as being around two years at the time of his birth) was also raised in the proceedings. There was a view that this diminished life expectancy meant that the higher risks of serious harm could justifiably be taken.

Fortunately the judge disagreed with the counsel for the defence and declared that the main issue in an already damaged child is to protect the child's valuable remaining potential. In other words, a small further restriction of any remaining developmental potential is highly significant in an already disabled child. Therefore, what may be a small risk to a fully functioning child becomes a large risk to a disabled child.

This case is a stark reminder of how dangerous obstetric factitious illness may be for the infant and of its links with subsequent MSBP abuse. It also serves to highlight the danger of different professions having varying understandings about the needs and abilities of children with special needs, especially where the child's level of function is very poor. Clear expression of some of the views above is unusual, but more often there may be subconscious feelings that the harm does not matter because of the child's limited ability to perceive it: clearly a human rights issue. It is our view that these sorts of feelings are unlikely to be articulated but may be present none-the-less, especially in those less experienced in child abuse issues.

Non-consent to medical treatment

There are cases where parental and/or child non-consent to treatment is the issue, raising thoughts of whether to consider child protection procedures with a child protection plan including obtaining appropriate medical treatment. A treatment order may also be considered. This only arises in circumstances where there are significant risks of harm if there is no treatment. These are particularly difficult cases, where the parental misconceptions about the benefits or otherwise of treatment are passed on to the child who also firmly refuses conventional treatment. The particular difficulties here arise where parental/child control of the disease management process has overtaken the doctor's ability to influence compliance with or acceptance of treatment. In some cases one is left feeling that there is a quality about the non-compliance – as if the parent is actively seeking not to help or save the child. Lack of treatment may be causing harm and may feel, at least to the doctor, to reach the threshold of abuse by neglect of treatment. However, doctors will also recognize that, if they feel passionately about the importance of treatment, the strength of their views may cloud their judgement about how perverse the parent is really being. An example is given below.

A teenage boy had severe dermatomyositis. Standard medical treatment was initially apparently accepted but adequate doses of steroids were refused, with subsequent severe deterioration of the child to a virtually untreatable position. The mother controlled the dosing of the teenager and stated the maximum acceptable steroid dose in her opinion. As this was an inadequate dose the effect was insufficient and the steroids were therefore deemed by the family not to have worked. In this case the child seemed to concur with the parents that the treatment was not working and therefore was not worth taking. Dietary manipulation by an extreme alternative practitioner was started and all drugs stopped on his recommendation. Legal advice was sought by the medical team who were advised that there were no grounds for over-riding the lack of consent to conventional medical treatment as this was also the child's wish – he was seen as being 'Gillick competent'. Thus issues about capacity to consent, alternative medicine and risk of harm all became intertwined. The boy is left with severe and irreversible muscle damage which is inconsistent with normal independent life.

Comment

Severe harm to the child has occurred and child protection procedures were not explored. It was the doctor's view that this child needed his parents now that he was so damaged and that to risk this relationship by trying to challenge the boy's acceptance of parental advice would be cruel to a child who had already suffered so much. Child protection procedures here were equated with removal of the child from home and a treatment order was not considered.

Non-consent to psychiatric involvement

This may occur for a number of reasons including a parental need to have the child remain ill. The treatments prescribed may not be given or other management defaulted from. This often includes psychological or psychiatric referral. The reluctance of parents to accept psychiatric referral may be due to the perceived stigma of such a referral, a misapprehension of what the treatment involves, or a fear of the involvement of other family members in the assessment. 'Stigma' here may refer to a shared and unexplored prejudice of doctor and parent. It may also be because the parents fear the truth of the situation will be uncovered. The lack of acceptance of mental health professionals' involvement with children does raise an interesting question in itself about failure to meet the child's needs. It may be that as a medical profession we accept the parent's right to refuse this intervention on their children's behalf too readily in some cases. Recently, however, parents' rights to take this course have been upheld in court (Dyer, 1998). In that case, of a child with chronic fatigue, the parental right to refuse psychiatric treatment based on cognitive behaviour therapy and exercise in favour of what was described as 'the more traditional form of treatment' (under a paediatrician's care), was upheld. This is despite the fact that only anecdotal reports exist of the success of 'traditional' treatment by comparison with published trials of the outcome of treatment with a cognitive behavioural approach (Wessely *et al.*, 1991).

Pitfalls of novel diagnostic labels in children with somatization disorders

Physicians are trained to diagnose, categorize or label illness with precision. This approach often fails to formulate a broader understanding of the dynamics of a situation. The physician may seek to place problems in diagnostic boxes rather than creating a larger formulation of the case with the physical symptoms as one part of a greater whole. It is possible for medical professionals to seek to create new diagnoses or hypotheses of illness rather than to seek to understand why a particular symptom is happening, what its meaning is to the family and what its function is.

When psychosomatic symptoms are present, diagnostic 'physical' labels may proliferate when physical changes occur as secondary phenomena. Thus, for example, when a child displays abnormal illness behaviour for whatever reason and ceases to use a healthy limb, treatment with limb splinting, pain amplification and secondary sympathetic changes may occur and result in temperature and colour changes to the limb and hyperaesthesia. As the secondary and tertiary symptoms are physical, the labels would reflect the desire to obscure the emotional element to the process. So, for example, the records could say 'reflex sympathetic dystrophy', 'neurovascular dystrophy' etc.

Another pitfall is to use a term such as 'pseudo-obstruction', which has a definite surgical application of apparent obstruction in the presence of an ileus. Applying the term inappropriately creates an impression of a clear physical diagnosis when one does not exist.

This 'over-physicalizing' by doctors not only misses the emotional issues of the case but may also sustain and support the patient's adoption of the illness role. When this need to be ill is transferred to a child, the first step in an MSBP abuse process may have started. Taylor (1979) has written extensively on this issue and notes the need for an 'ally' to a child's illness presentation (usually a parent) as well as a 'supporter'(a professional who maintains the 'illness' explanations).

The authors have experience of children presenting with pain amplification syndromes, reflex sympathetic dystrophy, 'ME' or chronic fatigue syndrome, and various presentations and refusal syndromes. The nature of the sick role is highly developed in some of these conditions and the perpetuating factors may include secondary gain for the parent.

Secondary gain may take many forms including having the company of the child at home and having a cause for which to fight. The 'cause' itself is interesting. The fight might include a crusade for a rare diagnosis to be made, or for eccentric treatments to be adopted. There may be an engaging battle with education authorities for home tuition, or battles with the housing department for rehousing or for expensive adaptations to be made. There may be the zealot-like campaigning on behalf of a self-help group (see below). The gain may come from having the child's illness as a problem focus in the family, detracting from the pre-existing family dysfunction. The shift to a physical illness focus may mask physical, emotional and sexual abuse, or other behavioural and emotional problems. When the gain for the family has become a financial one in the provision of various allowances or extra services for the family, there is a real incentive to keep the illness going. It may be necessary to resist the application for any allowances in these cases. The effect on the child may be similar despite the wide variation in the motives of the parents in the above examples.

There may be great extra attention and drama arising from the care of some of these patients, which may perpetuate the persistence as the parent is reluctant to lose this excitement. Thus we know of one patient, a girl who can now walk perfectly well after joint physical and psychiatric treatment of her pain amplification syndrome and (non-organic) inability to walk (a type of somatization disorder in psychiatric diagnostic terms). However, her mother will not let her out of the house unless she is in a wheelchair and is still refusing to send her to school. The girl accepts these limitations passively and is over-compliant in a way that is well described in patients with reflex sympathetic dystrophy. This over compliance is interesting in itself from an aetiological point of view. However, as a characteristic it may be dangerous as it implies that the child may be ill-equipped to withstand the parent's emotional pressure to remain ill.

Over-involvement with self-help groups

Over-involvement with and zealous acceptance of the doctrines of some self-help groups may reach a level which causes concern. Apparently well-intentioned advice may be used to justify quite extreme forms of 'treatment' in circumstances where parents, for a variety of understandable reasons usually, are motivated to pursue this to excessive lengths. The authors have experience of a self-help group where advice was reportedly being given out by a mother who had succeeded in obtaining treatment that was clearly harmful towards her own child (a child with pain amplification syndrome who had received over forty sympathetic guanethidine blocks – all without success: this the authors deem to be 'MSBP abuse'). The mother of this victim was encouraging another patient to demand the same treatment.

Another patient had a chronic bone disease, moderate learning difficulties and hyperkinesis. His behaviour was understandably difficult for his elderly parents to manage, despite successful use of methylphenidate (Ritalin), behavioural interventions and social work support. The parents always hoped fervently for a cure and, in their grief, searched widely. Following a parent support meeting for his bone disease, contact with an allergist was recommended to help with his oppositional behaviour. At substantial expense a course of twice daily injections commenced together with a rigid dietary regime. This only came to the attention of the 'conventional' medical practitioners when the boy attended for regular child psychiatric review. He was in an aroused and agitated state begging to have no more injections and so, in fact, was more oppositional and active than before. His parents were relatively easily dissuaded from the 'treatment', but neither the apparently reputable allergy clinic which had a hospital address nor the parent support organization who had recommended this treatment responded to letters of polite enquiry. This boy has done well subsequently. The persistent searching was judged to be due to parental grief combined with persistent hope that a cure could be found. Together these factors constituted a powerful belief system which, for a period, overwhelmed the parents' ability to weigh up the harm resulting from the injections against the benefits that had been promised but did not occur. This situation was harmful to the child but was recovered.

Common conditions and unusual reactions

Within clinic populations of common conditions will be those children whose parents have a reaction to the problem that is extreme or eccentric. This includes children with mild eczema where the parents have consulted widely with alternative practitioners and then apparently chosen the most extreme diagnosis and treatment to adopt. A further example of this is when behavioural difficulties (or parental management) are labelled in a way which is more acceptable to parents, e.g. 'total allergy syndrome'. Many unproven treatments appear frankly abusive. A report from *Hello* magazine (1990), 'Torment of a boy allergic to living', describes an active four and a half year old who cannot 'even walk down the street without becoming violently ill from chemicals common in everyday life'. The article explains how 'perfume, fumes from a car or mould in a dustbin can cause him to go red in the face, develop appalling headaches and nosebleeds and start running into things…at playgroup, "the colouring in the water makes him itchy and he gets bloated from the play dough (*sic*) and plasticine". Joe has to have three desensitizing injections three times a day'. Taylor (1992), in his paper entitled 'Outlandish factitious illness', which he describes as 'between Meadow's syndrome (MSBP abuse) and hysteria', reports a variety of cases where the parental reaction is unusual and has pointed out the link with parenting difficulties.

'The presenters show great favour to those physicians who seem likely to align themselves with their viewpoint. The physicians can then become over-involved – their reputations are at stake, and they will themselves then resist alternative explanations. This adds to the sense of ordeal, sacrifice and campaign which the parents are waging. The waging of the campaign on behalf of the child can then be a substitute for the ordinary care of the child, which was what was proving so problematic and the circle is closed.'

The 'Yes, but …' game: resistance to recovery

In the book *Games People Play*, Eric Berne (1964) describes interactions between therapist or doctor and patient where a series of possible solutions to a given problem are suggested only to have the repeated response 'Yes, but we have tried that', 'Yes, but that hasn't worked before', 'Yes, but we can't take any more time out of school', 'Yes, but …'.

The helplessness that arises in response to this psychological game should be a clue that the illness is necessary for some reason and that there is an active attempt to sabotage recovery. When persistent invalidism or a search for a physical illness label to justify a sick role is restricted to an adult's own health, then the issue of harm need not arise. However, when a child is involved and is apparently failing to respond to all treatments and where everything that the doctor can possibly think of has already been tried without success, the doctor should take a large step backwards and consider what is going on. This feeling of helplessness should not be ignored and should be the signal to call a halt to the relentless pursuit of a physical diagnosis. If this response is made early it is possible that the doctor may prevent the development of a more harmful case of MSBP abuse. This is the time to lay down a clear management plan centred on limiting investigation and treatment and scrutinizing the demand for medical attention. This is often best done by channelling all future consultations through the doctor who knows the case best (preferably the consultant or GP involved).

We have managed to retrieve a case where a very stressed and unsupported mother was presenting her baby frequently with multiple symptoms and 'bleeding'. The blood was only ever seen on the baby's cheeks in the presence of the mother and thought to be applied menstrual blood. Mother gave 'Yes, but …' responses to most interventions about the symptoms. The management planned at case conference was for one of the authors to be the sole doctor in charge of any subsequent paediatric management. By screening all future presentations and by developing a relationship with the parents the abnormal illness behaviour was contained. The mother rapidly calmed down, the father was encouraged to become more involved, which he did to the point of enjoying his role, and the whole family now functions in a more normal and supportive way. The infant's name has been removed from the child protection register but is still required to continue with a single medical carer. It is important to resist the urge to withdraw from these cases too early, and an outline of the overall management of cases of this kind is given in a later section of this chapter.

Special difficulties in adolescence

It is particularly difficult to deal with all kinds of unusual parental illness behaviour for children, both milder presentations and MSBP abuse, when the child concerned is an adolescent. The young person may be unaware of or trapped in the pattern of behaviour and the beliefs that maintain it; often with a very close, undifferentiated relationship. This has been described from the earliest factitious illness reports (Meadow, 1977) but remains difficult to manage. As insight and a wish for autonomy are likely to occur with development of maturity, it can be difficult to decide how to act in the best interests of the adolescent. Taking formal child protection procedures may distress the adolescent who is enmeshed in the relationship with the parents and probably less well separated than other adolescents of the same age and not yet able to distinguish their own needs and wishes clearly. Such young people may firmly resist an offer to test reality separate from parental views and perceptions.

Some of what is happening here is described by Taylor (1992):

'…the sicknesses created prolonged school absences and long interruptions in the normal process of child development. They involve the children supporting a belief system, a convention, about their health that they also know to be untrue, a circumstance which creates a profound and uneasy bond of silent conspiracy.

Such secret bonds have an echo of the dynamics of sexual abuse about them. They are reminiscent of the preparation of child sacrifices in ancient cultures. The secret rituals can become deeply personally meaningful.'

On the other hand, the adolescent may be trapped and feel very unsafe in the family and be desperate for help but unable to articulate this. It can be difficult, therefore, to obtain clues as to which way to proceed and the adolescent may resist even the gentlest encouragement to help them separate.

This situation blends imperceptibly into the dilemmas of many professional teams faced with a strong parental belief in maintenance of an invalid lifestyle for their child, when the professionals believe active rehabilitation would give a better quality of life. This again has similarities with what is expected in some religious cults. It is difficult to tease out what constitutes abuse in these circumstances but when the parent actively resists the child's recovery there is cause for concern, as in the example below. In such cases, strenuous efforts must be made to establish, if possible, what parental beliefs or fears underpin their views. It is also important to consult widely to attain professional consensus about progress and recommendations, for otherwise the situation may quickly become polarized with parents drawn into an anti-medical or anti-professional lobby, which obscures the real issues for the child.

A twelve year old girl currently under the care of the authors presented with a major pain amplification syndrome (a somatoform pain disorder), being wheelchair bound, unable to walk and also with florid symptoms of anorexia nervosa. With intensive physiotherapy and psychological treatment she made a rapid recovery. She became able to move normally during physiotherapy and yet was persistently confined to her wheelchair by her mother who refused to let her out of her sight or out of her chair when in public. This also extended to a refusal to accept any schooling. The dilemma is that, whilst emotional harm is occurring by exclusion from school and by being treated as a cripple, the emotional harm to the child, who is enmeshed in the abnormal relationship, may be greater should she be made party to lengthy child protection procedures when during therapy she has never given clues that she wants this. The strategy of the psychiatric team involved with her care has been to work on her autonomy and her hopes for the future whilst continuing to give her opportunities to identify any feelings of not being safe at home.

Strong arguments can be made for and against a strategy that involves monitoring progress rather than confronting serious issues directly. In each case this needs to be carefully thought about with the issues of harm and risk being consciously weighed.

Consulting with the adolescent

During the consultation involving an adolescent clues may arise that there is parental over-involvement in the child's illness. Examples include when the parent does not allow the adolescent to speak for themselves and appears to resent the doctor's attempts to engage the adolescent directly. Talking directly to the adolescent, alone if possible, is always helpful in consultations but particularly so in the context of concerns about MSBP abuse. Watching the parental reaction to these attempts is particularly informative as are the adolescent's reactions to the parental history. The adolescent's body language may betray their fear, anger, depression and resignation to the situation in which they are trapped.

In situations of this kind, parental psychopathology merits particular attention (see Chapter 3), for most mentally healthy parents do want the best for their children with somatization disorders. Such parents can often work with professionals if the pace can be adjusted and attention paid to their fears and beliefs in order to engage with them. If parents are mentally unwell, the situation may be easier to understand, though not necessarily to manage.

Desert storm syndrome

An adolescent girl was referred to the rheumatology clinic with vague aches and pains and complete school refusal. It was apparent that her mother had strong beliefs and it transpired that the mother was suffering from an organic psychosis and had delusions of physical illness (which followed amphetamine abuse). The adolescent was involved in a 'folie à deux' and believed her mother's formulation, which was that they had both contracted 'desert storm syndrome'. Both believed they were dying, with dates set for their death; both were spending most of the day in bed awaiting death. The adult mental health services did not consider that the mother constituted a sufficient danger to herself or others to warrant sectioning under the Mental Health Act (1983). She was able to conceal her abnormal beliefs and appear well enough whenever she was assessed. However, the child psychiatrists were very concerned that there was a significant risk of mother or daughter acting on their beliefs and that the girl's life might be endangered as a result. Child protection procedures were undertaken. The child protection procedures were further complicated by the junior social worker assigned to the case, who viewed his role as being to give equal care to the mother and daughter. This lead to his early withdrawal of supervision because mother requested it. This mother therefore managed to evade the very social work monitoring which would have helped to ensure her daughter's safety. The need for a subsequent case conference was only agreed when both child psychiatrist and paediatrician documented in writing their estimates of a severe risk of death to the adolescent if child protection procedures were not taken. Work with this girl involved moving her to foster care, resulting in her receiving normal inputs based on a more objectively tested reality. This enabled the girl to gradually accept that it was her mother who was ill and not herself. This experience of appropriate autonomy and being able to separate her own feelings from those of her mother enabled the daughter to feel safe from illness. Having lost the distorted, enmeshed relationship with her mother, she also lost the belief that she had an illness. She was then able to stand up to her mother safely and was returned home under supervision. She has done well ever since.

Summary: methods of dealing with situations of uncertainty

Thus far in this chapter a variety of difficult situations have been described, some of which constitute MSBP abuse, but in all of which, clinicians were concerned about the child's welfare. The process of taking the issue into another arena outside of the simple doctor–patient relationship, either through a case conference, panel of experts or through the courts, may free up all parties to reset their contracts with each other. For example, the parents may be able to see the situation differently through the view of other medical experts. The child may realize that the parents are not infallible in their decision making and be freed to consent as an individual. The medical carers may be freed from the pressure of negotiation for treatments and enabled to concentrate on the clinical issues of the case. Suggestions are now made about how the clinician may review such situations, to increase clarity about whether or not the situation is harmful at present or potentially so in the future.

Specification of possible types of harm

Moving forward in these sorts of cases depends on a clear awareness of where unnecessary harm is arising and defining the harm itself without being overwhelmed because of misapprehensions about the future care of the child. It is very difficult to judge the nature and severity of any harm to the child that results from different kinds of abnormal parental behaviour, and it can be hard to compare emotional and physical, and short and long term risks. Pearce and Bools in Chapter 11 of this book point out that secondary risks include losing professional control of the situation and, in children with severely handicapping presentations, this may still be a risk even though child protection procedures are not being seriously considered.

Rosenberg (1995) listed twenty-seven different types of harm (see Table 9.1). Weighing these up in the context of clinical management of a complex case is daunting. By virtue of the exhaustive nature of this list, even contemplating it in relation to a particular child clarifies the professional's thinking. This establishes the clinician's view of the extent of this particular child's vulnerability to each form of harm. Such clarity may subsequently be useful for discussing the case with colleagues, to see if they share one's assessment.

Table 9.1 The spectrum of harm*

Fear	Effects of surgery
Pain	Side effects of surgery
Suffering	Complications of surgery
Effects of drugs	Temporary disfigurement: physical effects
Side-effects of drugs	Temporary disfigurement: psychosocial effects
Complications of drugs	Temporary impairment: physical effects
Effects of medical tests	Temporary impairment: psychosocial effects
Side-effects of medical tests	Permanent disfigurement: physical effects
Loss of attachment	Permanent disfigurement: psychosocial effects
Loss of development	Permanent impairment: physical effects
Loss of growth	Other psychological problems
Loss of school time	Death
Loss of normal sibling and peer interaction	

Taken from Rosenberg (1995).
*With the exception of death, not in increasing order of severity.

Sharing concerns with others

Below are some helpful ideas in management when parental behaviour towards a child's illness is judged by a clinician to be incongruent and 'inappropriate'.

1. **Talk to a colleague**. It is invaluable to have an experienced colleague with whom to discuss difficult cases. An independent third party is often able to recognize a gap in the evidence, an important area of history that has not been obtained.

2. **Talk to a specialist**. A specialist in the field (perhaps a specialist in abnormal illness behaviour or MSBP abuse), a paediatric specialist in child abuse, or a paediatric liaison team (especially involving those familiar with this problem and those with substantial experience of adult psychopathology) may be sought out for an open confidential discussion. It is particularly important to cultivate an open relationship with a child psychiatrist, as they have particular skills in history taking and formulation of the dynamics of cases which can be enlightening.

3. **Discuss with a medico-legal expert**. In a difficult case which may involve preparation of reports and presentation of evidence in court, a medico-legal expert with experience in this field may be helpful in giving advice about how to present the arguments about a case.

4. **Involve an 'emotional abuse panel'**. An 'emotional abuse panel' may be helpful for discussion of difficult cases. In Nottingham such an 'emotional abuse panel' has been developed consisting of a consultant paediatrician, a social worker and a teacher. Professionals are able to bring difficult cases to the panel for discussion in order to clarify ideas and to decide possible management strategies prior to initiating child protection procedures.

5. **Involve a hospital ethics committee**. Some hospitals use the forum of the hospital ethics committee to air difficult cases. In the USA, use of a paediatrician (or small team including lay members), with special interest and training in ethics, is growing – a natural and perhaps healthy development in the face of the changes in paediatric medicine outlined in Chapter 2.

During the course of the discussions mentioned above, the clinician may need to undertake a more comprehensive review of what is known about the child and family, either to help in the decision about going to social services, or to be clear about whether one possesses sufficient information *not* to approach them. In effect this constitutes an early risk assessment.

Widening the knowledge base about the context

It is important to reflect on and consciously define what one's instincts are suggesting. If there is an instinctive feeling that there is more to the case than meets the eye, it is unwise to ignore these feelings. It is not possible, however, to build a case on the professional's feelings alone, however strong, and it is necessary to collect evidence. However, it is often the professional's instinct that signals the need to collect the evidence in the first place.

The question of what degree of risk is acceptable to take whilst building up a definitive case may be difficult. It may be necessary to act when one is sure that harm has occurred or is likely to occur in order to protect the child, even if this early intervention does jeopardize the collecting of evidence for a water-tight medico-legal case. In these circumstances the doctor will move quickly towards formal child protection and the process of preliminary assessment below will be abandoned. But in many less acute and very uncertain cases, the gathering of contextual information is of great assistance in clarification. In this case the risk assessment being described is part of Stage 1 and informs Stage 2 as well, rather than the formal risk assessment undertaken once a case has gone into legal proceedings and where the risk for the child of remaining with their family is being evaluated.

We describe a more general risk assessment process being undertaken before any formal proceedings are contemplated. It is a risk assessment nevertheless, as described in Chapters 11 and 13.

General considerations

1. The doctor must remember how significant his or her evidence will be as he weighs up whether to approach Social Services. Social workers, by the nature of their training and experience, will be uncertain about all medical terms, conditions and their implications. In contrast, once the case is fully within the legal arena, the court will be assisted by expert views on these matters. When one is still contemplating entering the child protection system, it behoves the doctor to have achieved great clarity about the facts as he or she sees them. The doctor also needs to be clear about his or her own appraisal of these facts and of his or her own current judgement of the risk of harm that this situation carries.

2. The risks considered are short term ones (physical harm and emotional distress) from factitious illness and from unnecessary medical intervention, and longer term risks, some of which are very serious. The latter include longer term physical and emotional harm from unnecessary medical treatment and experiencing distorted parental care, with emotional abuse being the more common form of abuse. It is important to distinguish the different kinds of risk.

3. No judgement of risk, however preliminary the stage or trivial the level of harm, can be made without high quality information. We have already alluded to the necessity for information to be corroborated with objective reports. It may be helpful to consider what is known of the circumstances under a series of headings (outlined below). It is important to bear in mind the good and poor prognostic factors in Figures 13.1 and 13.2 in Chapter 13.

Areas of information to be considered when weighing risks to a child's development

The child. The child's current state of health and his current functioning, emotionally, socially and academically, in the light of the child's inherent capacity and developmental norms in those areas. For example, for an adolescent, is the child able to pursue age-appropriate relationships with peers and other adults external to the family without undue dependence on parents? Is he or she encountering other sets of values apart from family ones, and tackling appropriate academic and peer group tasks?

To what extent is the developmental progress in these areas one that has been catastrophically interrupted? Has the child been on a similar trajectory over a long period? What intervention has already taken place to help the child attain normal milestones in all these areas despite or in consideration of any physical handicap that they possess?

The views of professionals with knowledge of this child, including teachers, health visitors and other family members including grandparents may be helpful in understanding the current position, and history.

The child's and siblings' histories

What is the history of the child's health, development, ill-health and illness behaviour including the pregnancy? Has the child had any psychological difficulties? Has there been intervention to address these and were the family able to engage with this?

The child within the family

What are the current family circumstances in terms of family relationships, family health, family beliefs? Is there a family pattern of health and illness, of health belief and illness behaviour? What is the current and past history of family relationships with other services, including health and social services, and the pattern of their engagement in relationships with those services? What is the history of development for this child and for other children in the family?

The parents: past and present

What are the parents' life stories in terms of physical health, social, educational and legal matters? What were the characteristics of their early life? Here, especially, it must be remembered that parents with emotionally abusive early lives may have idealized, forgotten, dissociated from or fabricated aspects of their own early experiences and, if possible at some stage, an independant witness to events should be sought. What is the mental state of the parents and what is the history of contact with mental health services?

What is the pattern of the relationship between the parent and between parents and children? In particular, what is the history of the relationship, and attachments, between this child and the parent who promoted illness and illness behaviour? Are trusting relationships formed between family members?

Family functioning

What is observed of current behaviour in the family towards the child and the child's health, and towards that of siblings and their health and illness behaviour? The parameters here include the management of children's behaviour, helping children to attain normal developmental and educational milestones, and appropriately encouraging friendships and moving towards independence. What is known and observed about other aspects of family functioning? Is there a history of abuse? Does the family live in an atmosphere of violence, substance abuse and disruption?

Relationships with professionals

Engagement with professionals from primary care/the community. Does the family have good relationships with their GP, health visitor, school, and school nurse? Contact with social services: have children spent time away from home? How has the family worked with social services?

Use and existence of more specialist professional help: are child mental health services and a specialist child protection team available? Have the family accepted their inputs in the past?

Having gathered information as far as possible from sources that enable the doctor to establish a relatively objective view of circumstances, the doctor must review his or her contemplation of the harm occurring to the child in the context of the new information. In making this judgement, which is essentially about whether to approach child protection agencies for a discussion of the case, the clinician needs to bear in mind first that past behaviour is the best single predictor of future behaviour. It is essential to remember this when considering plausible explanations by parents for aggressive physical assaults such as suffocation and poisoning. There is no evidence to suggest benign outcomes with a cessation of this behaviour (Southall et al., 1997; Bools, Neale and Meadow, 1993). Chapter 13 emphasizes that, even with substantial professional input, the risks involved with parents who have carried out such behaviours are high. Thus any previous harm which has occurred to children in this family must be considered with respect to future risk.

Reappraisal of the literature

The clinician's final step before integrating all he has learned so far, is to appraise the extent to which he or she is knowledgeable about the condition under review. This must include some knowledge of the literature of MSBP abuse, a study of which is difficult because many of the early clinical series contain heterogeneous mixtures of patients including parents who have carried out very basic physical assaults mixed with those who have invented stories. The evidence is not yet available that such heterogeneous groups of parents all have the same outcomes.

Thus, if early abuse including physical assault is seriously under contemplation, the risks of repetition and other adverse outcomes for children are high. This would encourage doctors to act protectively early on, and to discuss such cases with the child protection and police networks. The extensive series of Southall et al. (1997) supports this view.

Of much more relevance in most of the circumstances described in this chapter is the literature about the risk for children remaining in households when illness has been invented rather than induced. Again this is difficult to establish because of the heterogeneous nature of the series of studies reported, but follow-up studies (Bools, Neale and Meadow, 1995; McGuire and Feldman, 1989; again suggest caution particularly in families that are left with no monitoring or support.

The anecdotal literature on intervention (Nicol and Eccles, 1985; Loader and Kelly, 1996; Eminson and Postlethwaite, 1992) suggests that, with the protection of orders from the courts, children and families may be able, in certain circumstances, to be reunited safely. However, it must be emphasized that these are in circumstances where the parents can make an engagement with professionals and where other indicators give grounds for optimism. These include the availability of professional interventions, the ability of the family to acknowledge what has occurred and the presence of other family members who can protect the child. This literature gives little optimism for harmful cases without statutory intervention and would certainly encourage clinicians to move into a child protection environment in these circumstances.

Finally, the literature about the outcome for somatization disorders with parental support of an invalid lifestyle may need to be appraised. The literature on children is patchy and unsystematic and there is no certainty about the extent to which the adult literature about the outcome of, for example, fatiguing conditions, can be applied to this age group. Positive outcomes with active cognitive behavioural therapy and well-paced rehabilitative treatments are available for the adolescent age group and many clinical accounts support this (Nunn *et al.*, 1998). However, in all such studies it is evident that the ability of parents and children to collaborate with professional interventions is often a powerful predictor of a good outcome with an early return to active normal life (Vereker, 1992). Firm, unshakeable belief in a physical cause with antagonism to a psychologically informed and rehabilitative approach makes change difficult. Such a background, together with a belief that the condition involves many years of invalidism, is generally associated with an outcome which follows the self-made predictions.

Integration and formulation

Having appraised a case, filled in gaps in information about the family and the prognosis, appraised the possible risks of harm and talked to colleagues in the ways suggested in the preceding section, the clinician will, we hope, be more certain about how to proceed. He or she has to decide whether to approach social services or whether to continue to manage the situation without even considering moving into a strategy meeting and the procedures described further in Chapters 11 and 12. This decision can, of course, be revisited at any time.

Section A of this chapter deals with the circumstances where the clinician has decided he is definitely suspicious and concerned about harm and plans to approach the local social services department. A series of difficulties is discussed **prior** to a strategy meeting (methods to approach this **after** the strategy phase are discussed in Chapter 11). Section B of the chapter deals with the opposite 'limb' of the dilemma, namely where the clinician has decided that harm has not occurred or is insufficient to involve social services: this is not uncommon. An approach to the long term management of these situations is proposed.

Section A: Taking the case to child protection: possible situations

1. *How to deal with the varying practices, procedures and experience of the social workers dealing with a case of MSBP abuse*

These issues are addressed here from the perspective of the paediatrician. It is important to consider them also from the point of view of the child protection and legal systems, which are described in Chapter 12.

This is an area where a clear label is helpful, as uncertainties in medical diagnosis hamper the ability of the child protection team in making appropriate plans for the child. In the current climate of under-resourcing of social services departments in many districts, it may be that a social worker is only allocated to the case if the doctor is certain that abuse is occurring.

It is our experience that, in cases where the social work response is uncertain or seems inadequate in comparison with the level of medical concern, this may be because of inexperience on the part of the social worker allocated. We have found the following helpful.

- Ask the social worker to attend a professionals' meeting first, where it can be decided whether or not a formal case conference is necessary. If the social worker is insistent that parents are invited or informed, ask to discuss it with their line manager.
- Contact the social worker in writing as well as by telephone. In our experience telephone discussion is not adequate in these complicated cases.
- Ensure the social work representative at any meeting is at an appropriate level of experience. In cases of suspected MSBP abuse, it is appropriate to ask for a senior social worker or manager, just as in a complex medical case, the skill and experience of a consultant rather than a junior doctor is required.
- The term Munchausen syndrome by proxy abuse is familiar to social workers and may be used in order to describe the type of concern the professional has and to enable the social worker to understand the gravity of the situation, thus enabling a more detailed discussion of the issues.
- Once the social workers are familiar with the area of concern, concentrate on the issues of harm rather than the 'diagnosis'. This will hopefully prevent or precipitate responses that can occur in inexperienced social workers who are unfamiliar with the range of presentations and the difficulties of gathering evidence.

2. *What should happen when an opportunity is lost to clinch the diagnosis and legal evidence is missing? For example, in a case where poisoning is suspected but where drug levels were not taken, or were taken too late, or were lost in transit?*

Building up evidence. Sequential recordings of significant events is particularly important in nursing, where there is often reluctance to commit thoughts of concern to paper. These repeated concerns, if recorded, do over time build up into evidence which helps in recognition of factitious illness and will also constitute evidence in any subsequent legal proceedings.

Annotations of conversations. 'Word for word' annotations of conversations with parents can be invaluable later as evidence. If these discussions are not recorded contemporaneously, then they are lost as evidence, as retrospective notes are never as accurate and would be viewed as biased by subsequent events.

Further management

- If the history is very significant, this must be relied on alone and action taken to protect the child even if the legal case is subsequently weaker, for example because of lack of biochemical proof of poisoning. The paramount concern is to protect the child rather than winning a case in court.
- If the lost evidence was clinically certain then the doctors will be able to state their opinion.
- Monitor carefully for a repeat episode to replace the missing piece of evidence.

3. *How to deal with the vast differences in experience and perceptions between different members of staff, which may create tensions and potentially jeopardize appropriate handling of a case of suspected MSBP abuse*

- Hospital staff with many different professional backgrounds and levels of experience will often show an extremely wide range of responses to MSBP abuse. This is especially true if the abuse is the primitive, most taboo-breaking kind: for example, poisoning or suffocation of the child or interfering with the child's food. Reactions include: denial, refusal to consider issues of child abuse in the differential diagnosis, anger with the member of staff who is suspicious and has raised the possibility of induced illness, self doubt, feeling of betrayal, refusal to believe the evidence, loss of trust in all parents and over-identifying MSBP abuse, refusing to lie and being determined to be an 'advocate' for the family to the point of undermining the gathering of evidence. Chapter 14 describes pro-active and reactive systems to prevent and manage such reactions.
- Concern about the legal position: will the staff members be held responsible if further abuse takes place? Open discussion to consider this issue with staff and line managers.
- It is important that clear child protection procedures are in place which deal with lines of action, management and accountability both for medical and nursing staff. It is important to balance the need for an agreed management plan between the professionals involved in an individual case and the need for an individual professional to take responsibility for protecting a child at immediate risk.
- It is important to recognize that the mist of suspicion that can surround a case where there is difficulty in establishing the cause of a child's ill-health can lead to misinterpretation of innocent behaviour. The reverse is also true.

4. *How to achieve evidence that may require misleading the parents*

It is possible to achieve diagnostic evidence without lying to the parents. This issue is one of the reasons why we advocate the need to be clear with the parents that the uncertainty about the diagnosis does require different assessments (e.g. a psychiatric assessment) in order to fully understand what is occurring. It is useful to develop a variety of ways of telling the parents what is happening, much as one learns to use a form of words best suited to breaking bad news, or informing parents why referral to another service is needed. For example, 'I need to understand what is going on with your child in order to explain her symptoms'; 'Your baby's symptoms don't make complete sense from the usual medical diagnoses and we need to admit her/refer her to a special unit where we can watch her carefully to see if we can make sense of this'; 'We know that parents in this situation are often under a lot of stress/confused about how to deal with the child and we therefore have a child psychiatrist who is an expert in helping parents to take time to understand what may have happened to cause the symptoms'.

5. *How should we deal with gut reactions and instincts that something is amiss in the case, where there is no hard evidence to support the case yet but where there are real concerns about the child's safety? What is the best way to proceed when concerns have run ahead of evidence?*

- Refer to the section in Chapter 3 dealing with 'Dawning of private concerns in the mind'.
- Discuss your fears with a trusted colleague.
- Broaden your history taking to include any gaps in areas such as parental backgrounds, parental medical history, pregnancy and delivery history, child's emotional and behavioural history, contact with professionals.
- Make sure all clinical records are as detailed as possible, recording who is giving any piece of history and whether this is corroborated etc.
- Ensure that all nursing records note exactly who is reporting or witnessing each piece of information. Note details of significant telephone conversations, family visits and who was with the child when symptom arose.
- Meet with other family members to retake history from their point of view and note whether they spontaneously raise concerns for the child.
- It is crucial that the GP is involved. The health visitor/community paediatric nurses/school health service may have useful feedback about any other medical incidents and may fulfil a monitoring role. In these cases, it is vital that one doctor, preferably the consultant, is responsible for ongoing assessment and decisions about investigations etc. The GP would need to agree not to refer the patient to other teams but to route all referral decisions through the consultant until the diagnosis is clearly established.
- Remember that non-attendance at appointments can be evidence.

Section B: Management of cases where harm is deemed NOT to have occurred

On many occasions, clinicians find themselves managing cases where the extent of parental pursuit of sickness and health care for their child seems excessive and distorted, with evidence of incongruence. Presentation and persistence occur in the face of a healthy child (as described in Chapter 3) but the harm resulting is uncertain, or fluctuates, or is difficult to measure. Some cases will have been taken to a professionals' or child in need meeting or to a case conference, but registration or proceedings or even social work input has been deemed unnecessary. The clinician is left with the need to manage a difficult clinical situation so that any risk of future harm is monitored and curtailed. Various scenarios of the resulting situations are given below including revisiting each stage in the preceding section, including re-entering the child protection process.

Scenario 1

In a small proportion of cases, the process of invoking the case conference and bringing the child's health and well-being into centre stage is apparently itself sufficient to alter the pattern of parental behaviour. During the process, some formal acknowledgement of the difficulties encountered and the risk of harm to the child is made by the parent(s) and they begin to work with professionals to address issues. Usually this work is with parents in the main.

In a case of which one author (DME) had experience of over several years, the parents ceased to promote their daughters' imagined diseases when they were taken to case conference but were also offered help with parenting skills, so that they had help in managing the girls' (aged seven and five years) oppositional behaviour. A great deal of work was also done with the parents' beliefs and with medical staff who treated other family members and unwittingly increased parental illness beliefs. The complaints about the girls did not disappear entirely and have resurfaced from time to time but they no longer interfere with normal life for the children. Subsequent Children Act (and criminal) proceedings have taken place in this family, not affecting these girls, but because of harsh physical abuse of an older stepson. This we take as evidence that even such apparently treatable families often have a variety of difficulties and areas of poor parental functioning. Long term social work input may also be required.

Scenario 2

Another scenario with which the authors are familiar is the abrupt cessation of the particular type of abnormal illness behaviour which provoked the case conference, but without any acknowledgement that these presentations were invented or exaggerated: they simply disappear. Social work support and monitoring may have been introduced and the school, GP and/or health visitor are attentive to the family at this time. It is often easy for professionals to identify the social or psychological stress that triggered off the bout of abnormal illness behaviour. These cases are frustrating because progress with acknowledgement and other psychological work is simply absent. An example is included in the vignette. These families often present again, to secondary paediatric and mental health teams, perhaps similarly, perhaps differently. In the authors' experience, many of these families are poor, with limited education, much social disruption, numerous unstable partnerships and sometimes criminal involvement: a mixture of a neglectful and abusive background with massive social deprivation and disorganization.

> **Mysterious anticonvulsants**
>
> A single mother had two children aged twelve and eight years. The younger child had learning difficulties and epilepsy for which he was prescribed anticonvulsants. Both children began to cause concern when they became sleepy at school and on several occasions the anticonvulsant levels in the boy's blood were difficult to understand, apparently fluctuating wildly. On one occasion the girl's blood also contained traces of anticonvulsant, but she was said to have experimented with tablets. It seemed highly likely that the mother, who at this time had substantial somatization problems herself, had administered the medication to the children.
>
> A case conference took place and both children's names were placed on the Child Protection Register. There was a great deal of social work, education and primary care support: the mother declined further mental health input and denied administering tablets unnecessarily or inconsistently. All worrying symptoms in the children ceased and six months later the children's names were removed from the Register, though opinions at the case conference were divided. A further six months elapsed with no more evidence of illness induction but the daughter, now thirteen, has presented with a lacerated wrist and traces of amphetamine, dihydrocodeine and another unidentifiable substance in her urine. She denies experimenting and has accused her mother of poisoning her. The mother denies administration of anything except analgesics.

Often years of intermittent social work involvement has not been able to improve or alleviate the family's functioning, except in the short term. These cases probably have many features in common with those described in Chapter 7 dealing with presentations to community paediatricians, and the management outlined there (co-ordination between professionals over years, with repeated meetings of a core group) is appropriate. Deciding whether the situation is harmful or merely worrying is very difficult, as is deciding when to act decisively. Ultimately the decision taken at the Child Protection Case Conference will stand, however strongly the doctor feels that this decision is incorrect and that the 'critical threshold' has been crossed.

Scenario 3

A third pattern is seen in those with repeated, focused presentations of a particular physical complaint, as instanced by many of the cases described in Chapters 3–6 and 8 of secondary and tertiary paediatric hospital out-patients. These more organized and competent families often have a much greater drive behind their pursuit of a particular set of symptoms in a particular child, in comparison with the intermittent, less fixed manifestations described previously. The combination of greater intelligence, organization and drive puts much greater pressure on GPs and paediatricians to act, treat, refer and seek multiple opinions.

Management

- It requires a powerful professional, usually a secondary or specialist paediatrician or child psychiatrist, to insist on a pause and a meeting of professionals. The GP's attendance is essential.
- This meeting reviews the physical findings from an authoritative standpoint and decides if a further specialist opinion is required. The meeting up to this point is only for medical matters and parental presence is unhelpful at this stage. A further opinion, if necessary (which is rare), is undertaken as an opinion to the first specialist not to the GP or family: it is an opinion to inform and produce an agreed plan between professionals.
- The GP is pivotal. He or she must share the understanding of physical findings and a formulation of the pattern of parental behaviour, at least at some level. He or she must be agreeable to maintain an alliance with one paediatrician, with no other referrals without everyone's agreement.
- Systems must be set up to limit the extent to which new opinions can be sought from other partners in the practice, or through attendance at accident and emergency departments. This is a difficult matter for it interferes with the parents' liberty to seek opinions. Therefore the reasons for curtailing this liberty, and possible steps to review or appeal this decision, must be laid down clearly.
- This set of processes, which are there to develop a professional consensus with trust between the parties, must occur before the plan is shared with the family. It is presented to them as a way to manage a difficult clinical situation. If the family are very litigious and bullying, a conjoint presentation of the plan in writing may be better. The core group will probably need to offer support to whichever member comes under greatest pressure.
- If it subsequently transpires that these systems have been subverted and the child treated unnecessarily, it is almost axiomatic that child protection procedures should be introduced (or revisited).
- Very powerful families may subvert such systems and find their way to specialists who appear to have little understanding and respect for their colleagues' views and who take a highly interventionist route with reported symptoms.
- These families, who probably share the quality of unshakeable beliefs with many of those described in Chapter 8 (dealing with presentations in mental health settings), will often have been offered mental health consultation previously, either because of the child's core 'presented' symptoms (e.g. wetting, vomiting, failure to thrive, poorly controlled diabetes, headaches, abdominal pain) or sometimes, when maternal preoccupation is identified, in an effort to assess the abnormal illness behaviour patterns. The families rarely engage with these services and often denigrate them, but the assessment may produce insights for sharing with the other professionals. It may enable the mental health professional to give more specific advice and understanding to the core

group than is possible from note perusal and MSBP abuse expertise alone. The help of a child psychiatrist may be valuable to professionals even when the family decline to meet him or her.

• Sometimes the family can be engaged with mental health professionals.

Psychiatric treatment

Psychiatric management of these cases, which have not entered proceedings of any kind and are managed usually as out-patients or day patients, involves a more limited version of the processes outlined in Chapters 8 and 13 (to which the reader is directed). Loader and Kelly (1996) also describe similar work with a family as out-patients.

The painstaking gathering of the family history (and explanation of areas covered in the risk assessment section of this chapter) is usually the key to engagement of the disturbed parent. It should be therapeutic, in the broadest sense, in its own right. The sense of warm interest in the parent and lack of any judgmental quality is the cornerstone of psychiatric enquiry, and it proceeds through an understanding of the parent's past to exploration of the current family system and the interactions triggering factitious illness now.

Although the particular therapeutic techniques used will probably be those that represent the strengths of the particular mental health team, the underlying processes are likely to be common between mental health teams who work with abusive families. They will centre upon work with the parent, to enable her to examine her early life and make connections with her present thoughts, feelings and behaviour; upon rebuilding a relationship with the child; upon the child's needs (often through some direct work); and on 'systemic processes' in the family, including the role and position of any other parent or partner, the 'marital' relationship and family relationships as a whole. This is demanding work both psychologically and in terms of time, and requires the skills of a substantial multi-disciplinary child mental health team if it is to be engaged upon with enthusiasm by the family. Unfortunately, such engagement is the exception rather than the rule, and families with these difficulties often continue to avoid tackling their root problems.

References

Berg, B. and Jones, D.P.H. (1999) Outcome of psychiatric intervention in facti-
    tious illness by proxy. *Archives of Disease in Childhood* (in press).
Berne, E. (1964) *Games People Play*. Penguin.
Bools, C.N., Neale, B.A. and Meadow, S.R. (1992) Co-morbidity associated with
    fabricated illness (Munchausen syndrome by proxy). *Archives of Disease in
    Childhood*, **67**, 77–79.
Bools, C.N., Neale, B.A. and Meadow, S.R. (1993) Follow-up victims of fabri-
    cated illness (Munchausen syndrome by proxy). *Archives of Disease in
    Childhood*, **69**, 625–630.
Department of Health (1983) Mental Health Act (1983) HMSO, London.
Department of Health (1989) An Introduction to the Children Act 1989. HMSO.

Dyer, C. (1998) Parents can choose child's treatment. *British Medical Journal*, **317**, 1102.

Eminson, D.M. and Postlethwaite, R.J. (1992) Factitious illness: recognition and management. *Archives of Disease in Childhood*, **67**, 1510–1516.

Gray, J., Bentovim, A. and Milla, P. (1995) The treatment of children and their families where induced illness has been identified. In *Trust Betrayed? Munchausen Syndrome by Proxy, Interagency Child Protection and Partnership with Families* (Horwath, J. and Lawson, B., eds), pp. 24–46. National Children's Bureau.

Hello Magazine (1990) Torment of a boy allergic to living. Issue No. 113, 28th July.

Jones, D. and McGraw, J.M. (1987) Reliable and fictitious accounts of sexual abuse to children. *Journal of Interpersonal Violence*, **2**, 27–45.

Loader, P. and Kelly, C. (1996) Munchausen syndrome by proxy: a narrative approach to explanation. *Clinical Child Psychology and Psychiatry*, **75**, 57–61.

McGuire, T.L. and Feldman, K.W. (1989) Psychologic morbidity of children subjected to Munchausen syndrome by proxy. *Pediatrics*, **83**, 289–292.

Meadow, R. (1977) Munchausen syndrome by proxy: the hinterland of child abuse. *Lancet*, **ii**, 343–348.

Meadow, R. (1993) False allegations of abuse and Munchausen syndrome by proxy. *Archives of Disease in Childhood*, **68**, 444–447.

Moore, S.G. *et al.* (1998) Managing pervasive refusal syndrome: strategies of hope. *Clinical Child Psychology and Psychiatry*, **3**, 229–250.

Nicol, A.R. and Eccles, M. (1985) Psychotherapy for Munchausen syndrome by proxy. *Archives of Disease in Childhood*, **60**, 344–348.

Nunn, K.P., Thomson, S.L. *et al.* (1998) *Child Clinical Psychology and Psychiatry*.

Rogers, M.L. (1992) Delusional disorder and the evolution of mistaken sexual allegations in child custody cases. *Journal of Forensic Pathology*, **10**, 47–69.

Rosenberg, D. (1995) from lying to homicide. The spectrum of Munchausen syndrome by proxy. In *Munchausen Syndrome by Proxy. Issues in diagnosis and treatment.* (Levin, A.V. and Sheridan, M.S., eds). Lexington Books.

Schreier, H.A. (1992) The perversion of mothering: Munchausen syndrome by proxy. *Bulletin of the Menninger Clinic*, **56**, 421–437.

Southall, D.P., Plunkett, C.B., Banks, M.W. *et al.* (1997) Covert video recordings of life threatening child abuse: lessons for child protection. *Pediatrics*, **100**, 735–760.

Taylor, D.C. (1979) The components of sickness, diseases, illnesses and predicaments. *Lancet*, **ii**, 1008–1010.

Taylor, D. C. (1992) Outlandish factitious illness. *Recent Advances in Paediatrics*, **10**, 63–76.

Vereker, M.I. (1992) Chronic fatigue syndrome: a joint paediatric–psychiatric approach. *Archives of Disease in Childhood*, **67**, 550–555.

Wessely, S., Butler, S., Chalder, T. and David, A. (1991) The cognitive behavioural management of the post-viral fatigue syndrome. In *Post-Viral Fatigue Syndrome* (Jenkins, R. and Mowbray, J., eds). John Wiley and Sons.

10

Parental and adult professional gain from exceptional children: achievement by proxy*

Ian Tofler

Introduction

Whilst it is acknowledged that children of all strata of society are potentially at risk of neglect, abuse and factitious disorder by proxy (King, Noshpitz and Joseph, 1987; Newberger *et al.*, 1986), the most easily recognized presentations have been those of children from lower socio-economic groups with very damaged parents. However, recently, talented, high achieving and highly pressured children have been recognized and focused upon as a subpopulation potentially at significant risk for multiple forms of abuse and neglect (Cantelon, 1981; Donnelly, 1993; Ogilvie *et al.*, 1998). The new field of 'sport psychiatry' can offer a novel perspective on some of these issues (Stryer, Tofler and Lapchick, 1998; Tofler, Knapp and Drell, 1998).

The world's newspaper headlines seem to underscore an emerging societal awareness of the potential for abuse in high achieving children. What, actually, is

---

*The Editors have welcomed this contribution from an American perspective, for the light which it sheds upon an area of children's lives with potential both for enriching their development and also for abuse. Whilst the heavy promotion of sporting excellence is not yet so prevalent in the UK as in the USA, and the field of sport psychiatry has not yet arrived here, Tofler reminds us that all areas where parents promote the development of gifted children also provide the potential for parents' needs to be met as well. This situation in no way meets the criteria for inclusion in this book as a form of factitious illness involving the triad of parent, child and health care professional. It serves, however, to remind us that there are many other indirect ways of meeting parental needs that may risk the sacrifice of children's well-being – of which this is an example.

One of this book's aims is to alert health professionals to situations in which there are risks to children and where the professional may have a role in awareness and prevention of harm. This chapter is included not only for general interest but also because many health professionals may be involved, however tangentially, in these arenas.

it that is required to produce a six year old beauty queen, a seven year old pilot, a fourteen year old Olympic gold medal gymnast, a fifteen year old champion ice hockey player, a sixteen year old Rachmaninoff virtuoso, a twelve year old movie actor, or a seven year old golfing prodigy?

While these children and their parents may draw our collective admiration and wonder, and perhaps jealousy, they also elicit realistic concern about how their precocious talents were fostered. Were corners cut, or risks taken in the development of those skills? Could this have endangered that child in both a subtle and a serious fashion?

Initially, it may prove helpful to understand the individual, systemic and societal levels of behavioural distortions and abuses to which talented children are at risk. These behavioural patterns may be integral to the process of developing talented children. One can enhance comprehension of this field in terms of a general historical view of childhood, and the historical development of psychiatric and behavioural paediatric approaches to the problems of talented children in the sporting arena. A third goal is to understand how the interactive process between the normal and gifted child and his or her ambitious parents and mentors enables the children to reach the heights of success at an early age.

Finally, possible responses and management recommendations are considered which may prove helpful to paediatricians, nurses, physiotherapists, child psychiatrists and others interested in the child's welfare. These may prove useful to address the concerns about 'achievement by proxy' distortions in highly pressured, high achieving children, adolescents and young adults.

Some background factors

The developmental tasks of champions

Neither normal nor talented and gifted children develop in a vacuum. Like all children, their development is a highly interactive process between the child and the adult and adult systems within which they exist. On the one side there are trainable, genetically able, talented and resilient children, with the 'right stuff' of suitable temperament, right gender for the task, developmental suitability, malleability and obedience. An optimal interaction with experienced, ambitious, sufficiently adept, inspirational and charismatic adults and the systems within which they operate, may be geared towards focused training which develops that certain skill in the child to a sufficiently high level to achieve success. The child and adult mentors combine their talents in a relationship which, in association with opportunity, luck and other intangibles, culminates in that crucial moment when the potential is brought to fruition, the ability developed to a point where the talent is now a career worthy, marketable commodity. The relationships that occur in one particular field, the sport of elite women's gymnastics, provide a good illustration of how multiple individuals and systems may interact in the process of producing a champion. These are illustrated in Table 10.1.

Table 10.1 Achievement by proxy cascade for women's gymnastics

---

1. **The general public and media**

   Live and television audiences tend to view gymnastics and other elite sports, such as skating, largely as entertainment, leading the advertising industry to produce role models and advertising icons. The public shares responsibility for the exploitation of these children and adolescents through its support of such sports without demanding changes. All advertisers, sponsors and media involved in and benefiting from these sports should be obliged to contribute financially to the improvement of safety and medical and psychological health of these athletes.

2. **International Olympic Committee (IOC)**

   The IOC fosters the entertainment value of these sports for financial gain with minimal regard to any abuse potential or physical, medical or psychological dangers. Despite an awareness of these risks, as evidenced by increasing the minimum age of competition to 16 for the 2000 Olympics, they appear to be maintaining a position of 'plausible deniability'.

3. **International and national judging requirements**

   The 'International look' favoured by judges, that is the mesomorphic, prepubescent appearance, potentiates abusive training practices both explicitly and implicitly, by perpetuating its biases against competitors that don't meet this superficial standard. These guidelines need to be explicitly stated or revamped to regain credibility for this sport and to minimize its exploitative quality.

4. **National governments**

   National governments are large sponsors of gymnastics and other elite programmes. Tacit tolerance of abusive practices for national prestige reasons suggests that limits must be made at the IOC level with international enforcement of standards.

5. **International movements**

   Pro-active efforts to address some of the potentially harmful and abusive aspects of sport have been made in the USA and Australia. The USA gymnastics task force examining the Female Athlete Triad and the enquiry into abuse in gymnastics demonstrate some concern in this area. Nevertheless, gymnasts remain their 'product' and are thereby inevitably exploited as such. There needs to be more external objective supervision and greater funding for safety concerns.

6. **Medical supervision**

   This remains inadequate with insufficient controls to prevent injured child athletes from competing and risking serious permanent injury. There is insufficient medical, dietary, psychological and sexual education for these children and adolescents. Physicians and other medical professionals in the direct employ of sporting bodies are at risk of being ineffectual 'fans', over-awed and overruled by star coaches and athletes. They generally do not have ultimate say on whether athletes compete and may be co-opted into the system.

7. **Coaches**

   Coaches frequently have autocratic control not only over athletes but also over parents and national gymnastic movements because they 'get results'. Dubious techniques with potentially severe long term physical and psychological implications may be ignored if they produce short term benefits and champions. Coaches (both men and women) are at risk with respect to boundary violations and sexual involvement with athletes. The romantic attachment involved in the coach–athlete relationship (akin to any mentor relationship) is often abused with significant consequences.

8. **Parents**

   Parents may turn a blind eye to coaching abuses, and be able to rationalize or are oblivious to their own neglect and achievement by proxy abusive behaviours because of the potential long term benefits. They may live vicariously through their child, conscious of their own very real sacrifices in producing a champion.

9. **The athlete**

   The child involved may begin training at an extremely early age and frequently knows no other life, and accepts critical coaching and parenting as normal and acceptable. Children and adolescents with underdeveloped assertiveness skills, who are trusting of adults, may injure themselves deliberately to avoid competition. They may share and introject the goals of parents, coaches, gymnastics and Olympic movements, judges and media. These athletes lead extremely unbalanced lives with often inadequate social developmental skills, which become more noticeable and debilitating at the age of retirement in their late teenage years or twenties.

10. **Amateur level gymnastics**

    Elite athletes and coaches function as role models for amateur level peers who aspire to have the same levels of 'self-discipline' and control. Examples include amateur gymnasts also developing eating disorders and amateur coaches also using verbal abuse and destructive criticism as a technique to achieve the most from their athletes.

Taken from Tofler and Stryer Katz (1996).

Analogies between MSBP abuse and extreme forms of 'achievement by proxy'

The field of factitious illness by proxy and MSBP abuse allows us an opportunity to study the intrafamilial and societal processes and motivations whereby adults may submit children to potentially dangerous and even abusive situations. Children and adolescents are placed in these situations ostensibly for the purposes of 'a higher goal' such as in Olympic sports, entertainment or the arts, with little or no consideration for the potential consequences to that child: in effect, to achieve parental needs. This, it is suggested, is 'achievement by proxy'.

Recognition of this is not new. Most recently, Meadow included 'Victa

Ludorum by proxy' in his discussions on variations of Munchausen's syndrome by proxy (Meadow, 1995). This suggested a concern that ambitious parents could potentially damage their children by driving them towards apparently laudable goals.

Historical view

Complex human behaviours can be depicted as phenotypically similar to other traits, as proposed by the relatively new fields of evolutionary psychology, genetics and anthropology, which evaluate behaviour within the context of two million years of hominid existence. From this vantage point then, what may initially appear to be a pattern of cruel and exploitive behaviour, may actually conceal an evolutionary, adaptive form of 'chromosomal empathy' for future offspring. Perhaps it is our much more recently derived moral and ethical imperatives that are at odds with our biological, psychological and behavioural evolutionary historical base, and not the other way around?

United Nations enactments on child labour laws of 1973 remain essentially unenforceable in most countries. Overall then, despite dramatic increases in freedom, particularly in Western countries, the child has remained an instrument for the implementation of the parent's agenda, within an accepting social context. Inculcating the parental religious, educational, nationalistic, cultural or sporting imperatives continues to be an inalienable right. Similarly, a child provides a second chance to achieve lifelong parental goals and unfulfilled dreams. And what is wrong with this? It is clear that implementing parental agendas and goals leaves the door open for exploitation and abuse at many levels and of many degrees. That these abuses may occur, often in the name of love, support or altruistic parenthood, is ironic. When is a 'good enough child', to invert a Winnicott concept about parenting (Winnicott, 1958), simply not good enough for hard-driven parents?

Prior work in this field

Psychiatrists since Freud have long been aware of the risks of projection of adult goals on to young children. (Freud, 1957; Giovacchini, 1989; Gutheil and Gabbard, 1998). In their classic paper, Solnit and Stark reviewed the disappointment, indeed grief, experienced by the parent when his or her child is born defective (Solnit and Stark, 1961). The corollary to this thesis is that, in fact, all of us are born defective to some extent and, depending on their expectations, run the risk of disappointing our parents. At the time of our birth we may apparently be invested with unlimited potential, but our limitations and weaknesses, as well as our potential, are never more obvious than at that moment.

The Swiss therapist Alice Miller, drawing from many sources, further developed an understanding of this important dilemma in child rearing, which she described as 'the drama of the gifted child' (Miller, 1979; Miller, 1981). The most appropriate objects for (narcissistic) gratification are a parent's own children. 'The intuitive understanding a child has for his parents, and what he can do to

please them' is central to these ideas. She states '...in spite of excellent performance, the (specially gifted) child's own true self cannot develop' (Miller, 1979).
The conditional love that objectified, highly successful children can experience
often comes at a high price, the very authenticity of that individual.

Behaviour relating to children's achievement

Normal supportive behaviour and three levels of distorted behaviour are now
described, along with some insights into why such patterns emerge.

Normal range of 'achievement by proxy' behaviour: support-
ive behaviour

This refers to the adult pride and satisfaction experienced in supporting a child's
development while also nurturing that child's abilities, special talents and per-
formances. Although the parents and family may benefit financially and socially
from their child's success, this is not the primary goal of the adult. These collateral benefits are rather a pleasant side-effect of a more general altruistic behaviour. The child or adolescent's individuality is acknowledged, and the involved
adults have the ability to distinguish the child's needs and goals from their own.
Examples of adults taking normal pride in a performance include parents sharing
the triumph of a child scoring a goal in a youth soccer game despite the team's
loss, with which they are able to empathize on both an individual and team level.
Sometimes a parent may need to insist that a child decreases or even quits an
activity cherished by both, if the overall impact is deleterious to that child's
developmental progress. A well-rounded parent should be able to monitor their
own reactions, and know how to differentiate their own from their child's goals.
A child must never feel that the love of their parents is contingent on success in
one field of endeavour, be it an educational, sporting, career or social goal.

Similarly, a community experiencing tremendous normal pride in their representation is shown in the film and book *Hoop Dreams* (Joravsky, 1995), in which
the Chicago inner city project of Cabrini Green is represented by two teenage
basketball players pursuing the National Basketball Association 'dream'.

This normal range also includes an element of 'normal sacrifice'. Parents are
able to, desire to, and indeed are expected to make reasonable sacrifices, within
the cultural context of their lives. These sacrifices demand, in return, reciprocal
responsible behaviour and striving from children. There should not be any
excuse, however, for placing inappropriate and unacceptable pressures on young-
sters to achieve success in any area endangering their physical or mental health.

Distortion of 'achievement by proxy'

When parents' goals take precedence over children's, then normal pride in a
child's achievement, or 'achievement by proxy', may be distorted.

Achievement by proxy can be defined as follows: a child is placed, with his or her collusion, volitional or otherwise, in a potentially exploitative situation in order for a perpetrating adult or adult system to gratify *their own* conscious and unconscious needs and ambitions for the attainment of certain goals or achievements. Achievement by proxy constitutes child abuse when unacceptable physical or psychological harm is inflicted.

Children may be *intentionally* placed in situations where they must focus on a single activity to the exclusion of all others. In such cases, all other activities may be subordinated towards the achievement of certain goals, e.g. attaining Olympic, sporting, entertainment, music or educational success, often at the risk of physical and psychological well-being.

This vicarious experience of achieved success contains a conscious external motivation of obtaining collateral benefits, which may be manifold and may run parallel to the child's clear benefits. These include fame, financial gain, career advancement, peer recognition and respect, relationship with the child, social acceptance and improved socio-economic status. The vicarious success may be experienced on an individual, system, company, local or national level. Vicarious achievement of success also hints at an underlying transferential dynamic motivation for achievement by proxy distortions. Emotional and potentially economic 'nurturing' of the adult by the child may also result. While this is more prominent in 'achievement by proxy', role reversed nurturing is also possible in MSBP abuse.

Four stages of 'achievement by proxy' were mentioned – the first within the normal range of behaviour as described above (supportive behaviour) and three in a potentially pathogenic range. There may, of course, be overlap between normal achievement by proxy behaviour and all the achievement by proxy components. The general trend, however, is from benign to potentially abusive.

Risky sacrifice

This involves a mild loss of an adult's ability to differentiate between their own needs for success and achievement and a child's developmental needs and goals.

At this level of behaviour, a family or a system may construct conditions for a child or adolescent whereby there is increasing pressure, of a subtle but easily comprehended nature, that they must 'perform'. A parent may take a second or even a third job to support a child's career, families may move closer to a gym or training facility, or may allow a thirteen year old to make the decision to travel to a different state to live at a training facility or even be adopted into the custody of a coach. Plausibly deniable rationalizations, which may be emotionally compelling, become major conscious and unconscious defensive strategies at this stage. Parents may appear helpless and even passive with comments such as: 'I want my child to train less but she loves it. If she insists on training eight hours a day, six days a week, how can I say no? I love my child'. Children and adolescents collude with their parents' and coaches' goals with comments of encouraged pseudo-autonomy such as, 'It is *my* decision to play injured, no one forces me to'. When the child gets injured, neither the parent nor the coach need feel responsible. An adult's, and particularly a parent's, role to protect the safety of their child may be abrogated. The level of sacrifice demanded from a child surpasses defensible 'safe' levels.

Reaffirming normal parental decision-making autonomy (for example, when parents insist that a child misses practice to complete a school assignment) may produce unpleasant situations where an awe-inspiring, charismatic coach threatens to remove the child from his roster, with comments such as 'there are others who are more serious and may be more worthy'. The sacrifice is now not only expected, it is demanded. To resist this external and internal pressure requires not only insight but also painful parental courage.

Objectification

This refers to the moderate loss of the ability of the adult to differentiate their own needs and goals for success and achievement from that of the child: the child is treated as an object, a means to the adult's ends, rather than as a unique individual. At this stage, the intensity of the pressure on the child is further increased. With increasing social isolation, a child or adolescent becomes increasingly defined by one activity in which they are able to perform well – the so-called 'uni-dimensional identity' (Gould, 1993). This focus causes increased social isolation and potentially compromises multiple developmental possibilities (while opening others) within the social, physical and emotional spheres. With this objectification, comes the loss of ability of adult caretakers to distinguish their own needs and goals from that of the child (Eminson and Postlethwaite, 1992). This leads to rationalizing of routine risk taking. This has parallels in more familiar child protection arenas, such as states of abusive neglect, for example when a mother severely burns her child to teach them that they should not play with matches. A child may be encouraged or even forced to train at levels that are potentially endangering to health. She may be advised to use pathogenic forms of weight control, which may lead to life-endangering eating disorders. Parents, coaches, and sometimes entire systems, the media and governments turn a blind eye to, or actively as well as passively encourage and support pathogenic behaviours.

Clearly, to involved adults, 'the end justifies the means'. The objectified child becomes the means to achieve those ends. Once objectified, it is much more difficult for the parent to empathize with that adolescent's pain or experience. This is a point that may be driven home to, and easily accepted by, emerging young, talented and malleable entertainers, actors, musicians and sports stars, who may emotionally distance themselves from their own feelings and collude in this objectification of themselves. This is a process not dissimilar to Anna Freud's concept of 'identifying with the aggressor'. A good example is the gymnast who assumes full responsibility at age fourteen years for training with a broken wrist, with the full knowledge of coach and parents. The child prodigy's body and mind become, even to themselves, vessels to be driven and exploited in the pursuit of a 'worthy' goal. 'She can leave at any time' is a frequently heard statement, not only from parents and coaches, but from cult leaders!

Potential abuse

This scenario involves a severe or complete loss of the ability of adults to differentiate their own needs and goals for success and achievement from those of the involved child. At this level, the child is at risk of simply becoming an objectified and exploited instrument of the involved adult's goals. These goals are pursued without regard for short and long term potential physical and emotional morbidity or mortality. An adult, be it parent, mentor, coach, sponsor or system, may often appear to be perfectly attuned with the child ('she is my best friend') – but all the features of sacrifice and objectification are present. A child may become, in essence, an adult's meal ticket. If badly injured in practice, it is because 'she is a dare-devil' (conditioned from age four years to ignore pain and to take risks). If permanently injured representing her country, team doctors may have colluded with her competing with catastrophic injuries. Here, the national team system is an important component of a potentially abusive process. The media and ourselves as spectators and consumers are also part of this cascade.

Management: recommendations and interventions

Recognition and general societal awareness of these very real potential risks to children and adolescents is a critical first step in the management of 'achievement by proxy' distortion issues.

'Psycho-education' of parents, mentors and coaches is designed to harness their responsible 'observing egos' to frequently re-evaluate their own and other interested adults' goals, motives and agendas in encouraging the professional development of a child.

It is important to recognize the 'red flags' of achievement by proxy when we or others are being over-directive and too goal oriented with our children. Examples of these include:

1. Parents making life decisions based on a child's activity. For example, selling up and moving to another city, getting a second or third job so that their child can work full time as a gymnast, quitting regular school.
2. Parents may allow the coach to make ALL decisions in their child's life, they may even suggest that the coach take custody of the child, so that the child can 'live and breathe the sport'.
3. The parents, the thirteen year old competitor, the coach, the orthopaedic surgeon and the team manager are all aware of an injury, but all agree that the decision to compete with a broken wrist is the child's to make.

'Self-help tips' can be provided to parents, educators and coaches, enabling them to fulfil their obligations to children, and to both recognize and respect their individuality and separation from the involved adult. This can be accomplished without denying outstanding children and adolescents the opportunity to succeed at any level. Some examples include:

1. Balancing career goals with developmental goals and requirements. An adolescent may spend the summer on vacation with friends and family. As a result this may entail missing acting classes. This may be against both the child's

wishes and the acting coach's *orders*. Being able to *be a parent*, and to some-times resist pressures from the child as well as internal ambitions and external professional pressures, is a vital skill. This involves the ability to say 'no'.
2. Learning how to examine objectively one's own motivations for encouraging or pushing a child to develop a skill or a talent. This involves asking questions such as: 'Am I doing this for my child or myself'? If I am doing this a little for myself, where does the child fit into this equation?'.
3. Knowing when to consult a family therapist, counsellor or other mental health professional. When the risks and benefits of a child's involvement in an activity are great, it can be very helpful to obtain a more objective view of the child and other family members, including siblings. For example, when a parent feels themselves trusting a charismatic coach over their own instincts, it is essential to seek a second opinion.
4. Learning how to recognize 'risky rationalizations' such as 'plausible deniabil-ity' and 'pseudo-autonomy'. When care givers rationalize dangers to our chil-dren in the same manner in which a government spokesman responds to a war situation, we need to be aware of it and respond appropriately.

A bio-psycho-social model which is flexible developmentally and systemically, and culturally informed, enables therapists to help the involved adults ascertain the progress of a certain child within an acceptable framework. Ethical dilem-mas raised by that child's involvement in professional activities such as acting or sports training can be addressed, and the potential risks of regression in key developmental areas, social isolation from peers, or other physical and psycho-logical morbidity can be fairly gauged. Does the trauma or illness induced in the service of this hitherto worthy professional goal justify that child's contin-ued involvement? Emerging research may markedly alter our understanding of the risks versus benefits of certain activities. Monitoring any possible changes in goals, motivations or agendas of the many participants in the system sus-taining the child's career may alert us to immediate reasons for freezing, dimin-ishing or even discontinuing the child's involvement in that professional activity.

Any therapist for the child or family or 'outside' consultant to the system must establish boundaries clarifying his or her primary role. This should prevent any countertransferential motivations impairing one's sense of fully protecting the child from abuse or unnecessary risk taking which could lead to potential abuse.

Anticipation is perhaps the best method for avoiding, or at least minimizing, the damage of directly confronting the dangerous collusional rationalizations of parents, governing bodies and children. All parts of the system need to be aware that, much like the suicidal adolescent, confidentiality ceases when the child is at significant risk. Any abuse must be reported to local authorities.

The risks of systemic collusion through non-communication of important information are obviously greatest where the potential benefits increase expo-nentially such as at the time of the Olympic games. Examples could include a national gymnastics organization encouraging, hiding or turning a blind eye to chronic injuries, eating disorders or analgesic abuse, or sexual or physical abuse of minors. National pride and patriotism are invoked and seem to justify any expediency. Similarly, representing one's country, as a minor, seems to confer a form of honorary adult status on that individual, at least in terms of the refusal of supervising adults to take ultimate responsibility. Do we need to wait for a child's death during Olympic competition before we respond to this crisis? Because of the abuse potential, rigorous history taking must be conducted from the child and other collateral sources. As in all psychiatric evaluations, this must be accompanied by a focused mental status examination and special investigations, which can include physical and psychological testing, blood work, cardiac work-ups and other physiological and radiological investigations, as required. Toxic screens for substances of abuse and performance enhancing drugs may be necessary. Forensic assessments may sometimes be required, as may mandated reporting in situations when abuse is suspected.

Standardized achievement by proxy interviews for the child, parent, coach or mentor, and risk/benefit scales currently being developed (Tofler and Butterbaugh, 1998) should contribute further to our understanding of these conditions.

The role of the child psychiatrist as a physician advocating the safety of children at all levels of endeavour in society, demands that high achieving children and adolescents not be excluded from this area of concern.

Because of the enormous risks for exploitation, there is a growing need for legal protection of the rights of professional children, including the development of enforceable laws to limit hours of work and training, and the removal of loopholes that suggest that these working professionals are 'simply enjoying themselves and having fun'. Changes in the rules concerning Olympic routines are needed, to eliminate dangerous routines and to minimize the unrealistic and health-risking aesthetic demands of judging. Age limitations are required which favour, or at the very least do not sabotage, adult participation.

Case examples with suggested clinical strategies (Ogilvie et al., 1998)

GD, a fourteen year old Asian American female is badly injured in a vaulting routine, sustaining spinal cord injuries at the C6–7 levels. Father, AD, is a forty year old professional soldier and has been instrumental in her involvement in gymnastics despite no training himself. He was her first coach. It was his ambition initially that she become an Olympic gymnast.

Mother, MD, a thirty-nine year old executive, is only minimally involved in her daughter's gymnastics and seems to be somewhat marginalized during GD's recovery. DC, GD's thirty-five year old coach has been working with GD almost daily for the last six years and is her major role model, confidante, 'big sister', even mother, travelling with her to all competitions. DC believed that GD would reach the elite level and possibly Olympic standard. She attends all therapy sessions during the hospitalization, giving advice to staff members.

Some quotes from those involved are given below.

Fourteen year old: 'I don't feel sorry for me, and I don't expect others to be either, I don't feel sorry for them (coach and family).'

Father: 'Of course I was in shock at the beginning, but you've got to adapt … I guess I was ready for something like this, having my mother in a wheelchair most of her life … you've got to adapt and adapt quickly. I am certain my daughter will improve and I won't be surprised if she returns to gymnastics at a competitive level; if not she will be a success at whatever she puts her mind to.'

Coach: 'As soon as it happened I felt, and I know this sounds selfish, that this was the end of my chance to coach a champion. I was upset about the loss of her and my own future. It doesn't matter any more … all I care about now is will she be able to walk again, will she have a functional life? Everyone wants me back coaching, but I'm not ready yet; none of the other children have quit…'

Tim has been training with a tennis pro since the age of fourteen years. He had demonstrated unusually precocious talent for his age. He was regularly able to defeat high quality opposition two to three years his senior. Physically mature for his age, Tim experienced no disadvantage in this area. While Tim's family were of modest means and private lessons were a burden, his tennis pro was able to offer a 'solution'. Convinced that Tim was a future champion, he offered to continue lessons with the fifteen year old at no charge to the family, but with the stipulation that he have full control over Tim's career. The family, including Tim, felt they could not refuse this Faustian bargain.

For Tim (and, to a less profound degree, for his family) there gradually evolved an increasing sense of loss of personal freedom and control. First, there was a dramatic shift in priorities, with the teaching pro becoming almost dictatorial. These priorities were felt as extremely intrusive, especially by Tim. Tim nevertheless played exceedingly well at the Junior National level, seeming to justify the coach's new strategies. His tennis professional/manager/guardian then responded by becoming almost obsessively possessive and even more controlling in regard to every aspect of Tim's training and life.

After two years Tim's mother telephoned the author to discuss her feeling that she was losing her own relationship with her son. He had become increasingly remote and rarely communicated with her and other family members. He began to express attitudes and extreme forms of behaviour that were characterologically atypical. At eighteen he seemed to be in a constant state of rebellion. There had been a dramatic change in his on court behaviour during competition. Mother commented that 'he is just not the son that I had thought I had raised'. It was suggested that resolution of her conflicting feelings could best be achieved by arranging a meeting with her son, husband and coach. This attempt at a resolution failed because the father refused to attend. Still caught up by Tim's success and public recognition, he was unwilling even to talk about the possibility of foregoing his own vicarious satisfaction in favour of his child's welfare. One could imagine his fantasies of Tim at the French Open, Australian Open or on Centre Court at Wimbledon.

The coach's relationship with Tim also contained elements of exploitation. It was apparent that he had lost any sense of the importance of maintaining boundaries and emotional differentiation from his student. He appeared driven by both conscious and subconscious needs for both personal and vicarious fame and financial success, with an increasing objectification of the adolescent in question. This resulted in destruction of family harmony with the father continuing to support the coach against mother and Tim's wishes. Years later Tim remained extremely bitter that he had not attained the level of success he felt his considerable talent should have commanded.

A number of complex factors may have contributed to the destruction of this young man's career. These included the parents' lack of wisdom in acceding to the teaching professional's demands for total control. The mother's awareness of not having set appropriate limits for her son's relationship with the coach also contributed, and at least suggested some belated empathic concern on her part and the ability to reconsider earlier errors. This perhaps reflected upon power differential issues in the parental relationship. Tim's active ambition and participation in an 'achievement by proxy' distortion masked a passive collusion with the adults' plans for his future. The parents' and the coach's involvement with powerful achievement and materialistic motives caused them to ally both actively and passively to allow the coach's tacit adoption of this adolescent for mutual personal gain and exploitation of his abilities. This type of situation is likely to become an ever-increasing issue that sport psychiatrists will confront, as youth sports adapt to a more professional model with huge potential financial rewards for the successful few.

Possible clinical interventions

1. The importance of anticipatory case finding methods is illustrated in the above scenarios. In the first case, psychiatry had not been involved but was able to be of benefit in immediate and longer term management. Establishing credibility within school systems and sports medicine facilities and with parents in teams can only occur over time.
2. Engaging in therapy may take many forms, including intermittent long distance telephone involvement.

3. Be prepared to slowly work with and try to comprehend maladaptive coping strategies, along with the potentially more adaptive 'positive denial' strategies. Do not prematurely interpret child or parental behaviours as this may result in the family fleeing therapy. In the first case, an 'over-achieving' father's maladaptive and goal-directed adaptive strategies may actually facilitate this child's resilience during her long, slow, painful recovery towards a fuller physical life, while also limiting her tolerance of and ability to express her own affect. This may lead to masked and unrecognized psychopathology in both the short and long term, with potentially severe consequences including major depression and suicide.

4. It is important to establish rapport and alliances with all members of the 'extended family', which may include both parents and a coach and even the coach's family in surrogate parental or family roles, after full permission has been obtained. When biological parents refuse or are reluctant to engage in therapy themselves, the surrogate parent/coach may be an acceptable avenue for ongoing contact with the child or adolescent and their parents, albeit in a displaced therapeutic fashion.

5. Deal with trauma issues in both an anticipatory fashion and as they present themselves. In the first scenario above, the coach's individual issue regarding the trauma of witnessing and supervising an athlete during a life-threatening and life-changing event cannot be minimized, and both short and long term trauma-related psychotherapy may be helpful. The coach may be able to model her own fairly adaptive coping skills for this child recovering from and dealing with ongoing, lifelong physical impairment in the adolescent developmental framework. Hopefully, the biological mother can also be engaged at a later stage in therapy with the child.

6. It is desirable to broaden the alliance with the parents and coach through empathetically being able to understand the reasons why a parent (or parents) may be covertly (or overtly) creating extra and possibly unacceptable pressure on a child. Both the father and the coach appear to be straddling the 'risky sacrifice'/'objectification' levels of achievement by proxy in the first vignette. The mother was apparently less attached and involved from an achievement by proxy standpoint.

7. Understanding the child's, the parents' and the coach's needs and goals is critical and requires skills in dealing with potentially strong negative countertransference. Attempt to take all of their perspectives into account. This may facilitate willingness to accept the existence of problems and the subsequent benefits of psychotherapeutic intervention. Unfortunately, many are not willing to engage and may disparage the 'weakness' of any involvement with psychosocial supports. If parents and coach are covertly creating pressure to produce achievement by proxy, try to empathize as much as possible with the individual parents. This should assist them in finding their own various alternatives and strategies for accomplishing their needs, aside from the vicarious pride, success and achievement from and through their child, and in a less abusive way.

Conclusions

Children have historically been exposed to the risks of exploitation and abuse whenever there is the possibility of financial reward or other collateral advantage accruable to involved adults. So called 'enlightened' times have not diminished this social phenomenon which may serve an evolutionary behavioural need.

Primary prevention, through outlawing the most flagrant abuses, and secondary preventive strategies, through minimizing risks, anticipatory guidance and psychotherapeutic interventions including psycho-education, are the best available methods for minimizing the pathogenic dangers of achievement by proxy distortion. The authors have described normal supportive achievement by proxy behaviour – the positive, nurturing pride, altruism and voluntary adult sacrifice for their children. Placed within a historical perspective, pathogenic achievement by proxy distortion behaviour is also described. This occurs when a child is placed, with his collusion, volitional or otherwise, in a potentially exploitative situation in order for a perpetrating adult or adult system to gratify their own needs and ambitions for the attainment of certain goals or achievements.

This overview has included examples of the three descriptively defined stages of 'achievement by proxy' behaviour: (1) risky sacrifice, (2) objectification and (3) potential abuse. Such information should increase awareness of this field, thus facilitating communication and enabling child psychiatrists and other professionals to identify the 'red flags' which can lead to abuse and exploitation of children and adolescents. It should also further contribute towards psycho-education of 'self-help' skills, especially in relation to the understanding of parental and other adult motivations behind distorted behaviours and risky rationalizations, in addition to proposing prevention strategies. We have a powerful obligation to educate parents, teachers and legislators of the potential risks and potential abuses of current and future generations of gifted and high achieving children.

References

Cantelon, H. (1981) High performance sport and the child athlete: learning to labor. In *Career patterns and Career Contingencies in Sport* (Ingham, A.G. and Broom, E.F., eds), pp. 258–286. University of British Columbia.

Donnelly, P. (1993) Problems associated with youth involvement in high performance sports. In *Intensive Participation in Children's Sports* (Cahill and Pearl, eds). American Orthopaedic Society for Sports Medicine.

Eminson, D.M. and Postlethwaite, R.J. (1992) Factitious illness: recognition and management. *Archives of Disease in Childhood*, **67**, 1510–1516.

Freud, S. (1957) *On Narcissism: An Introduction*. Hogarth Press.

Giovacchini, P.L. (1989) *Countertransference Triumphs and Catastrophes*, pp. 20 Jason Aroson.

Gould, D. (1993) Intensive sport participation and the prepubescent athlete: competitive stress and burnout. In *Intensive Participation in Children's Sports*

(Cahill and Pearl, eds), pp. 19–38. American Orthopaedic Society for Sports Medicine.

Gutheil, T.G. and Gabbard, G. (1998) Misuses and misunderstandings of boundary theory in clinical and regulatory settings. *American Journal of Psychiatry*, **155**, 3.

Joravsky, B. (1995) *Hoop Dreams: A True Story of Hardship and Triumph.* Harper Perennial.

King, R.A., Noshpitz, J.D. and Joseph, D. (1987) Child physical abuse. In *Pathways of Growth, Essentials of Child Psychiatry, Volume 2: Psychopathology*, pp. 678–679. Wiley.

Meadow, R. (1995) What is, and what is not 'Munchausen syndrome by proxy'? *Archives of Disease in Childhood*, **72**, 534–539.

Miller, A. (1979) The drama of the gifted child and the psychoanalyst's narcissistic disturbance. *International Journal of Psychoanalysis*, **60**, 47–58.

Miller, A. (1981) *The Drama of the Gifted Child.* Basic Books.

Newberger, E.H., Hampton, R.L., Marx, T.J. and White, K.M. (1986) Child abuse and pediatric social illness: an epidemiological analysis and ecological reformulation. *American Journal of Orthopsychiatry*, **56**, 589–601.

Ogilvie, B.C., Tofler, I.R., Conroy, D.R. and Drell, M.J. (1998) Comprehending role conflicts in the coaching of children, adolescents and young adults. Transference, countertransference and achievement by proxy distortion paradigms. *Child and Adolescent Psychiatric Clinics of North America*, **7**, 879–890.

Solnit, A. and Stark, M. (1961) Mourning and the birth of a defective child. *Psychoanalytic Study of the Child*, **16**, 523–537.

Stryer Katz, B., Tofler, I. and Lapchick, R. (1998) A developmental overview of child and youth sports in society. *Child and Adolescent Psychiatric Clinics of North America*, **7**, 697–724.

Tofler, I.R. and Butterbaugh, G. (1998) The Achievement by Proxy Interview Schedule. (Unpublished).

Tofler, I.R. and Stryer Katz, B. (1996) Recommended standards for elite level gymnastics. International Society for Sports Psychiatry Working Paper for Gymnastics. Presented at the American Psychiatric Association Conference, May 6th.

Tofler, I.R., Knapp, P.K. and Drell, M.J. (1998) 'The achievement by proxy' spectrum: historical perspective and clinical approach to the pressured and high achieving child or adolescent. *Child and Adolescent Psychiatric Clinics of North America*, **7**, 803–820.

Winnicott, D.W. (1958) Transitional objects and transitional phenomena. In *Collected Papers: Through Pediatrics to Psychoanalysis.* Basic Books.

11

The child protection process

Dymphna Pearce and Christopher Bools

Introduction

The chapters which precede this one have been concerned with a range of presentations from parental abnormal illness behaviour through to factitious illness.
This embraces a spectrum of behaviour from harmless exaggerations through
benign and then less benign, more risky fabricated stories and signs, and on to
more persistent and harmful inventions and then to illness induction. Other chapters have also dealt with situations analagous or related to MSBP abuse, and with
procedures for establishing whether factitious illness of various kinds has taken
place. From this point onwards, the book is dealing with circumstances where
harmful factitious illness by parents (MSBP abuse) is taking or has taken place,
to the point where the child protection procedures are considered and invoked,
and with the events that may follow this. In terms of the stages outlined in
Chapter 1, Stage 1 (identification of paediatric fabrication) ends with the start of
this chapter, which is concerned with Stage 2 (information gathering), Stage 3
(judgement phase) and, to a certain extent, Stage 4 (management and treatment
after legal proceedings).

Available evidence indicates that the outcome of fabrication of illness (MSBP
abuse) for the child victim who remains with the fabricating parent is likely to be
poor if the parent and family are both untreated and not monitored (Gray,
Bentovim and Milla, 1995; Gray and Bentovim, 1996; Jones and Bools, 1999). In
this chapter an attempt is made to inform the management of MSBP abuse
drawing upon what is known about behaviours and psychiatric disturbance that
have been identified in fabricators. The recommended approach to management
aims to provide protection for the child using an intervention under the Children
Act (1989). This has to be at an appropriate level dependent on the assessed risk,
and combined with psychiatric treatment for the fabricator in a family context.
The initial focus is on the procedures and personnel involved in assessment in the
short and medium term. Consideration is then given to ways in which the involvement of a psychiatrist may be of assistance.

The initial case conference is the central event in child protection work.
However, the stages before the conference are particularly important when a case
of MSBP abuse is suspected. For this reason, brief overviews of the Children Act
1989 and the early stages before the case conference are presented.

The child protection framework in England and Wales

The Children Act 1989 has been the major development in the law relating to children and has provided the framework for child protection work since 1991. The Act applies mainly to England and Wales, with Scotland largely having its own legislation and procedures. The Act focuses on the responsibilities of parents (rather than, as in previous legislation, their rights), the provision of services for children 'in need' and protection for children who may be suffering, or are likely to suffer, 'significant harm'. This new phrase and the concept of 'significant harm' is central to intervention, including legal processes, and will be considered in more detail later in this chapter and in the following chapter. The Public Law Orders and Private Law Orders will be considered in more detail in the following chapter.

Shortly after the arrival of the Children Act, the document 'Working Together Under The Children Act 1991: A guide to arrangements for inter-agency co-operation for the protection of children from abuse' was issued. There is a strong emphasis on a high degree of co-operation between parents and local authorities, between professionals and between agencies. Duties are placed on each Area Child Protection Committee, and this includes the establishment and monitoring of inter-agency guidelines on procedures to be followed in individual cases. Each area will have a local handbook which will set out procedures including the local services available. Information about types of abuse, including MSBP, will be provided. All professionals in England and Wales will need to consult their local handbook, which should be available to the general public. There is an intention in the Children Act and the 'Working Together' document that, as a result of the emphasis on partnership with parents and improved procedures, less cases will be taken to court.

Duty of the local authority

The statutory duty of the local authority to investigate the circumstances of a child applies when there is reasonable cause to suspect that the child is suffering, or is likely to suffer, significant harm. The duty includes assessment of the needs of the child and of the family, including the likelihood of significant harm and the need for protection.

The doctor in the early stages

In the majority of cases of suspected MSBP abuse the professional notifying the local authority social services department will be a paediatrician, and this will be the beginning of a long period of working closely together. For any case of suspected physical abuse medical opinion will be crucial, and for almost all cases of MSBP medical opinion will be central and will remain so throughout the assessment and monitoring period. At some stage highly specialized medical opinions may be required, in addition to those of the local paediatrician and general practitioner.

Communicating the concerns of professionals about child protection to parents early on is encouraged as good practice. However, this matter may be particularly difficult in suspected examples of MSBP abuse and it is helpful to consider the advice to doctors regarding their approach to situations involving possible abuse addressed in the addendum to 'Working Together': 'Child Protection Medical Responsibilities' (Department of Health, 1991). There will often be uncertainty in the early stage of any suspected child abuse and possibly greater uncertainty than average in most suspected cases of MSBP abuse. The doctor is advised to discuss concerns with an experienced colleague (possibly the designated doctor for child protection) to decide if the critical threshold of professional concern has been reached. The critical threshold will be a matter of individual professional judgement. Preliminary consultation 'is a means whereby thoughts and information can be clarified amongst experienced professionals when child abuse is a consideration or during the early stages of its recognition ... It is not the beginning of an investigation'. It comes before any strategy discussion.

Medical practitioners will be concerned about the confidentiality of their patients. Such concerns about confidentiality are clarified in 'Child Protection Medical Responsibilities': 'in the context of child protection it is the child whose interests are paramount'. Essentially, the breaking of confidentiality will depend on the decision regarding the critical threshold.

The strategy phase

A strategy discussion is a multi-disciplinary discussion to decide if the available information is sufficient and serious enough to warrant undertaking a child abuse investigation and how to conduct it. The strategy discussion may not require a single meeting, and may be a series of discussions, and hence the alternative term of strategy phase. 'Working Together' reminds us that both civil court proceedings and criminal prosecution could possibly follow and this needs to be kept in mind early on. It is at this stage that an investigation may need to be planned carefully to maximize the chances of acquiring suitable forensic evidence (as discussed in Chapters 4 and 5), for example, with heart and breathing recordings in suspected smothering, toxicology in suspected poisoning and laboratory findings after dilution of milk. Many cases of MSBP abuse involve infants and children who are not able to talk. However, if the child victims are older and are able to talk, an interview with the child should be considered. The child may have already been interviewed by the doctor. For example, in the unusual case of a boy who had been smothered from an early age and was still being smothered at age 3 years, the boy was able to describe to the paediatrician what had happened to him.

Only so much may be achieved before moving to a situation in which concerns of the professionals are put to the mother and family. One of the tasks of the strategy phase will be planning how to present the concerns of professionals to the fabricating mother and her partner.

Table 11.1 shows the various stages involved for the clinician and the order in which they usually occur.

Table 11.1 Stages for the clinician

Private concerns in the mind
Preliminary consultation with colleague(s)
Referral to social services
Strategy phase
Investigation in process
Presenting concerns to parents
Initial child protection case conference
Child on Child Protection Register
Core group in operation
Comprehensive assessment
Legal processes
Review child protection case conference

Putting concerns of the professionals to the fabricator

Various ways of presenting concerns to the fabricator are possible. The discovering paediatrician may be the most appropriate professional to confront the fabricator, supported by the knowledge of a plan of multi-disciplinary action formed in the strategy phase. Depending on the seriousness of the situation, a social worker may be present at the initial confrontation or nearby to interview the fabricator. There may be an opportunity for a psychiatrist to become involved at this stage and possible roles at this point are discussed below.

In view of the possibility of a criminal investigation, sometimes the police may become directly involved at this stage by interviewing the fabricator. In cases of suspected smothering when video surveillance has been used the police will already be involved, having set up the surveillance operation in co-operation with the hospital staff. In this situation, police officers will be on the ward at all times according to the surveillance protocol for suspected smothering.

When presented with concerns, the usual reported response of the fabricator is complete denial – almost by definition for the classical or prototypical presentation. Fisher (1995) discusses those who do not deny accusations, whom he refers to as 'help seekers', as suggested by Libow and Schreier(1986).
The two main concerns at this stage will be:

- The continuing protection for the child and siblings.
- The mental health of the mother.

The abnormal dependency of the mother on the child, or at least the 'illness' state of the child, may be very strong (Bools, 1996). The risk of further unusual physical dangers to a child will need to be kept in mind. Other concerns and difficulties are discussed below in the section regarding the case conference.

It may help to acknowledge the distress of the mother at the same time as expressing concern about actual or possible harm to the child. This approach may, however, be more successful in establishing a working relationship and be acceptable to the mother when dealing with a 'help seeker'. The main concerns about the mental health of the mother at this stage are regarding the possibility of self harm as well as the risk of escalation of fabrications. The mental health of the mother is further discussed below.

The initial child protection case conference

Key functions

The initial case conference is an essential stage in the organization of multi-disciplinary working. However, its timing, if delayed, should not lead to a delay in work that needs to be carried out. There are three key functions:

- To facilitate communication between professionals and the family.
- To make an assessment of risk in the short and medium term.
- To make recommendations for action.

Communication

Key professionals and family members will be invited to attend or to submit a written report. The question of excluding parents from a case conference may arise. As a matter of principle and practice, exclusion of parents should be kept to a minimum. However, 'Working Together' mentions specific reasons for such exclusion, e.g. safeguarding of confidential information for a specific purpose, the likelihood of violent behaviour. Exclusion may be for the whole, or part, of the conference. The decision ultimately rests with the Chair. Participants at the conference may wish to discuss concerns with the Chair prior to the meeting. On a few occasions MSBP abuse may be one special case for exclusion of the parents from the initial child protection case conference at the early stages of an investigation.

Assessment of risks to the child

At this stage the assessment will focus on risks in the short and medium term, which will lead to recommendations and, therefore, determine the early management of the case.

In the process of assessment of MSBP four areas will require particular attention:

- Gathering and collating medical information regarding the child and any siblings.
- Assessing the mental state of the fabricator.
- Difficulties in forming a partnership with the parents (fabricator and partner).
- The role of the extended family.

One way of approaching the assessment of risks is to consider the physical risks and emotional risks separately. This area has already been discussed in certain respects in Chapter 9. Emotional risks are usually more complex for a number of reasons, including the problem of assessing emotional harm already caused, as well as attempting a prediction of the possibilities in the future.

Gathering and collating medical information concerning the child

Medical information will be available in a combination of written records and the opinions of medical practitioners. Gathering information and opinions from recently involved doctors and nurses, especially those involved during the time of the fabrications, should be straightforward, and the importance of first-hand reports is stressed. However, even at this stage it may be useful to have access to older records which certainly will be needed for the later comprehensive assessment. It will be important to access enough information to decide whether it will be necessary to separate the child from the fabricator and, if so, the degree of supervision at contact, if this is considered to be safe.

Assessing the mental state of the fabricator

The importance of recording observations and the findings of investigative enquiry, such as interviewing relatives, cannot be over-emphasized in terms of contributing to the assessment. Such information may not be given due weight in the psychiatric assessment because of the limitations of traditional examination of the mental state by means of interview with the subject.

Forming a partnership with the fabricator and partner

There are potential difficulties in forming a partnership with a fabricating parent for a number of reasons. The ability to lie and deceive may be well developed with a plausible appearance; there may be an overtly uncooperative and even antagonistic approach; sometimes the mother may find that separation from the child generates a very high level of anxiety which is almost intolerable to her because of the extreme and inappropriate degree of dependency on the child (or at least dependency on the illness state of the child, especially if there has been a chronic fabrication); the fabricator may self harm, move to further somatization in herself or exhibit symptoms of depression. Although a rare occurrence, the possibility of abduction of the child should be considered (Fisher, 1995).

The stance taken by the partner at this stage, and as the picture evolves, will be one of the critical factors to be considered in the assessment of risk and possibilities for therapeutic work. As with most aspects of MSBP abuse the range of responses is broad.

The extended family

Extended family members, at least early on, may not be able to accept what has happened to the child, may have no, or very little, knowledge of MSBP and, therefore, may not appreciate the seriousness of potential risks to the child. The usual principle of giving high priority to the possibility of placement with a close relative will be challenged in such a situation.

Recommendations at the case conference

One of the concluding decisions of the initial conference will be whether to place the child on the 'at risk register'. Registration of MSBP abuse will usually be under the category of 'physical injury'. This will certainly be so for all cases of induced illness (with associated physical harm). Alternatively the category will be 'emotional abuse' if there has been persistent verbal fabrication leading to actual or likely severe adverse effects on the emotional and behavioural state of the child. If registration occurs, the initial plan will include a comprehensive assessment.

The pre-birth child protection case conference

It is necessary for the social services department to be alert to the risk of a mother known to have fabricated illness in one child causing similar harm to a subsequent child, including during the pregnancy (Jureidini, 1993) if she has made insufficient or no progress in her understanding of her role in the first child's illness. This potential situation highlights the important role of attempting to continue therapeutic work pro-actively with a fabricator following permanent separation from one child (Bluglass, 1997) for the benefit of a second child.

For example, in the case of a family in which a child incurred near fatal poisoning, that child was removed permanently from the family and the case was closed by social services who were unaware that the mother was again pregnant. The mother then changed her general practitioner and health visitor, and began to poison the second child. In another case, a mother had been poisoning her small son's milk in his bottle both at home and in hospital. When the boy was taken into care and placed with foster parents the second child, who had been well until that point, suddenly became ill with the same symptoms. When she became pregnant with the third baby, this third baby became the subject of a pre-birth child protection (CP) conference.

The function of the pre-birth conference, as for the initial CP conference, is to discuss and decide on the level of risk being posed to the child by the mother, and to formulate an action plan to safeguard his/her welfare. The conference will decide at this point whether the child can be sufficiently protected by staying within his own family but with the support of the various services. Alternatively, the child may be at too great a risk to be in his mother's care for even a short while and therefore will need to be separated from her at birth or within a few days of the birth.

There may be a situation in which a number of years has elapsed since the presence of the mother had been deemed to be significantly harmful and the child had been removed permanently from her care. After this passage of time the mother becomes pregnant again, although in the intervening years she appears to have functioned better. A pre-birth conference should still be called, but in this instance, it might be decided that there should be a reassessment of the mother's mental state and attitude during the pregnancy, which may in turn give some indication about the level of risk to which the new baby would be exposed if he remained in his mother's care after birth. Pre-birth conference members usually agree to meet again as soon as this preliminary assessment is completed so that they can plan for the baby's care directly after the birth. If the mental health assessment can identify sufficient positive changes in the mother's functioning and situation for it to be felt that the baby does not appear to be at least at immediate risk, the mother and child could be discharged home from the hospital, although on the understanding with both parents that there would be very regular monitoring of the baby's physical progress and care, that a comprehensive assessment would be undertaken, and that there would be regular meetings of the core group (see below). The comprehensive assessment would update the information obtained about the family when the first child was removed. If the assessment of the mother during her subsequent pregnancy raises concerns of a re-emergence of her distorted attitudes and functioning, the baby may be most safely protected by becoming the subject of care proceedings at birth and removed from the mother's care at this stage.

After the case conference

Placement and contact

Depending on the assessment of risk, and in the absence of a voluntary agreement or the granting of a court order, the options for the child will be to:

- Remain with both parents.
- Reside with the non-abusing parent.
- Reside with another family member.
- Be placed with foster parents.

The placement decision will need to take into account not only the risk of what may happen, based on what has already happened (the primary risks), but also the risk of not being able to adequately control the situation (one of the secondary risks). When fabrication has occurred without direct harm being caused to the child, and placement with the fabricator is under consideration, the assessment of the secondary risks (of being able to maintain sufficient control) becomes more relevant.

Under certain circumstances, for example, if the family are able to co-operate fully, if the child is placed with the father and the mother leaves the home to live with another family member, it may be considered safe to negotiate conditions of contact with the fabricator and her family and avoid the need for a court order. Usually, however, this will be considered a high risk strategy, leaving open the possibility of allowing the fabricator to avoid having to face the detail of the fabrications as they would be presented in court, and also giving insufficient control to the local authority. It is more often the case that the court order will need to be changed at this time, for example, from an emergency protection order to an interim care order or interim supervision order.

If mother and child are separated, the issue of contact will need to be negotiated with the mother and other family members. Decisions will need to be made regarding the frequency and duration of contact and the level of supervision. If there is disbelief by family members and/or separation problems exist for the mother (as discussed earlier), then a high level of caution and vigilance will be needed. We are aware of family members (aunts and uncles) who have allowed contact additional to that agreed. In another situation a mother achieved unsupervised communication with her child by befriending one of the domestic staff of a local authority facility and then sent notes via the staff to her daughter who was of school age. If the child remains with the family the core group will become the cornerstone of the monitoring and support for the family.

Establishing the monitoring system – the core group

The core group will comprise the key worker for the family, usually a social worker from the social services department (or other child care agency with statutory powers such as the NSPCC), and other professionals having direct contact with the child such as the health visitor, GP, school teachers and school nurse (where the child is of school age and well enough to attend). The paediatrician for the child will provide information to the group. The family member(s) caring for the child would also be invited. The attendance of the fabricator would depend on a number of factors affecting the risk to the child at that point in time, including initial co-operation and progress. If the fabricator has a psychiatrist, then his opinion will be important for the group in their understanding of the fabricator and the ongoing risk she presents. The psychiatrist will have direct knowledge of the fabricator's state of mental health and pattern of behaviour in her relationship with her child and in her working relationships with professionals. Only in the more unusual cases where the child/young person is of an age and understanding to participate in his/her own protection would serious consideration be given to their participation in the core group.

It is the task of the core group to put into operation a detailed child protection plan. This involves the core members regularly and vigilantly reviewing the risks of further abuse and noting areas of concern specific to the MSBP, as well as reviewing all the more usual issues such as basic care and the observed relationship (as evidence of the attachment) between the mother and child. In situations when the child has remained with, or been returned to, the fabricator this could include whether the child has been taken to a different hospital or if medication has been sought from a locum doctor for misperceived illness, and having targets for positive change, such as weight gain after failure to thrive due to the dilution of the baby's milk. Other aspects of the situation may be more complex and less easily measured, especially the changes in behaviour and complex psychological states that will be encountered; nevertheless, here too an attempt will need to be made to agree on measurable targets.

It is essential that every member of the core group has a working knowledge of MSBP abuse and is aware of the fabricator's ability to deceive and present as caring and concerned whilst continuing to fabricate illness. It is known that the successful management of this type of case is dependent on the perceptions and co-operation of the professionals involved (Neale, Bools and Meadow, 1991). It is recommended that an independent chair of the core group, again with knowledge of the syndrome (although with a working distance from the child and family), is appointed. Such a person will be in a position to offer an overview and guidance for the group. This means that the local authority will need to commit two experienced social workers throughout work with the family.

The core group ensures that a comprehensive assessment of risks and the needs of the child is completed by the time of the child protection review, which is held a maximum of six months after the initial conference, although often sooner for the first review.

The comprehensive assessment

Role of the local authority

The purpose of the comprehensive assessment is to put together information from the multi-agency members of the core group and other specialists (such as the mother's psychiatrist), as well as the child and family themselves, so that decisions about future actions are made with as sound a basis as possible. This process should be distinguished from the initial assessment used for short term planning and the immediate protection of the child.

The key worker is responsible for co-ordinating and then writing up the assessment which is a complex, multi-faceted piece of work requiring regular updating between reviews as the child, fabricator and family react in the aftermath of the medical confrontation. There are times when the assessment is used as the basis for an application for court intervention if it is felt that the child is at too great a risk without legal proceedings.

The 'Guide for Social Workers Undertaking a Comprehensive Assessment' (Department of Health, 1988) provides a framework for social workers to carry out the assessment. It is recognized that this is not an all-inclusive document; however, it does identify the aspects of the child, family and family life that need to be understood and evaluated before long term decisions can be made about a child. It recommends aspects to be looked at under the general headings of: causes for concern about the child; the child's developmental needs; the composition of the family; the family's financial resources and physical environment; the personality, strengths, attitudes and problems of the parents (parent and partner); family interactions, including the adults' relationship with each other and the children, and their ability to meet the children's needs; the child and family's network of relatives, friends and links with professionals; what led to the causes for concern; the extent of the parents' acceptance of responsibility for concern about their child, their wish to bring about change and their ability to do so; and the help that the family are likely to require and the time-scale needed for changes to occur.

The key worker involved in cases of MSBP abuse may be faced with difficulties in gathering information for the comprehensive assessment, and the 'Guide for Social Workers' does not recognize these difficulties. The list of suggested harm to a child does not specifically include MSBP abuse, which does not fit readily into the categories of harm listed in the guide, although it may include some aspects from the lists of harm, such as physical and emotional abuse, and comments could be made about the physical problems exhibited by the child.

Having considered the child's behavioural or emotional problems, and the parents' perception of the child's routine and care, the social worker is advised to gather information about the child's early history. Lynch (1976), discussing risk factors in a child, stresses the significance of the information concerning this part of the child's life because 'statistical studies showed six factors to be highly significantly over-represented in the biography of abused children as compared with their siblings: abnormal pregnancy, abnormal labour or delivery, neonatal separation, other separations in the first six months of life, illness in the first year of life, and illness in the mother in the first year'. Another factor that could be added to Lynch's list is when there are expectations that are unrealistic, which may have their origins even before conception, and the child fails to live up to the parent's expectations, or the mother fails to fulfil her expected maternal role. Disappointment in either respect can contribute to the risk of a child being harmed.

Information about the history is sought from the parents, but interpretation of this history may be particularly difficult in cases of MSBP abuse when it is given by an accomplished deceiver and liar (the mother) whose perception of events has been shaped, and skewed, as a result of her abnormal psychological functioning. A preliminary understanding of the mother's functioning is likely to be available from the mother's psychiatrist at this stage and should be noted, not only whilst history taking, but also in gathering information about her perception of herself, her role as a mother and her relationships (both with other members of the family, including her husband/partner, and outside the family, perhaps at work or friends). Asking identical questions of the father and the mother (even close relatives and any friends) could elicit different answers, which would be worth comparing to identify the different perceptions.

Medical contributions to the comprehensive assessment

Whilst assessment is a process which may be ongoing for a considerable time, it is helpful and practical to consider the contribution of medical assessment and opinion in two discrete stages.

In the first stage the presence or absence of fabrications will be established, and their nature and extent will be clarified. Usually this will involve both the paediatrician who discovered the fabrication and a second paediatrician who will be able to give an expert opinion on the particular area of medicine in question, for example, respiratory medicine, gastroenterology or neurology. A high level of suspicion, or knowing for certain that there has been fabrication of illness, may mean that, in a review of all the available medical records, other episodes of illness in the child may come under suspicion. The quality of notes will be critical in attempting to collate information. It may be helpful to interview the authors of some of the notes to clarify what has happened in more detail.

In the UK, because of the way in which the National Health Service is organized, general practitioners almost always act as referrers to specialists. The result is that, at the minimum, there will be copies of referral letters in GP records and usually either out-patient clinic notes and/or hospital discharge summaries. Using the GP notes as the first point of reference, it should be possible to obtain all the hospital records relating to a child. It will be useful to examine the overall pattern of consultation not only regarding the index child but also in relation to the consultations with any siblings and the mother herself. For example, when gathering information about a child suspected of being the subject of fabrications by examining in parallel the GP records of a mother and her two children (both the index child and a sibling), it became evident that the mother had consulted with a general practitioner concerning one or other member of the family about once per week for a period of about two years. As well as providing information about fabricating behaviour relating to the child primarily under consideration, the possibility of a similar behaviour pattern with the sibling was revealed. In addition, information was obtained which was useful in the second stage of the assessment when the psychiatrist assessed the behaviour and emotional state of the mother. The role for the psychiatrist in the first stage is limited. However, it may be possible to commence the second stage in overlap, although caution is advised until the medical facts are established, with the danger of under-recognition of risks. The exception is when the fabrications are of a psychiatric nature (Fisher, Mitchell and Murdoch, 1993).

Moving into legal processes

One may view a change from a voluntary agreement to court proceedings as essentially a failure of the parents and the local authority to work in partnership. This failure of partnership may arise for a variety of possible reasons.

The fabricating parent and/or their family (partner and the grandparents of the child) may feel unable to co-operate with various conditions set out by the local authority; for example, the conditions of residence of the child, restrictions of contact with the child and participation in the comprehensive assessment. Since denial of fabrication is the usual response (an integral part of the classical presentation by definition), it may be useful to some degree to consider the question of 'co-operation' as a separate issue from the denial of the fabricated nature of the illness and harm caused. For example, a mother may not be able to acknowledge publicly what she has been doing in order to fabricate illness in her child; however, there may be co-operation with the conditions of residence regarding the child and the agreed contact, together with co-operation with the assessment process to the extent of attending appointments with social workers, psychiatrists etc. The co-operation may indicate a useful degree of 'acceptance' of problems, although falling short of acknowledgement. In this situation, depending on other risk factors, it may be possible to proceed with the assessment without the need to enter the court process at the beginning. The result of the assessment, however, may lead to a decision to proceed in to the court process. Alternatively, there may be a substantial lack of co-operation involving marked oppositional behaviour, possibly with outbursts of temper, or avoidance by retreat into claiming to suffer from physical illness. For example, a child had been admitted to a paediatric ward and the paediatrician began to become more suspicious of fabrication of bleeding. The mother seemed to become aware of the concerns and was admitted to the gynaecology ward of the same hospital with a history of bleeding which was almost certainly fabricated.

In situations that are considered to be high risk because of particular aspects of the mental state of the mother at this time, for example erratic behaviour including self harm or threats to others, clearly seeking a court order will be appropriate. In such situations, or if depressed mood or florid psychiatric illness is suspected, an urgent assessment by an adult psychiatric team will be appropriate. In some situations this will lead to admission to a psychiatric ward.

Once allegations of MSBP abuse have been made, parents will usually consult their lawyer(s). The local authority will already have consulted their own legal department. Thus, depending on the situation and the participants, legal processes will commence which will be more or less adversarial. These are described in the next chapter.

Difficulties in carrying out an assessment with local resources

The local authority may experience difficulties in being able to offer all the required elements of an assessment that include appropriate expertise. This may be as a result of lack of experience or training in the local social services department combined with difficulties in access to appropriate additional resources or expertise, especially in the early stages of an assessment. This situation is not surprising in view of the rarity and lack of recognition of MSBP abuse, although as time goes by most departments will have dealt with at least one case and expertise will develop. There are implications from such difficulties both for training and resourcing in social services. With regard to training, in one area a group of professionals formed an interest in MSBP abuse after two cases had proved to be a challenge to local knowledge. With regard to resources, family centres are potentially very useful as a resource for carrying out an assessment of a mother–child relationship. Not every area, however, will have a family centre and in a situation involving MSBP abuse a high level of supervision and safety will be needed. This may be beyond what some centres can provide.

The management of a case of MSBP abuse has major implications for liaison between social services and other local services, in particular with child and adolescent psychiatrists and specialists in adult psychiatry (general adult, forensic or psychotherapy) and their multi-disciplinary teams. In some parts of the country the local child and adolescent psychiatry team may be inadequately resourced and unable to meet the demands of even more mainstream referrals. In addition, there is a national shortage of consultant psychiatrists in both child and adult services. There may be a lack of suitable specialist resources; for example, there are very few in-patient facilities for children and families across the whole of England and Wales. There may also be difficulties in finding a suitable outside expert who is able to allocate the time needed to offer what is required. Remedies for some of the difficulties outlined above may be possible by clarification of local arrangements by negotiation at commissioning level and by liaison between local managers of the services.

The guardian ad litem

Introduction

The guardian *ad litem* (GAL) is appointed by the court in care proceedings as an independent person whose paramount concern is the child's welfare. Guardians are generally social workers, divorce court welfare officers, or probation officers with a significant number of years of post-qualifying experience of which a substantial proportion should be in working with families and children. GALs are grouped into 'panels' whose working areas correspond with county boundaries or unitary authority boundaries (depending on the panel or panels on which they serve) and are co-ordinated by a panel manager (although this system is to be reorganized in the next few years). It is essential that they are seen to be independent of the local authority. There are National Standards for Guardians to which they have to adhere in their working practice.

Duties of the guardian ad litem

The duty of the GAL is to inform the court of the child's wishes and feelings about his situation, to interview and gain information from all those people who have been involved in the child's welfare and to read any records made by relevant agencies such as the social services department. With permission or a direction from the court, the guardian may also have access to the medical records of the parent and/or child. If there are aspects of the child's or parent's functioning that need further, specialist understanding, the guardian will recommend that an 'expert' in that field is appointed to make an assessment and provide a report to the court. It may even be that more than one 'expert' is involved in the same hearing. This may be because there is more than one issue to be taken into account – for example, an adult psychiatrist to assess a parent, and a child and adolescent psychiatrist to assess the child. It could also be because a parent so totally disagrees with the opinion of one expert that the court has granted permission for that parent to seek a second opinion. For reasons of using court time more efficiently, and the additional cost, the use of a second expert to consider exactly the same area of concern as the first is now rarely accepted practice. If more than one expert is used, a 'meeting of experts' is often arranged following the filing of their reports, the purpose of which is to identify areas of agreement and disagreement between them. These meetings are formal, usually organized by the GAL and her solicitor (being independent), with minutes being taken and agreed at the end of the meeting. If an expert has clearly changed his or her opinion about a matter from that written in his original report, it would be helpful and clearer for the court and all parties if that expert could explain, in writing, the reason for the change of opinion.

Ultimately, for the final hearing, the guardian conveys her views through a report. Written interim reports may already have been produced for interim hearings where specific issues are being addressed or if the interim order is being contested. In the final report, the guardian records and comments on the concerns raised about the child, and the child's wishes and feelings, with further comments on the child's ability to understand his situation, taking into account his age or level of functioning. There will also be an assessment of the child's developmental needs and of the parent's capability of meeting these needs with specific reference to the opinion of any experts. The guardian considers what help or support has been available to the parents and/or child both before the proceedings began and during the time of the proceedings and concludes by considering the variety of orders available to the court that could arguably be made to protect the child and enhance his welfare. It may even be that an order is not necessary to achieve this if, during the court proceedings, substantial progress has been made.

The guardian must ensure that there is minimal delay between the initial hearing in the proceedings and the final hearing. When guardians were first involved in proceedings it was not unusual for cases to take a matter of weeks. The evidence needed in present proceedings, with the use of statements (which are a consequence of the 1989 Children Act), has meant that proceedings can now continue for many months, sometimes even twelve or more. During the course of this time, there will be continuing assessments of the child and parents in response to initial work or to gain a greater understanding of the exact nature of the concerns. It is essential for a detailed care plan to be submitted concerning the child at the final hearing (usually by the local authority). The court has increasingly indicated a wish to have the final care plan at an advanced stage so that delays do not occur subsequently because the social services cannot find a suitable placement for the child or do not immediately have the personnel or financial resources to implement the care plan.

Specific problems in the role of the guardian ad litem in MSBP abuse

Allegations made by the local authority are critically reliant on medical evidence and usually the parent actively refutes the allegations. In such circumstances court proceedings commence and the GAL is appointed. With the primary focus being the welfare of the child, the guardian is at the interface between people with conflicting positions. There is the mother, whose view of the child's needs is likely to be distorted; the father, who may or may not be beginning to acknowledge the medical concerns; the social services department, who again may or may not have understood the seriousness of the alleged concerns; and the court, with its authority.

The GAL will have an understanding of MSBP abuse through reading the available literature, talking with an expert, and (now more often the case) through direct experience of previous cases, before she begins her investigations. The guardian is very likely to encounter a number of strongly felt responses to the allegation that the mother has been harming her child, not only through the denial and incredulity of the mother herself, and sometimes from the husband and other relatives, but also through those who have known the mother and been encouraged to see her as a caring, perhaps even ideal, parent in the concern that she has shown towards her sick child. The health visitor and the general practitioner may have only observed her apparent compassion towards the child, and the social services department may have doubts about the concerns being expressed by medical staff when, in many other ways, this mother appears to demonstrate a parenting ability that is not often found amongst other families with whom they work. If she is articulate and persuasive it is not unusual for those working with her to find themselves doubting the evidence initially presented to the court.

In cases newly allocated to a guardian, it is general procedure to see the child first, where practicable or possible, followed by the parents and then the authorities concerned about the child's care. The reasoning behind this practice is that, if the guardian is to be seen to be independent, then she should interview the children or parents without preconceived views from others. If the guardian adopts this customary procedure in cases of MSBP abuse, she must hear the mother's explanation and opinions whilst being alert to what is known about fabricators and their presentation.

There is strong argument for the GAL to begin her investigation and assessment by understanding the nature of the concerns being expressed about the child. If a very detailed medical report has not already been produced for the court by the child's paediatrician, it is essential for the guardian to interview the paediatrician and view any available videotapes very early in the proceedings. Further information should be ascertained from the ward staff who had (and may still have) care of the child during his stay in hospital. They will have observed the mother's interaction with and care of the child, and it is likely that they will also have gained an impression of the personality of the mother, as well as that of the father or mother's partner.

The guardian must see the child and elicit his wishes and feelings about his circumstances. Clearly, if the child is very young and unable to communicate these with any degree of clarity, information about the child's needs can be learned from those directly involved with him and from observing his interaction with 'significant others'. These include the mother (during supervised contact sessions), father/mother's partner, grandparents and even particular nursing staff with whom the child may have developed a relationship during his stay in hospital. Where the child is older and able to convey his views, the guardian must take these into consideration whilst making an assessment (and ultimately her recommendation) about the child's welfare, having regard for his age and level of understanding of his circumstances. There are situations where the child has clearly been able to express a view, even at a very young age (such as the child referred to earlier, aged 3 years, who was able to say what his mother was doing to him). There are also situations where an older child and mother have developed a mutually dependent bond so that separating the child from the mother is likely to lead to emotional problems. In such a situation the balance of factors (when considering benefits and problems created by separation) will need to include the child's ability to protect himself from his mother's need for him to be ill. If the child does not have sufficient understanding of the problems, and is not able to protect himself, then this factor alone could be persuasive in deciding on the separation issue.

The GAL will investigate the perpetrator's perspective on the allegations that the child has been harmed. Inevitably there are a variety of ways in which mothers respond to these allegations, ranging from fierce anger and denial to, occasionally, some acknowledgement of a need for help. The mother will often maintain that she has provided good care and concern for her child and may seek the support of relatives, neighbours, friends, health visitors and sometimes even nursing staff to confirm their observations of her as the caring and attentive parent. Assessment of the mother's parenting may be difficult because she can present with a general ability to look after the child. She may present with a façade of coping: neglect of the child and chaotic disorganization are not often featured, although this is sometimes the case. The guardian must be alert at all times to the different perspectives and views being put forward in these cases and the reasons for these views. She must also be alert to the potential wide variety and degree of severity of the mother's psychopathology (Bools, Neale and Meadows, 1994). The guardian may become aware, in the course of her enquiries, of collaborative evidence (particularly from relatives) with respect to the mother's lying, of illegal activity (police records of convictions), or of the mother's unusual interest in medical matters or animal cruelty, such as the injuring or killing of pets.

The guardian considers this information from the mother, together with that gathered during the comprehensive assessment, in the light of a psychiatric assessment. The appointment of a psychiatrist to assess the mother and open up possibilities for therapeutic work with her should be done very early in the proceedings, ideally at the first hearing, if the mother is not already under the medical care of a psychiatrist. If she is, a report will be requested from this psychiatrist according to a letter of instruction set out by the mother's solicitor. Ideally that letter would include issues that other parties (the local authority, the father, if separately represented, and the GAL) would also like to be addressed in the report on the mother. If the mother was not previously a patient under the psychiatric services, it would be very useful at this point in the proceedings to engage a psychiatrist with specialist knowledge of MSBP abuse to assess her, if she is agreeable, under a joint instruction from all the parties. The complex issues involved in the possible roles for psychiatry are discussed elsewhere in the chapter. It is not necessarily the case that those who fabricate illness have an overt mental health problem, and a standard psychiatric assessment may not be helpful except in the small number of cases where the perpetrator has a mental illness. A psychiatric assessment that considers a very wide range of issues, especially personality functioning, dangerousness of the mother and risk to the child, will be more useful.

The father/partner of the mother, the grandparents, aunts, uncles and teachers, playgroup leaders and health visitors can all provide helpful information about the family's functioning, the relationship between mother and child, and the role of any other siblings in the family. Some of these, and particularly the father, may still be incredulous about any suggestion of fabrication, and will remain supportive of the mother and her position. The extent to which the father is prepared to reconsider his views in the light of increasing evidence of the mother harming her child gives some indication as to his ability to change and become a protective parent. The role that the father is able to take becomes crucial in situations that are considered to be borderline in terms of the psychopathology and stance of the mother. A protective and caring father, who is able to balance the needs of the child and support for his wife, and to appreciate potential risks to the child, can make a critical difference in the assessment of risk and the potential for a good outcome for the child.

The GP has usually been approached by the consultant paediatrician by the time the GAL is appointed, but where this has not happened it is often very enlightening, with the mother's permission or under the direction of the court, to obtain the medical records of both the mother and the child. The notes will need to be reviewed by an appropriate medical practitioner. A paediatrician will be the best person to study and summarize the notes of the index child and siblings to facilitate forming their opinion. A psychiatrist may find reviewing the notes of the mother to be essential for contributing to decisions about diagnosis and, subsequently, risk to the child. The GP notes, combined with the hospital notes, provide information about the frequency of, and reasons for, either the mother's or child's attendance at the surgery. It may also become apparent in searching for the notes that the mother has changed medical practitioners and hospitals an unusual number of times and apparently without reason.

Upon the filing of all the medical experts' reports, the GAL and child's solicitor will carefully elicit all the points of agreement and disagreement in the reports, and send copies of these to the experts. It is good court management for the experts' meeting to be arranged at the time of appointment of the experts themselves, such that the date is scheduled in their diaries from the beginning. Not to do this when many medical practitioners are involved could lead to lengthy delays whilst finding a meeting date convenient to all. Following the meeting, a summary of the points agreed and disagreed should again be circulated amongst the medical experts, either for their acceptance or alteration if there are errors. Reference is made above to the need for an expert who fundamentally changes an opinion to be allowed to file an addendum report explaining his reasons. The final document is then filed before the court, and it is clearly essential that the social services department have access to it before they decide their plans for the future care of the child.

Having completed her investigations, the GAL submits a report for the final hearing in which she makes a recommendation for the future welfare of the child. This takes into account all that has been said to her during interviews, and the content of statements and other records and information available. The guardian considers the threshold criteria, including the needs of the child and the parents' capability of meeting those needs, and the concept of past and future significant harm.

The guardian also considers the type of order that would best protect the child's future welfare. In cases of MSBP abuse, it is unlikely that the child would be protected by no order if placed with the mother, or if the mother is nearby. There may be situations when a residence order is made to the father, grandparents or other relative, if the court is satisfied that this relative can be relied upon to protect the child from the mother. There may occasionally be situations when a supervision order is made on a child. However, as this gives the parent or carer the responsibility for protecting the child, only requires the local authority to assist, advise and befriend the child, and lasts for a maximum of three years, it does not provide sufficient protection for a child who is still young and vulnerable and whose carer may be susceptible to influence from the perpetrator. A care order offers a child the greatest protection, as it is the duty of the local authority under this order to safeguard the child's interests. In deciding how this can best be achieved, the local authority can consider whether the child is sufficiently protected if returned home with the protection of the order or whether the child should be placed away from home.

Consideration of placements and contact

The Guardian must also consider the issue of contact when the child is not to be rehabilitated. When a child is to be placed for adoption, because the risk would be too great if the child was returned to the mother or father, there is unlikely to be a recommendation of direct contact, however infrequent, because (by inference) the mother is such a cause for concern that the child might continue to be at risk. Indirect contact, therefore, is likely to be recommended, through updated photographs and possibly birthday or Christmas cards. Even these may need to be strictly monitored to ensure that there are no emotive messages likely to have negative consequences. Arranging for the child to have updated information about his birth mother is intended in part to reduce the development of fantasies about the past.

When the child is older the care plan can include placement in long term foster care, possibly with relatives, or otherwise with carers under the auspices of the local authority. This is an option when the older child has a strong attachment to the mother and is clearly expressing a wish to remain with the mother. The risk from regular contact (intended to maintain the mother/child relationship) in this situation, is that the mother is unable to moderate her need to be over-dependent, over-involved and over-controlling of the child. The result is that the child becomes highly anxious and the foster placement is disrupted with the risk of it ending. The mother may be more concerned with possession of the child than being able to offer genuine affection.

Finally, under the auspices of a care order, the care plan may include placement of an older child, who has a close attachment to the mother, in a short term fostering placement. The child learns to separate from the previous collusive relationship with the mother and gains some independence whilst contact is minimal and closely monitored. If the process is successful, the contact can then be increased as there is a move towards rehabilitation. In such a situation, it is anticipated that the child can avoid any physical risk his mother may pose in the future, both because of his age and his increased awareness – being able and willing to report any attempts to harm him that may be made as part of fabrications.

Roles for the psychiatrist

Introduction

There is a range of possible roles for a psychiatrist depending on speciality (child and adolescent, general adult, forensic or psychotherapist), location of work (teaching hospital, district general hospital, community service or specialized facility) and level of experience and expertise in this form of abuse.

In the following account the assumption is made that the child is admitted at some point to an acute paediatric ward. This is the central point of initial intervention. The role with the chronic exaggerator, who sometimes adds in lying and who tends to remain in the community, has been considered in Chapters 1 (in the 'Primary care' section) and 9.

The potential roles for the psychiatrist can be broadly categorized as: assisting the investigation, informing the child protection plan with psychiatric knowledge, perpetrator treatment, victim treatment and staff support. It may be necessary, although very difficult, to attempt some element of all of these roles at the same time in order to facilitate the eventual treatment of the perpetrator. It may be necessary to work with colleagues to share out these functions, although this introduces the problem of the need for a great deal of communication.

Early involvement

By early involvement we are referring to the phase before professional concerns are shared with parents (see above). Throughout the assessment and management process, a psychiatrist may be able to contribute either by direct work with the family or by indirect means.

Indirect work by consultation and liaison with professional colleagues in health, social services and education is a method of working often used by child and adolescent psychiatrists. In addition, a number of consultants have a special interest in paediatric liaison work. In practice, usually this means providing a service to the staff of an acute paediatric ward and the associated community services. If an adequate psychiatric–paediatric liaison service exists through good planning and appropriate funding, the ward and associated liaison service should be in a good position to manage the presentation of a case of MSBP abuse. If this is not the case, then local professionals will need to consider service development and may need to involve the Health Authority who are responsible for the commissioning of services. The Health Authority employ consultants in public health and also seek medical advice from doctors providing clinical services.

There are a number of ways in which a liaison service may be helpful: Chapter 14 gives further detail of some of these examples.

- Contributing to the continuing professional development of ward staff with a focus on child and family psychiatry which may include specific information about psychiatric aspects of MSBP abuse.
- Assistance in assessing the behaviour of a suspected MSBP fabricator, and child, perhaps including direct observation if this is possible.
- Contributing to planning the confrontation, focusing on the mental health of the fabricator – liaison with adult mental health services.
- Support for staff during the stressful experience of suspecting, diagnosing and confrontation.

An early task that is likely to be most useful is a one to one discussion with the suspecting paediatrician, followed by discussion with other paediatric staff. In addition to assistance with the issues as listed above, issues raised or evident may include differences of opinion amongst staff, and the fabricator forming inappropriate social relationships with staff (see Chapter 14 and Fisher, 1995). Subsequently, by collecting information from the medical notes supplemented by accounts from paediatric medical and nursing staff, it may be possible to begin to formulate hypotheses about the mental state of the suspected fabricator, the relationship with the child and the workings of the family, all of which will inform the initial risk assessment.

The issue of whether, in a small number of cases, it may be possible to do direct work with a parent early on, whilst the child is on the paediatric ward, is also addressed by Fisher. The psychiatrist may become involved following referral from the paediatrician and with the agreement of the suspected fabricator, on the basis of, for example, helping the mother cope with her anxieties about the health of the child. Through engagement and rapport building, the first objective is to present an opportunity for the mother to respond to support and unburden herself by expressing problems of not coping, if this is perceived to be the case. The further objective is to stop the need for progression along the fabrication spectrum. Thus the approach could be considered to be an unusual form of preventative medicine. This approach probably has limited potential and is only likely to be helpful in less serious cases, or in examples where 'help seeking' predominates. If there is a degree of engagement, however, the psychiatrist will also be in a more useful position to contribute to the overall assessment of risk to the child, by examination of the fabricator's mental state as an individual and in the relationship with the child. The enhanced value of observation and assessment (informed by a psychiatric training) at this time results from it being as contemporaneous as is possible with the period that is most pathological in the mother–child relationship, and in terms of the mother's abnormal relationship with the medical system. The value of this cannot be overestimated when compared with the very different situation after confrontation, when child protection procedures have further progressed and changes in the mental state of the fabricator are likely.

Putting concerns to the suspected fabricator: confrontation

If it has proved possible to form a rapport with the fabricator, the psychiatrist may be in a position to assist at the time of confrontation. How the confrontation with the fabricator is carried out will be a matter for the child's paediatrician to decide, in consultation with the local social services and the psychiatrist. The police may also have a role if they have already been involved in the monitoring on the ward and wish to interview the fabricator. The psychiatrist may be able to assist in predicting the likely reaction of the fabricator, which could in extreme cases range from anger and aggression, requiring protection for the child and staff, to suicidal thoughts and behaviour, requiring urgent intervention by the local adult psychiatric team.

Assessment after confrontation

The importance of planning a strategy and co-ordination of case management from the beginning cannot be over-emphasized. This means carrying on with the process of information gathering despite avoidance and challenges by the fabricator, ensuring the physical safety of the child at all times, and protecting the child from possible increased psychological and behavioural disturbance by the mother during the early phase of the assessment process. Engaging other members of the family in a working partnership becomes extremely important whether or not there is co-operation from the fabricator.

Whilst it is theoretically possible and would be very useful for a psychiatrist to remain involved after the pre-confrontation work in order to contribute to the full assessment, the fabricator may not agree to see this psychiatrist, who is perceived as being allied with the accusing paediatrician. In practice, therefore, the social services, often via their legal department, will need to commission a psychiatrist to undertake this piece of work.

It is worth emphasizing the point that an assessment can be thought of as a two-stage procedure. In the first stage, the issues will be the physical medical evidence regarding what has happened to the child and whether this constitutes harm and to what degree. In the second stage, the psychiatrist has a major role which is to provide an opinion about what will be the best options for the child, whether ultimately this be with the natural parents or in alternative care. In attempting to formulate such an important opinion, the key area of attention is the risk of further harm to the child in the context of the quality of the mother–child relationship. In addition to consideration of the situation at the time of the fabrications, the focus will be on the future and the assessment of the prospects for positive change.

Psychiatric contributions to the comprehensive assessment

Assessment may be undertaken in a number of settings, with corresponding resource implications:

- In the community – at home or during attendance at a day centre.
- Hospital in-patient unit with mother and baby facility.
- Hospital family unit.

The first decision will involve consideration of the safety and adequacy of carrying out an assessment in the community without in-patient observation of the family. It is practical to commence an assessment in the community and consider referral for in-patient work if community assessment becomes unsatisfactory. This is likely to mean that situations in the middle ground of risk, or of significant uncertainty, are likely to benefit from in-patient assessment. Examples of such situations include:

- If the prospects for rehabilitation look good, but some doubt remains and in-patient work will provide extra information and therapeutic momentum for the family.
- If there is disagreement between agencies about rehabilitation.
- If there appears to be good co-operation, but clever deception is suspected.
- If a great deal of therapeutic work needs to be done which is beyond community resources and expertise.

Situations which are assessed to be at the mild end of the spectrum of risk may be managed in the community. By contrast, at the other end of the spectrum of risk there is little point in referring families for in-patient work when the risk is very high and combined with inadequate co-operation, and there is therefore little prospect of rehabilitation. In-patient resources are scarce and it is realistic to make the best use of those that are available. Considerations for in-patient assessment and treatment are discussed in detail in Chapter 13.

Combining roles

There are a number of roles that a psychiatrist could take at this stage. Roles involving direct contact with the mother may include being the therapist for the fabricating mother (Coombe, 1995; Parnell and Day, 1988), working in a variety of ways (with or without the addition of work with the partner, or family work including children), or being an assessor, contributing towards the comprehensive assessment and ultimately the court process. It is complex to carry out therapeutic work from which the therapist(s) also provide reports to the court process. There are potential problems both in trying to separate the two roles and in combining them. Black and Hollis (1996) address this issue in their account of work with a couple after MSBP abuse. There may be conflict for the professionals in terms of balancing the wish to preserve a degree of confidentiality and providing sufficient information to the court for decisions to be made fairly. Disclosure considered to be excessive by the fabricator may lead to a loss of confidence and make ongoing therapeutic work difficult or impossible. The fabricator may try to use the sessions for persuading the professional of their point of view rather than taking the opportunity to use the time therapeutically. Working to maintain a balance will be a continuing theme.

Continuing the indirect role

Alternatively, the psychiatrist could continue indirect work by consultation to the social services department – for example, with advice regarding the ongoing strategy of the investigation, informed by indirectly monitoring the mental state of the fabricator and the psychological state of the children (especially for older children). The psychiatrist should be able to work closely with the local paediatrician. One of the tasks for the local paediatrician, and perhaps most suitable for one with a special interest in and time allocated for child protection work, will be to put together a chronology of all medical events, together with family information about the birth of children, moves of house etc. Whilst the paediatrician will be able to interpret the physical medical aspects, the psychiatrist will be able to apply a complementary perspective, and together this will be of great assistance in the risk assessment. Adding to the chronology from any other reliable records, such as social service files and police reports, will be invaluable (Precey, 1995). A further invaluable task is to complete parallel chronologies for all children in the family and the mother, which can be viewed at the same time.

Seeking an external opinion

It may sometimes be more appropriate, for the court process, to seek the opinion of a psychiatrist who is not local: an 'external' opinion. The circumstances in which this should be considered by the local psychiatrist are listed in *Child Psychiatry and The Law* (Black, Wolkind and Harris Hendricks, 1989) as follows:

- It is a complex or rare problem outside their competence.
- Their therapeutic relationship with the family may be jeopardized if they have to state an opinion in court.
- Their long term relationship with other agencies may be damaged.
- Their relationship with the family has already broken down, or the family has split up, or the local psychiatrist may be perceived, with or without reason, as acting partially.
- The NHS service would be jeopardized unreasonably by the time that would be taken up by the case.

The adult psychiatrist

Consideration of the individual psychopathology of the perpetrator, both in terms of type and severity, should indicate the sort of psychiatrist best suited to carry out a more extensive assessment. It may be useful, or essential, to have more than one expert opinion, and the complementary approaches of an adult psychiatrist (general, forensic or psychotherapist) and a child and adolescent psychiatrist are likely to be a useful combination.

When the variety of fabrication is persistent and severe, and the parent clearly displays very abnormal behaviour (for example, with other evidence of antisocial behaviour or a serious lack of co-operation), the forensic consultant may be the appropriate choice for an opinion. A forensic psychiatrist may also be the best professional to offer individual treatment. The forensic psychiatrist has special expertise in the management and treatment of people with significant personality disturbance and will have access to the most appropriate resources.

The question of one or more expert witnesses

The process of involving the best professional or combination of professionals may be complex. As soon as the local authority take the case into the court process, the situation may become more polarized and adversarial. This can then become an unusual and difficult situation for a doctor. Until recently, the legal representatives for the different parties in the court proceedings instructed experts independently, so that it was possible to have one expert witness instructed by the local authority, another instructed by the GAL and a third by the mother (and possibly a fourth by the father or grandparents). This situation has now changed so that, led by the proactive court, the neutral position of the doctor is reinforced from the beginning, so that he or she is better able to inform the court and all parties. The usual arrangement, in cases managed in this way, is for instructions to be put together by all parties in a letter of joint instruction. This is helpful in that:

- The questions to be asked of the expert have to be carefully considered and agreed by all parties.
- The family do not have to attend multiple interviews which are essentially for the same purpose.
- Any children old enough to be aware of what is happening are exposed to only one or two experts (even if they are not directly interviewed).
- The assessment may be carried out more quickly.
- There is more efficient use of expert witnesses.

There are possible disadvantages with the above situation, however:

- The situation is perceived as being out of control, and possibly biased, by the parents and their legal representatives, who are not able to select their own expert witness.
- Having two opinions allows for debate between different opinions and approaches in complex situations.

An approach to assessment

A developmental and ecological perspective is a widely accepted framework in which to consider child maltreatment, and it is also the foundation for assessment and intervention (see Chapter 13). The psychiatric assessment must therefore:

- Be integrated with the perspective of other disciplines, i.e. be multi-disciplinary – a common approach in child and adolescent psychiatry.
- Consider and integrate difficulties at the various levels of complexity.

In practice this means that an assessment will consist of a combination of assessments, including appraisal of:

1. Individual psychopathology of the perpetrator and other significant adults, both in terms of psychiatric diagnosis and the relationship with, and parenting of, the child.
2. The parent couple, both in terms of their parenting together and their wider relationship – for example, looking at transactional processes, adaptations to married life and parenthood, and consideration of the life cycle of the family.
3. The extended family – for example, are there unresolved intergenerational issues that could be usefully worked with? Do the grandparents perceive the problem in a way that will allow a balance between support and protection?
4. The local social and cultural influences surrounding the family, including the professional resources available.

Treatability

The issue of treatability is paramount and will include considerations at the levels outlined above, which can be summarized briefly as the intrapsychic, interpersonal and cultural elements. Treatability requires consideration of psychological conflict, denial (especially pertinent in MSBP abuse) and the possibility of forming a treatment alliance (Fitzpatrick, 1995). In practice, the fabricator should have the potential for acknowledgement that caretaking problems have occurred and for ownership of their contribution to the problems. There should be some internal motivation for change and an ability to see professionals as helpful.

Therapy or assessment?

Maintaining a therapeutic approach through an extended assessment process will be necessary and a challenge. The broad approach described by Reder and Lucey (1995), which they term 'therapeutic assessment', is recommended. The key issue is that the 'capacity to benefit from treatment and resume adequate care of their children only becomes evident over the course of a lengthy assessment process'. This is contrasted with the 'trial of therapy', which will 'occur over a small number of sessions, perhaps two or three, during which the assessor clarifies whether good treatment indicators are present and introduces the person to the process of therapy'.

The balance will need to be maintained between ongoing challenge by the assessor/therapist (which may be required because of the lack of recognition of difficulties, in some cases with dissociation, and lack of internal motivation to look at problems) and maintaining a therapeutic approach. A risk is that the balance between essential challenge and being perceived as therapeutic may be too difficult to tolerate. In one situation, a mother who had persistently fed diluted milk to her baby continued to perceive various medical problems including problems with feeding. The treatment plan included the therapist, regularly informed of what had been happening by the core group, being prepared to challenge the perceptions of the mother in an attempt to 'reconvert' the medical problems into real life problems. If successful, these problems could then be dealt with, rather than allowing them to be maintained as somatized presentations with the child.

Issues that will arise include who should be included in the therapeutic assessment and for how long should the therapeutic assessment continue.

The psychiatric report

The essential element of the report by the child psychiatrist will be an integration of information concerning the effects upon the child of what has happened so far, and what may happen in the future. There will be a range of possible courses and consequences that will need to be addressed. The likely implications for the future will be based on the assessed needs of the individual child, integrated with the conclusions of the four levels of assessment listed above (as points 1 4) in the section on 'An approach to assessment'. The focus from the psychiatric perspective will be the opinion regarding future risks to the child if reunited with the fabricator, with consideration of the response, or predicted response, to treatment of the fabricator and family. The issue of risk is further considered below.

There are many more issues to be considered in the production of a report and it is suggested that further publications be consulted, notably the books *Child Psychiatry and the Law* (Black, Wolkind and Harris Hendricks, 1989) and *Good Practice for Expert Witnesses* (Tufnell, Cottrell and Georgiades, 1996).

Looking ahead

Reunification and the specific risks

The process of reunification should be considered in the context of risk management, and therapeutic work will have as one of its primary goals risk reduction. It is unlikely that risks will be considered to be reduced to zero in most cases. In order for risks to be managed and reduced, the future risks must be estimated specifically, both in terms of type and severity. For example, the most dangerous risk in one situation may be a physical risk – the risk of further suffocation leading to brain damage or death. In another example, it might be an emotional risk – the risk of an attachment disorder and emotional neglect as a result of failing to meet emotional needs, or emotional abuse by keeping the child in an inappropriate sick role. All of these very different risks may co-exist in the same family.

For the child the risks of remaining with the fabricator must always be considered together with the risks of separation and alternative care. Both courses of action may carry very significant risks for the child and siblings, and it is the balance of the risks that will always need to be considered.

The importance of a long term strategy

Whenever a child remains with or is returned to a fabricating parent, the risks should be considered to be long term, unless there has been very substantial change during the treatment of the fabricator. The importance of long term management cannot be over-emphasized for the child and siblings. It is recommended that a long term strategy is implemented which will include medical and social services oversight. This has implications for agencies working together over long periods of time. The limitations of the time-scale of a supervision order have already been discussed.

De-registration – removal of child's name from the At Risk Register

Not infrequently the stated aim of any parent with a child on the At Risk Register is to have the child's name removed from that register. There can be considerable tension around the time of each Child Protection Review as the parents learn what will be said about their care of the child and whether there has been sufficient progress for de-registration.

Whilst the issue of de-registration must be considered at every review, in examples of MSBP abuse it should not come about simply because the extended three year supervision order has come to an end, or because there has been co-operation from the family towards those working with them, or as a gesture of encouragement to the family. As fabrication of illness by its nature has the potential to be a long term problem, de-registration should only be agreed when the programme of intended work with the family has been addressed or the child's circumstances have changed so that the child is no longer at risk. It is essential that de-registration only occurs with the complete agreement of all the key medical and social services personnel involved with the family, ideally including the professionals who have been most closely involved throughout what may be a lengthy process.

Rarely it may be the case that, after many years of having support from different agencies because their child's name is on the Register, the parents do not want de-registration, as they have become dependent on the help available. Such an unusual view would need to be taken into account in making the final decision.

References

Black, D., Wolkind, W. and Harris Hendricks, J. (1989) *Child Psychiatry and the Law*. Royal College of Psychiatrists.

Black, D., Wolkind, W. and Harris Hendricks, J. (1989) Clinical and forensic child psychiatry: forensic second opinions. In *Child Psychiatry and the Law*. Royal College of Psychiatrists, pp. 1–5.

Black, D. and Hollis, P. (1996) Treatment of a case of factitious illness by proxy. *Clinical Child Psychology and Psychiatry*, **1**, 89–98.

Bluglass, K. (1997) Munchausen syndrome by proxy. In *A Practical Guide to Forensic Psychotherapy* (Welldon, E. and Van Velson, C., eds), pp. 89–97. Jessica Kingsley, Publisher.

Bools, C.N., Neale, B. and Meadow, R. (1994) Munchausen syndrome by proxy: a study of psychopathology. *Child Abuse and Neglect*, **18**, 773–778.

Bools, C. (1996) Factitious illness by proxy: Munchausen syndrome by proxy. *British Journal of Psychiatry*, **169**, 268–275.

Coombe, P. (1995) The in-patient psychotherapy of a mother and child at the Cassel Hospital: a case of Munchausen syndrome by proxy. *British Journal of Psychotherapy*, **12**, 195–207.

Department of Health (1988) Protecting Children. A Guide for Social Workers Undertaking a Comprehensive Assessment. HMSO.

Department of Health, British Medical Association, Conference of Medical Royal Colleges (1991) Child Protection: Medical Responsibilities. Guidance for Doctors Working with Child Protection Agencies. Addendum to 'Working Together Under The Children Act 1989'. HMSO.

Fisher, G.C. (1995) The role of psychiatry. In *Munchausen Syndrome by Proxy. Issues in Diagnosis and Management* (Levin, A.V. and Sheridan, M.S., eds), pp. 369–397. Lexington Books.

Fisher, G., Mitchell, I. and Murdoch, D. (1993) Munchausen's syndrome by proxy. The question of psychiatric illness in a child. *British Journal of Psychiatry*, **162**, 701–703.

Fitzpatrick, G. (1995) Assessing treatability. In *Assessment of Parenting: Psychiatric and Psychological Contributions* (Reder, P. and Lucey, C., eds), pp.102–117. Routledge.

Gray, J. and Bentovim, A. (1996) Illness induction syndrome: Paper 1. A series of 41 children from 37 families identified at great Ormond Street Hospital for Children NHS Trust. *Child Abuse and Neglect*, **20**, 665–673.

Gray, J., Bentovim, A. and Milla, P. (1995) The treatment of children and their families where induced illness has been identified. In *Trust Betrayed? Munchausen Syndrome by Proxy, Interagency Child Protection and Partnership with Families* (Horwath, J. and Lawson, B., eds), pp. 149–162. National Children's Bureau.

Home Office, Department of Health, Department of Education and Science, and Welsh Office (1991) Working Together Under the Children Act 1989. A guide to arrangements for interagency co-operation for the protection of children from abuse. HMSO.

Jones, D.P.H. and Bools, C.N. (1999) Factitious illness by proxy. In *Recent Advances in Paediatrics*, Vol. 17 (David, T.J., ed.), pp. 57–71. Churchill Livingstone.

Jurcidini, J. (1993) Obstetric factitious disorder and Munchausen syndrome by proxy. *Journal of Nervous and Mental Disease*, **181**, 135–137.

Libow, J.A. and Schreier, H.A. (1986) Three forms of factitious illness in children: when is it Munchausen syndrome by proxy. *American Journal of Orthopsychiatry*, **56**, 602–611.

Lynch, M. (1976) Risk factors in the child. In *The Abused Child* (Ballinger, M.H., ed.) quoted in Department of Health 1988.

Neale, B., Bools, C. and Meadow, R. (1991) Problems in the assessment and management of Munchausen syndrome by proxy abuse. *Children and Society*, **5**, 324–333.

Parnell, T.F. and Day, D.O. (1998) *Munchausen by Proxy Syndrome: Misunderstood Child Abuse*. Sage.

Precey, G. (1995) On first encountering Munchausen syndrome by proxy: a guide for beginners. In *Trust Betrayed?* (Horwath, J. and Lawson, B., eds), pp. 24–46. National Children's Bureau.

Reder, P. and Lucey, C. (1995) *Assessment of Parenting: Psychiatric and Psychological Contributions*. Routledge.

Tufnell, G., Cottrell, D. and Georgiades, D. (1996) 'Good practice' for expert witnesses. *Clinical Child Psychology and Psychiatry*, **1**, 365–383.

12

Munchausen syndrome by proxy – legal aspects

Vera Mayer, Lesley-Anne Cull and Christopher Bools

The framework of the Children Act 1989

The Children Act 1989 provided a new framework for the welfare of children. The Act represented a fresh start for lawyers and professionals working with children and families. It established a new range of orders for the benefit and protection of children, with new criteria. The central concepts of the Children Act are that:

1. The child's welfare is the court's paramount consideration for any court in deciding any question with respect to the upbringing of a child (Section 1(1)).
2. Any delay in deciding issues involved is likely to prejudice the welfare of the child and should be avoided if possible (Section 1(2)).
3. A court cannot make any order in respect of a child unless it is satisfied that the making of the order would be better for the child than making no order at all (Section 1 (5)).

The key words in Section 1 are 'welfare' and 'paramount'. Welfare is a concept that is easy to recognize but hard to define. In framing the Children Act 1989, the Law Commission used the following definition (Walsh, 1998):

'Welfare is an all encompassing word. It includes material welfare in the sense of adequacy of resources to provide a pleasant home and a comfortable standard of living and in the sense of adequacy of care to ensure good health and due personal pride are maintained. However, while material considerations have their place, they are secondary matters. More important are the stability and security, the warm and compassionate relationships, that are essential for the full development of the child's own character, personality and talents.'

Section 1(3) sets criteria that the court must take into consideration when making a decision whether or not to grant a local authority a care order in respect of a child. The list is not exhaustive and not the only consideration the court must have reference to, but it provides a framework for the decision-making process.

Section 1(3) is commonly referred to as 'the welfare checklist' and sets out the following issues:

1. The ascertainable wishes and feelings of the child concerned (considered in the light of his age and understanding).
2. His physical, emotional and educational needs.
3. The likely effect on him of any change of circumstances.
4. His age, sex, background and any characteristics which the court considers relevant.
5. Any harm which he has suffered or is at risk of suffering.
6. How capable each of his parents, and any other relevant person in relation to whom the court considers the question to be relevant, is of meeting his needs.
7. The range of powers available to the court under the Act in the proceedings in question.

In those cases where a local authority is making an application for a care order on the basis of evidence suggesting that the child is a victim of Munchausen syndrome by proxy (MSBP) abuse, the court must have particular regard to the question of significant harm. This will be explored further below.

The 1989 Children Act reflected in part a wide range of concerns around state intervention in family life, and it forms the basis of law relating to children and their welfare. The emphasis on welfare can be recognized in the Act's central principles of the importance of working in partnership with children and families and of reaching agreements (wherever possible) in planning for children. The emphasis is on keeping children with their families and it sets out a range of duties on local authorities to provide services and facilities for children in their area. Accompanying the Act is a multitude of guidance notes, regulations and circulars encouraging professionals to negotiate with, to inform and to empower parents and children. The Act supports the keeping of statutory proceedings and emergency interventions to a minimum; for example, Section 1(3) specifically requires the court to consider whether an order needs to be made in respect of a child who is the subject of proceedings.

There are cases however, where intervention to protect a child's welfare is necessary. Suspected cases of MSBP abuse usually fall within this category. The criteria for state intervention under the Children Act is that the child concerned is suffering, or is likely to suffer from, significant harm (Section 31(2)(a)). Therefore, under the Act, intervention can be made on the basis of a prediction of what might occur or might be likely to occur to the child in the future.

The assessment of actual or likely significant harm has become a central concern around which proceedings are frequently based. In addition, methodology of assessment, and interpretation of medical findings and reports, may themselves be contested. Given the nature of allegations in MSBP abuse, and the consequences of any decision for the future of the child concerned, it is essential that the court is provided with sufficiently informed evidence on which to base a decision. Therefore in cases involving allegations of MSBP abuse, forensic (i.e. medical) evidence is necessary.

The critical issue of harm and significant harm

In care proceedings, the level of proof required is a balance of probabilities, not beyond reasonable doubt as in the criminal court. However, paradoxically, there may in fact be more difficulty in reaching the necessary standard in those cases where the nature of the allegations is particularly serious. The *House of Lords in Re H and R (Minors) (Sexual Abuse: Standard of Proof, 1996)* 1 All ER 1 addressed the issue of the standard of proof required to establish that a child has suffered significant harm in the past. Lord Nicholls, who delivered the majority opinion, stated that the correct standard of proof required for proving the occurrence of significant harm in the past, is the balance of probabilities. Accordingly, the court should be able to reach a finding that 'on the evidence, the occurrence of the event is more likely than not'. (per Lord Nicholls at p16). This appeared to be a move away from previous case law whereby the more serious the allegations the more cogent the evidence required to prove them.

However, Lord Nicholls went on to state that:

'When assessing the probabilities the court will have in mind as a factor ... that the more serious the allegation the less likely it is that the event occurred and, hence, the stronger should be the evidence before the court concludes that the allegation is established on the balance of probability ... The more improbable the event, the stronger must be the evidence that it did occur before, on the balance of probability, its occurrence will be established.'

The reality is, therefore, that the courts will continue to require more cogent evidence where allegations are of a more serious nature.

The second part of the decision in *Re H* regarding the standard of proof relates to the likelihood of future significant harm. The House of Lords held in *Re H* that where there was insufficient evidence to establish (on a balance of probabilities) significant harm in the past, the same evidence could not establish a likelihood of future significant harm to a child.

This restrictive approach, which appears to leave the child in the position that the more serious the risk, the more difficulty the local authority will experience in obtaining a care order, is in contrast to the relaxation of the rules of evidence in hearings involving children. In particular, where expert evidence has been obtained by any party to the proceedings, that evidence is not protected from disclosure by legal professional privilege. For example, where a report is unfavourable to the parent concerned, this must still be disclosed in the proceedings: *Oxfordshire County Council v M* [1994] 2 All ER 269. This was confirmed by the House of Lords in *Re L (A Minor)(Police Investigation: Privilege)* [1996] 2 All ER 7 (Fortin, 1998).

The complexity of the issue of significant harm where MSBP has occurred

In cases involving identification of MSBP abuse the issue of significant harm to a child may be a subtle one. A mother who presents her child at hospital frequently may not have caused physical harm, but may be exposing the child to persistent examinations, which in themselves often involve intrusive physical techniques. In addition, arguably, there is an element of emotional harm by exposing a child to continued intervention unnecessarily. In many of these cases, however, the issue will be one of future significant harm and thus the ability to predict and extrapolate from present data and present diagnosis of the adult into future significant harm to the child, be it physical and/or emotional.

In a recent case, a father himself was diagnosed as suffering from a factitious illness. The whole family functioned within the home as if the father was gravely ill. The issue of MSBP abuse was brought to light when the father presented one of his children at hospital. As a result of what the father told doctors, the child underwent ten days of intrusive tests. It became clear that there was nothing wrong with the child and it was strongly suspected that the father had falsely reported the child's symptoms. The issues were whether the child had suffered significant harm and, more importantly, whether he was likely to suffer significant harm in the future. The question of significant harm related not only to whether the child had suffered physically as a result of needless medical tests but also whether the father's psychopathology made him a risk to the child in the future. This case raises an important point in relation to MSBP abuse. Professionals in a case may become too focused on the fabrication of illness in the child and fail to recognize that other aspects of the relationship between the perpetrator and the child may in themselves constitute emotional neglect and/or abuse, with a risk of significant harm.

The legal personnel

Local authority legal department

As stated earlier, the local authority has a duty to work in partnership with parents and to facilitate the care of children within their own families. However, where sufficient concern leads to the application for a care order, the local authority must consider and focus upon the specific issues upon which the application will be based. These include the evidence needed to support the application, the proposed care plan and the likely time-scale for concluding the court case in the light of the complexities involved and the ages and needs of the child. The local authority will have the burden of establishing the likelihood of significant harm to the child.

Guardian ad litem (GAL)

Where there are public law proceedings the court must appoint a guardian *ad litem* (GAL) for the child concerned. The GAL's duties are prescribed by the rules of the court and include the main duty of safeguarding the child's interests (see Chapter 11). One duty is to appoint a solicitor to represent the child. The appointment of a GAL is made as soon as practicable after the commencement of proceedings or the arrival of transferred proceedings if the transferring court has not already made the appointment.

The Guardians *ad litem* and Reporting Officers (Panels) Regulations 1991 provide that any GAL appointed under the Children Act 1989 must be selected from a panel established by the local authority. There are currently 54 panels in England and six in Wales. In some areas voluntary agencies such as Barnado's or the Children's Society provide a guardian *ad litem* service on behalf of the local authority. A GAL is appointed to a panel for a maximum of three years. When that time expires, he or she must reapply. The guardian proposed in a case can come from any panel in England and Wales, unless they have a particularly close connection with the local authority bringing the case. When appointed, the court may specify the length of the appointment; otherwise the appointment will last until terminated by the court. The latter is the more usual course.

Under the Children Act 1989, Section 41(2)(b), the GAL is under a duty to safeguard the interests of the child in the manner prescribed by the rules of the court. However, if a care order is made, the GAL has no role in relation to the way in which the local authority performs its duties under the order, and the court has no power to direct the continuing involvement of the GAL.

The duties of a GAL are set out in the Family Proceedings Rules 1991 and include the following:

- Ascertaining the wishes and feelings of all parties, especially the child and his or her siblings, in relation to each alternative.
- Giving appropriate advice to the child and giving instructions to the child's solicitor on all matters relevant to the child.
- Notifying everybody who should be made a party to the proceedings in order to safeguard the child's interests.
- Attending all the hearings and giving advice to the court.
- Preparing a written report whenever asked to do so and always for the final hearing.
- Serving and accepting documents on the child's behalf and, if the child is mature enough, telling the child what is in the documents.

In carrying out the investigation, the GAL must have regard to the welfare checklist. In particular, he or she must interview a number of people, such as the child and family and relevant professionals. In addition, he or she must inspect relevant records and seek professional assistance from expert witnesses if this is appropriate (or the court directs it). For example, the GAL has the right to examine and copy all social services files relating to the child, as well as all local authority, voluntary organization and children's home records.

In the report, the GAL must address several issues including the child's level of understanding (including his or her ability to refuse a medical or other examination), the options available to the court and a recommendation as to the most appropriate order he or she considers should be made.

Solicitor for the child

The GAL is expected to bring to the attention of the court any conflict between his or her views and those of the child (*per Wall in Re M (Minors) (Care Proceedings: Child's wishes)* [1994] 1 FLR 749, at p754). This would include the duty to advise the court whether the child is capable of instructing her solicitor independently (the guardian may then, with leave, be granted separate legal representation). In such circumstances, the child's solicitor can only take instructions from the child alone if satisfied that the child is 'able, having regard to his understanding, to give such instructions on his own behalf...' (FPR [1991], r.4.12(1)(a)). However, it is important to note that a child deemed to have sufficient understanding to instruct a solicitor will be served by an adult whose duties are far more restricted than those of a GAL. A solicitor acting for a child in these circumstances is under no legal duty to provide her client with any emotional support, to mediate between the child and her family, or indeed to provide the court with any information about the solicitor's perceptions of the child's best interests. Obvious judicial misgivings about these changes led to two rapid developments, both aiming to concentrate supervisory powers over children instituting legal proceedings in the High Court judiciary. First, there was a practice direction issued in 1993 indicating that all applications for leave brought by children under Section 10(8) of CA1989 were more suitable for determination by the High Court and would be transferred there if started any lower (Practice Direction [1993] 1 All ER 820). Second, case law established that the courts have the final word over whether children have sufficient capacity to instruct a solicitor to initiate or carry through legal proceedings without the services of a GAL (*see Re T (A Minor)(Child: Representation)* [1993] 4 All ER 518).

Barristers for all parties

Barristers usually become involved in a case at some stage during the proceedings. That stage is as often determined by the workload and experience of the solicitor who has conduct of the case as it is by the ability and expertise of the barrister who is instructed by the solicitor. Since children's proceedings have always been in chambers (i.e. not in open court), solicitors have had right of audience for many years and quite a few have had an opportunity to practise advocacy skills in a manner similar to that of the Bar. Thus, often solicitors deal with many of the preliminary applications in a protracted public case, and no doubt would deal with final hearings if it were practical for them to spend two to three weeks in court, and on top of that run a busy solicitor's office!

The reality is that the majority of contested High Court litigation is conducted by specialist barristers. They are people with many years' experience in dealing with similar matters, versed in the likely difficulties and familiar with the subject matter and with practical aspects of the cases. Family proceeding courts and county courts see more and more solicitor advocates. Some local authorities use in-house advocates for interlocutory and indeed final hearings; they may, however, require legal opinion to advise whether there is merit in pursuing an application in a given case. For this they would often instruct a barrister.

Once instructed in proceedings, the barrister works with the client and solicitor through to the final hearing of the matter.

The Official Solicitor (OS)

The Official Solicitor (OS) to the Supreme Court is appointed by the Lord Chancellor to look after the interests of children, the mentally ill and others who are unable to represent themselves in court. The OS is a barrister who works independently of the government and local authorities. He has a team of about 130 staff, about 10 per cent being qualified lawyers. Most of the OS staff are civil servants who specialize in particular areas of work and about half of the staff have day to day conduct of cases under the supervision of senior lawyers.

The OS acts as a GAL or 'next friend' in family proceedings in the county court (i.e. private proceedings or adoption) and the High Court. Where the OS acts for a child, his main duty is to make recommendations in the best interests of that child. In this role he investigates the child's wishes and views and conveys them to the court, giving advice on options for the future. In complex cases, the help will be sought of a consultant psychiatrist, psychologist or paediatrician.

The OS may be appointed in the following circumstances.

1. In Public Law proceedings under the Children Act, the OS may be appointed in and by the High Court where:
2. the child does not have a GAL in the proceedings; and there are exceptional circumstances which make it desirable, in the interests of the welfare of the child, why the OS should be appointed. For example, where there is a foreign element, where there are several children, where there are other High Court proceedings in which the OS is representing the children, or any other exceptional circumstances the court thinks are relevant.
3. In Private Law proceedings under the Children Act, the OS can act in the High Court or county courts (but not family proceedings courts). In most cases, a child's interests are sufficiently safeguarded by a CWO report. Only where this is not so, would the question of appointing the OS arise and even then the appointment should be exceptional rather than automatic.
4. The OS will accept appointments in those exceptional cases in which it has been established that a child's interests might not be adequately protected by a court welfare report and when it is desirable that the child should be separately represented. Such exceptional circumstances include those where: there is a substantial foreign element; there are exceptional or difficult points of law; there are unusual features, such as if one parent has killed the other or one parent is a transsexual; there is conflicting or controversial medical evidence; a child is ignorant as to his or her true parentage or is refusing contact with a parent, thus indicating a need for psychiatric assessment; he is acting for the child in other proceedings.

5. The OS will almost invariably accept the appointment in the following cases: where a child wants separate representation but he or she is not thought competent by the court; where a child is separately represented but the court needs the assistance of the OS either as GAL or 'next friend' or *amicus curiae* (an advisor to the court); where there are difficult issues such as medical confidentiality; in special category cases such as in sterilization or abortion cases, which come under the inherent jurisdiction of the High Court.
6. The OS may act as the 'next friend' of a child who wants to get a court's leave to make an application under the 1989 Act or in other family proceedings. He can also accept appointment in respect of a child who is a mother of a child involved in family proceedings (Lord Chancellor, 1991).

Preparation for court in care proceedings

As soon as an application in respect of a child is made by the local authority, a directions appointment is set for all the parties and their legal representatives to meet. A range of issues must be addressed by all the parties at this stage. For example, whether there should be a split hearing, timetabling for statements and the instruction of expert witnesses. The local authority is expected to have set out the issues within a comprehensive care plan in order that the parties know what case they have to meet. The basic principle is that the earlier matters are considered and acted upon by the parties and their advisors, the better the court process can serve the interests of children.

Appointment of expert witnesses

In any case, the court must give leave before a medical or psychiatric examination or other assessment of a child can take place. There was a growing trend over recent years for an increasing number of experts to be instructed in a case, thus increasing the adversarial nature of proceedings and the length of time it took for final hearings to be completed. It was eventually felt necessary to set down guidelines in order to limit this practice and in *Re C (Expert Witnesses)* [1996] 2 FLR 115: Bracewell J set down the following points as good practice when instructing experts:

1. Generalized orders for leave to disclose the papers to an expert should never be made. The area of expertise, the issues to be addressed and the particular expert should be identified in advance of the appointment.
2. The court has a duty to inquire into the information provided by the advocate, in particular the category of expert evidence sought to be adduced, the name and the availability of the expert and the relevance to the issues of the case.
3. Experts' reports based solely upon leave to disclose documents in a paper exercise are rarely as persuasive as those reports based on interviews and assessments as well as documentation.

Additional guidance can be found in the case of *Re C (Expert Evidence: Disclosure: Practice)* [1995] 1 FLR 204. The court stated that, in contested cases, it should be a condition of appointment of any expert that he or she be required to hold discussions with other experts instructed in the same field of expertise in advance of the hearing in order to identify areas of agreement and dispute. These meetings should be chaired by a co-ordinator, such as the guardian *ad litem*.

With regard to the content of letters of instruction and provision of information to experts appointed, Bracewell J stated that:

1. Medical experts asked to give reports must be fully instructed.
2. Letters of instruction should identify any relevant issues of fact to enable each expert to give an opinion on each set of competing issues, so that the court, on determining the facts, can consider the relevant expert opinion.

The experience of the experts and the courts has been that the bulk of expert reports were brought into being before the facts of the case had been established and so were often premised upon a wrong factual base. However, following the guidelines set down by Bracewell J, it is hoped that expert reports are now more likely to address the relevant issues of each case.

The expert witness report

In most cases of MSBP abuse the expert witness is a psychiatrist or a psychologist. The ideal is of an expert witness as an unbiased authority simply reporting findings from the perspective of his or her professional judgement. This does not, however, reflect the practical difficulties that can be experienced in a case. Although there may be consensus between all the experts in a case, frequently there is not. There can be a number of reasons for the differences. For example, areas of expertise or different theoretical orientations may result in disagreement. It is clearly of use to the court, where there are different expert opinions, to have an understanding of the ways in which assessments were undertaken, and the status attributed to different methods of interviewing and so on. For this reason, there are certain duties that an expert owes when writing a report for use in court and when giving evidence. The following should be noted:

- The expert report as presented to the court must be, and must be seen to be, the independent product of the expert, uninfluenced by the instructing party.
- An expert should provide independent assistance to the court by way of objective, unbiased opinion in relation to matters within his or her expertise and should never assume the role of an advocate.
- In his or her report, the expert should state the facts or assumptions upon which his or her opinion is based and should not omit to consider material facts that could detract from his or her concluded opinion.
- The expert should make it clear when a particular aspect of the case is outside his or her expertise.
- If the expert's opinion is not properly researched because it appears that insuf-

ficient data are available, he or she must say so, indicating that the opinion is no more than a provisional one (*Re J (A Minor) (Expert Evidence)* [1991] FCR 193).

- When an expert advances a hypothesis to explain a given set of facts, he or she owes a duty to explain to the court that what he or she is advancing is a hypothesis, and to inform the court if the hypothesis is controversial. The expert also has a duty to place before the court all available material that contradicts the hypothesis.
- If an opinion is based, wholly or in part, on research conducted by others, the expert must set this out clearly in his or her report, identifying the research relied on. The expert should state the relevance of the research to the points in issue in the case and be prepared to justify the opinions he or she expresses.
- If, after exchanging reports, an expert has a change of mind on a material matter, he or she should inform the other parties and the court (Practice Note, 1990).

The role of the expert in court

In some cases there will be a consensus between the experts. In others there will be a narrowing down of the issues in the meeting prior to the final hearing. However, even supposing this to be the case, it is not unusual to find that areas of disagreement remain. These may relate to conclusions reached by each expert as to whether the threshold criteria under Section 31 are met, or there may be disagreement as to the future course to be adopted for the child's welfare and safety. What is a judge to do when faced with the problem of experts who disagree? What is the role of the expert in this situation? This issue was addressed in *Re AB (Child Abuse: Expert Witnesses)* [1995] 1 FLR at 191 by Mr Justice Wall, who stated:

'...it is not for the judge to become involved in medical controversy except in rare cases where such a controversy is itself an issue in the case and judicial assessment of it becomes necessary for the proper resolution of the proceedings. Whilst the judge has knowledge and experience from practice and previous cases, he or she rarely has more medical knowledge than the intelligent lay person: the judge, almost by definition, is not an expert in the field about which the expert is giving evidence.'

The judge brings to the inquiry forensic and analytical skills and has the unique advantage over the parties and the witnesses in the case, that he or she alone is in a position to weigh all its multifarious facets.

Mr Justice Wall went on to state that:

'...the dependence of the court on the skill, knowledge and, above all, the professional integrity of the expert witness, cannot be over-emphasized.'

The expert, therefore, informs an assessment and expresses his opinion within the particular area of expertise. The judge, however, has a unique overview of the case, and it is his or her role to decide particular issues in the case.

Can an expert report on a case where he or she has carried out a 'paper' investigation? In MSBP abuse cases, there is an argument for saying that an expert may give valuable evidence on the papers and that such an investigation may, in fact, be more valuable than interviewing an alleged perpetrator. This could be true with respect to assessment of the risk as well as regarding the possibility of successfully treating the perpetrator. It is true that the court may find reports of this nature valuable, particularly in the case of MSBP abuse, on a preliminary point. However, when comparing the strength of evidence in contested hearings, there is no doubt that greater weight is likely to be given to those experts who have actually interviewed the alleged perpetrator. Even more compelling, arguably, is a report based in part on observation of interaction between the alleged perpetrator and the child.

This leads to a consideration of the weight given to expert evidence in care proceedings. It was once considered that the expert's role was merely to say whether evidence was consistent or not consistent with child abuse. However, it was stated by the Court of Appeal in *Re M and N (Child Abuse: Evidence)* [1996] 2 FLR 489 that 'in cases involving child abuse, the expert evidence may relate to the presence and interpretation of physical signs. But it may also relate to the more problematical area of the presence and interpretation of mental, behavioural and emotional signs. That evidence often necessarily includes, if not a conclusion, a strong pointer as to the expert's view of the likely veracity of the [interviewee] ... indeed the diagnosis and the action taken by the local authority may depend on the conclusion reached'. The judge may therefore rely on expert opinion when considering the issues, while never losing sight of the fact that the final decision with respect to the child rests with him or her.

The case for split hearings

Courts and practitioners need to be alert to identify those cases that are suited to a split hearing. In general they are likely to be cases in which there is a clear and stark issue, such as sexual abuse or physical abuse. It may be that MSBP abuse cases would fall into this category, although for slightly different reasons. In cases of non-accidental injury (NAI), there may be a number of possible perpetrators. The purpose of a split hearing is for the court in the first hearing to make findings as to the occurrence of NAI and the person responsible. Generally in MSBP abuse cases, the identity of the alleged perpetrator is clear. The purpose of a split hearing would be to decide whether abuse has taken place. As indicated earlier in this chapter, the issue of whether the child has been abused may not be obvious, particularly where fabrication has been verbal. In the case described above, the father had not administered substances to the child, nor had he smothered him (two frequent presentations of MSBP abuse). However, by lying to the medical staff, the father had caused the child to undergo a series of unnecessary tests. In such a case, a split hearing would mean that the court could make findings as to whether abuse had occurred. The second hearing would then be able to focus on the future for the child by considering assessment of risk and the potential for change in the perpetrator. Local authorities and GALs can and should give assistance to the court in identifying such cases in order to prevent delay and the ill-focused use of scarce expert resources. The court is asked in the first hearing to make findings with regard to the perpetrator of the abuse. Following this, a further hearing is set down for consideration of the best way forward in the interests of the child. An example can be found in the case of *Re S (Care Proceedings: Split Hearings)* [1996] 2 FLR 773.

The facts were that on 30 March 1995, S (then aged 10 months) was admitted to hospital having suffered serious injuries which were non-accidental. An application for a care order in respect of S was made on 10 April 1995. The full hearing commenced on 18 June 1996. Although the issues had been clear at an early stage of proceedings, the local authority could present no definitive care plan as the factual issues required determination. In the long period between application and hearing, various assessments had been carried out by separately instructed experts; not all the experts had received all relevant information, and no meeting occurred in advance of the hearing. Neither the experts, nor the local authority, nor the GAL were able to make recommendations as to the outcome at the time of the hearing.

Criticizing the conduct of professionals in the case, Bracewell J stated that, as soon as the medical evidence was obtained by the various parties, it should have become clear that the area of factual dispute related to the identity of the perpetrator. This involved an investigation of the causation and timing of the injuries, the pattern of movements of S between two households, and statements and explanations given by the adult carers. Until those issues were resolved, any consideration of the outcome for the child was neither feasible nor desirable. In her judgement (given in open court), Bracewell J made a care order and issued the following guidelines:

1. Judges and practitioners should be alert to identify those contested care proceedings cases that would be suited to a split hearing.
2. Identification should be made of cases where there was a clear issue of sexual and/or physical abuse.
3. The identified cases should then have an early hearing to decide factual issues. The substantive hearing would then be able to focus on the welfare of the child with greater clarity.
4. Experts in the same field of expertise should meet in advance of the preliminary hearing to identify areas of agreement and dispute, which should then be incorporated into a schedule for the court.

A further example of the advantage of split hearings can be seen in the case of *Re CD and MD (Care Proceedings: Practice)* [1998] 1 FLR 82. The facts are that in November 1996 a one month old baby was admitted to hospital with severe head injuries. Diagnosis was of at least two non-accidental incidents. The baby (CD) was discharged into the care of her grandparents. MD (the brother of CD), aged two years, remained living with his mother. Social services began an investigation of the family but were met with hostility from both parents and grandparents, who all refused to co-operate. However, the local authority did not apply for any order until February 1997. It then applied for a care order in respect of CD and a supervision order in respect of MD. There was evidence that the family had concealed domestic violence. After intervention by the GAL the local authority changed its application in respect of MD to a care order. There were four amendments to the local authority care plan for CD, the last being only two days prior to the final hearing. It was proposed by the local authority that CD should be adopted outside the family.

The court found in this case that the threshold criteria in Section 31 Children Act 1989 were satisfied in respect of both CD and MD, and care orders were made in respect of each child. Bracewell J made a number of critical observations on the conduct of the case. Firstly, the delay by the local authority in bringing proceedings. This was seen as extremely detrimental to both children. In the absence of admissions by the parents, there was no basis upon which any assessment could be undertaken. Care proceedings should have been commenced in respect of each child by late November 1996. The case was a clear example of one where an early split hearing could have resolved the disputed issues of fact – an application for a split hearing should have been made at the first directions hearing.

There are clearly a number of cases for which split hearings are appropriate. The more easily identifiable cases could include, for example:

- Physical injury where causation is denied.
- Physical injury where there is a dispute as to causation between medical experts.
- Sexual abuse cases where the allegations are denied.
- Failure to thrive cases with a documented medical history.
- Neglect cases where there is a documented history of parenting failure.
- 'Risk' cases that depend on factual determination being made on the basis of historical information.

It is possible that MSBP abuse cases could fall into a number of these categories; prima facie these are ideal for split hearings. However, professionals should be careful not to rush into requests for split hearings, as these cases are much more complex than the relatively straightforward non-accidental injury cases. For example, the evidence regarding significant harm is likely to rely on more than merely physical medical expertise. It could be argued that in MSBP abuse cases, the totality of evidence needs to be examined, including the admission of psychiatric evidence. In *Re CB and JB (Care Proceedings: Guidelines)* [1998] 2 FLR 211, however, Wall J stated that, when a split hearing is ordered, it is unlikely that evidence of propensity of character will be relevant to the issue of fact to be determined. In addition, he stated that it would rarely be appropriate for expert psychiatric or psychological evidence of the parents' propensity to injure a child or the likelihood of their having done so to be adduced. Certainly, the incidence of MSBP abuse has to be proven on the basis of facts and coincidence of circumstance. The abuse is almost always denied and it is essential for facts to be established in order to be able to go on to consider future plans for the child.

Split hearings in MSBP cases

There are cases, however, where the medical (forensic) and psychiatric issues are so intertwined that it may well be impossible, or perhaps inappropriate, to separate the psychiatric factors from preliminary questions of a pure factual/forensic nature.

A hydrocephalic child was in hospital as a result of complications with an external drain draining cerebrospinal fluid. The hospital became suspicious of the mother's behaviour and thought she was tampering with the child's equipment so as to harm him and attract sympathy and attention. The child suffered an above average number of disconnections of the drain and an inordinate number of infections, which the local microbiologist thought impossible to have occurred without external intervention (a view, incidentally, disagreed with by an equally eminent biologist). The nurses described some strange and extremely worrying behaviour on the part of the mother. For example, she told stories which were highly elaborate but had no roots in reality. She had reported deaths within the family (parents, sister) which were completely untrue. In addition, she reported attending different hospitals with one of her other children and indeed on behalf of herself, some of which was untrue and some of which was unnecessary. Certainly the local psychiatrist felt that the mother was exhibiting many features commonly associated with MSBP abuse. None of this evidence was considered by the trial judge, since the first part of the split hearing dealt with forensic issues only. It was clear that the medical evidence was so disputed as to not enable the judge to come to any conclusions based on balance of probabilities. The case concluded before any psychiatric evidence was introduced. It left some participants wondering whether the exclusion of all psychiatric evidence did serve in the best interests of the child. This example lends support to the argument that each case has to be considered on its own facts and there should not be a uniform approach.

In considering the appropriateness of a split hearing in MSBP abuse cases, it may be that, where findings are made with respect to the threshold criteria, this enables some parents to move to an acknowledgement and acceptance of the need for help. This lends further weight to the argument for split hearings in MSBP abuse cases. Once the court has established what happened to the child, psychological or psychiatric evidence can be presented at the second hearing regarding the perpetrator's potential for change. In the last chapter, the implications of whether a parent was able to accept his or her responsibility in harming the child and the relevance of treatment for such a parent, were examined. These issues clearly have a significant impact on the nature of the care plan and ultimately the order made at the second (final) hearing in respect of the child's future. However, even when a parent or both parents are unable to accept a court's findings, the court and the parties involved will at least be able to embark upon a properly focused 'welfare investigation', with the consequent advantage of being able to identify and establish a timetable for appropriate and necessary assessments.

References

Allison, D. and Burrows, D. (1997) Care proceedings and the recovering parent. *Family Law*, December, p. 809.

Department of Health (1989) The Children Act 1989. Guidance and Regulations Volume 1 – Court Orders. HMSO.

Fortin, J. (1998*) Children's Rights and the Developing Law.* Butterworths.

Hardy, S. and Hannibal, M. (1997) *Law for Social Workers.* Cavendish Publishing.

Lord Chancellor's Direction 7 October 1991.

Parton, N. (1998) Risk, advanced liberalism and child welfare: The need to rediscover uncertainty and ambiguity. *Journal of the British Association of Social Work*, **28**, 5–27.

Practice Note 27 (July 1991). 1 FLR 291, *Best Practice Guidance*, June.

The Hon Mrs Justice Bracewell, District Judge Anthony Clearey, His Honour Judge Nigel Fricker QC (Eds) (1998) *Family Court Practice.* Family Law, Jordan Publishing.

Walsh, E. (1998) *Working in the Family Justice System – A Guide for Professionals.* Family Law, Jordan Publishing.

13

Management, treatment and outcomes

David P. H. Jones, Gerry Byrne and Caroline Newbould

Introduction

What options are there once severe MSBP abuse has been identified? Are the options restricted to parent–child separation and subsequent considerations about what to do about contact? Or is it safe for parent and child to remain together, or to be reunited following a period of time in foster care? What is the situation for the siblings of the index child? What too of future, as yet unborn, children – how safe will they be?

This chapter considers these issues in relation to severe MSBP abuse: the reader is referred to Chapter 9 for consideration of cases where less harm to the child and/or less severe parental problems occur. First, the chapter provides an orientation to MSBP abuse that is embedded in a developmental and ecological approach to child maltreatment. Next, the assessment of risk in MSBP abuse cases, which informs the approach to management, is discussed. Such management is then considered in the situation of severe cases.

The management of cases identified as MSBP abuse has principally concentrated on diagnostic issues and the subsequent confrontation of parents, with the child protection issues which follow (Meadow, 1985). The severity of abuse in the cases first described and the degree of parental personality disorder and capacity for persuasive subterfuge (Schreier and Libow, 1994) did not auger well for family reunification. Follow-up studies of abused children who generally have not received systematic intervention from a psychiatric point of view are sobering, both in terms of high rates of re-abuse and poor outcomes for behavioural and emotional problems, and with respect to and educational difficulties among the children (Bools, Neale and Meadow, 1993; Davis *et al.*, 1998). Added to these observations concerning poor outcomes in untreated cases, psychiatric teams have sometimes had difficulty accepting the harm inflicted on children, instead falling prey to the fabricator's allure (Schreier and Libow, 1994; McGuire and Feldman, 1989). The present authors advise that mental health teams recognize these potential difficulties, and makes recommendations for preventing and countering them. Family reunification should only be considered for certain cases involving MSBP abuse, and even then only with a full appreciation of the risks involved and a multi-disciplinary care plan to minimize such risks (Parnell and Day, 1998).

A developmental/ecological model of child maltreatment

One aspect of MSBP abuse is the child abuse dimension (Jones and Bools, 1999). The developmental/ecological perspective is a widely accepted framework through which to integrate various factors that are known to contribute to or be associated with the predisposition towards and occurrence, precipitation or perpetuation of child maltreatment (Belsky, 1993; Cicchetti, 1989; National Research Council, 1993; Jones and Ramchandani, 1999). There are two themes to this framework, the developmental and ecological. The developmental perspective emphasizes that, as the child grows, he/she becomes increasingly organized and integrated, each stage laying the foundation for increasingly complex development (Cicchetti, 1989). Maltreatment can lead to disruption of this progressive build up of competence. The extent to which the child is affected by this, or recovers, is dependent upon a wide range of influences, which may be either compensatory or ameliorative. These influences occur within domains of successively more complex social arrangements that influence the child. At the closest, they include the influence of the main care giver and the quality of child–parent(s) relationships, extending outwards with increasing social complexity to include family, extended family, networks of friendship, school, neighbourhood and work influences, together with the still broader influence of the culture within which the family live. This model is diagrammatically represented in Figure 13.1.

The potential harm of MSBP abuse and any accompanying factors that either ameliorate or potentiate the outcome for the child will be considered using this framework. One important implication that derives from this is the variety of routes through which MSBP abuse can occur, as well as the different possible outcomes, dependent upon the particular mixture of intervening factors and the effect of transactions between them subsequent to the maltreatment itself. We will now use this general framework to consider MSBP abuse more particularly

Application to MSBP abuse

In MSBP abuse a parent or carer feigns an impression or produces a state of ill-health in a child they are looking after. The key elements are two-fold: parental falsification or deceit and, secondly, a triangular series of interactions between the parent, the child and the health professional. In this triangular interrelationship the health professional is misled by the parent, a parental need is somehow satisfied (at least partially) and the child is harmed (see Chapters 1 and 2).

Figure 13.2 illustrates these potential contributions to the final common pathway of MSBP abuse. Although it has not been systematically explored, the author's own clinical work has emphasized the importance of parent–child attachment difficulties as part of the process through which MSBP abuse can

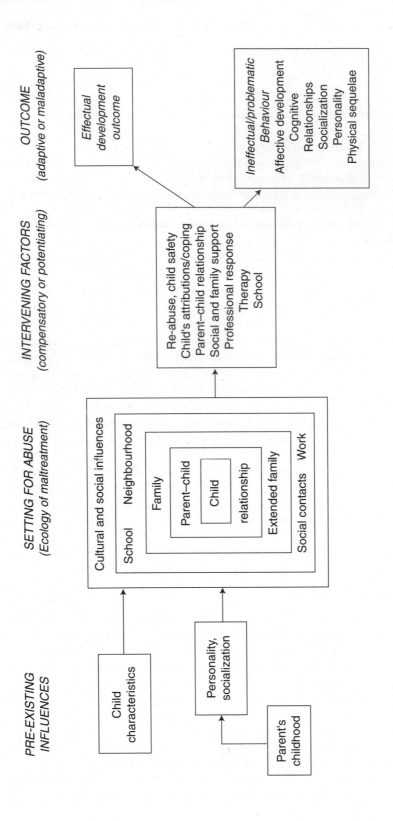

Figure 13.1 A developmental and ecological perspective on child maltreatment. (Reproduced from Jones, D.P.H. and Ramchandani, P. (1999) *Child Sexual Abuse: Informing Practice from Research*, Radcliffe Medical Press, with kind permission from the publishers)

occur. This is not unexpected because the central place of attachment disturbance has been noted in child maltreatment cases more generally. Thus it is of little surprise that such attachment disturbance features so prominently in MSBP abuse cases (Jones and Bools, 1999). Attachment difficulties in turn are linked with parental childhood histories of abuse and deprivation, parental personality difficulties and functional illnesses such as depression. The identification of parent–child attachment difficulties has important implications for intervention, particularly in view of the outcome literature in child maltreatment, where persisting parent–child attachment difficulties combined with evidence of psychological maltreatment on follow-up are consistent findings (Jones, 1998).

The assessment of risk

The theoretical perspective outlined above guides our approach to the assessment of risk. In view of the fact that MSBP abuse can be a life-threatening phenomenon, and can give rise to significant morbidity, the first consideration must be the child's immediate safety. The relevant procedures for the exploration of the child's safety are thus necessary for all cases. In England and Wales this would comprise a child protection conference to draw together the different professional groups in order to evaluate the risk of further harm to the child and to make an appropriate plan to reduce this to the absolute minimum. Normally this will lead to separation of the child from the fabricating adult in all but the mildest cases, while risk and prognosis are being fully assessed (Jones and Bools, 1999). It is best to err on the side of caution in the initial child protection plan, while undertaking a full assessment, in cases where the child has suffered physical harm.

The developmental/ecological framework described determines the domains for assessment which are relevant to recurrence of MSBP abuse and its continuation, as well as other forms of maltreatment, severe parenting difficulties, and other influences on the child's development (Jones, 1997). These domains of assessment are: child, parent, parent–child, family, social and professional. Within each domain, some factors are associated with a more positive outcome while others are more likely to potentiate difficulties (Jones and Bools, 1999). The emphasis here is on the particular mixture and transaction between different factors in the individual case. The first task for the practitioner is to obtain sufficient data about each domain, which will involve both historical and contemporary understanding, so as to obtain a comprehensive picture of the child within his/her ecology. It is tempting to rush this initial assessment, but the significant morbidity and mortality involved in MSBP abuse cases dictates against this. Table 13.1 sets out factors involved in MSBP abuse according to this scheme, considering each domain of assessment and the factors that raise or lower the risk of child maltreatment recurring.

Initially, the main risk considerations will be: the type of abuse (induced illness being more severe than invented); the extent of other forms of child maltreatment; the level of parental acknowledgement; the potential for co-operation in treatment and social casework; whether a focus for psychological treatment work

Transacting domains	Child	Fabricator	Family/Social	Health care
Predisposing factors		Early deprivation, abuse	Parenting, problems, family violence	
			Somatization in family members	
		Illness/illness behaviour problems in childhood	Collective illness behaviour in family	Care for complaint presented but psychological state not addressed
		Somatization (adolescence/ young adult)		Frequent attendee at GP and A&E departments
		Capacity for dissociation		
		Personality difficulties or disorder		Somatization is not confronted, or treated
		Self harm		
	Unwanted pregnancy		Parental couple disharmony	
		Prenatal attachment problems	Partner remote and preoccupied	
Precipitating	Premature	Somatization to self	Social isolation	Hospital provides sanctuary
		Foetal MSBP abuse	Lack of partner or family support for mother and child	
	Neonatal problems	Postnatal depression, mental illness		
	'Different'			
	Parent–child attachment difficulties	Parent–child attachment difficulties		Sick role increasingly attractive, by proxy
	Feeding, settling problems	Exaggeration of child's symptoms		
Manifestation	Significantly harmed	Maltreatment of child		Search for diagnosis Multiple investigations by several doctors
and	Direct/indirect harm	**MSBP abuse**	Family sympathy to parent of sick child	
	Child now 'really' sick and requires treatment	Improvement in personal well-being while child in sick role		Treatment and care for child and parent Comfort from paediatric services
maintenance of MSBP abuse	'Assists' parent with MSBP abuse	Satisfaction in child's ill-health		
	Adopts sick role	Repeat MSBP abuse		

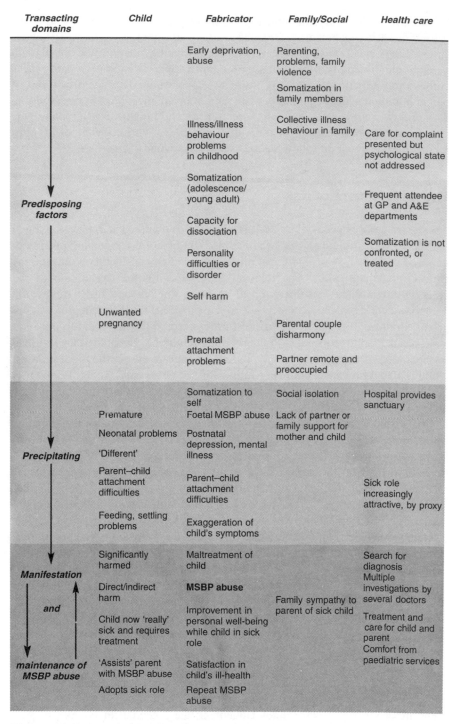

Figure 13.2 Pathways and transactions in the development of MSBP abuse

Table 13.1 Prognostic factors in MSBP abuse

Domain	Poor prognosis	Better prognosis
Abuse	Induced harm Sadistic element Accompanying child sexual abuse or physical abuse Deaths of earlier children Harm to animals	Fabrication Shorter duration of MSBP abuse
Child	Developmental delay Physical sequelae of MSBP abuse Development of somatizing behaviour	Absence of delay or sequelae of abuse
Parent	Personality disorder Denial Lack of compliance Alcohol/substance abuse Abuse in childhood – unresolved	Personality strengths Acknowledgement of abuse Compliance Treatment-responsive mental illness Adapted to childhood abuse
Parenting and parent–child interaction	Disordered attachment Lack of empathy for child Own needs before child	Normal attachment Empathy for child
Family	Domestic violence Multi-generational abuse	Non-abusive partner Supportive extended family
Professional	Lack of informed resources	Partnership with parents Long term psychological treatment and social casework
Social setting	Violent, unsupportive neighbourhood Isolation	Local child support facilities Social support

emerges and is deemed feasible; and whether there is the prospect of finding other families/friends who might be supportive and assist in the management of the case and reduction of risk. Cases involving suffocation and poisoning, and where the abuse has been life threatening, would only be considered for family reunification in exceptional circumstances and where there are many other positive features. Equally, some cases which, on the face of it, 'merely' involve fabrication may be embedded in such extensive evidence of other forms of parenting breakdown and child maltreatment, that treatment with a view to reunification is not feasible. Nonetheless, from these evaluations of risk an initial decision can be made as to whether a child care and psychological treatment approach can be envisaged without parent–child separation, or not.

Risk assessment now progresses to evaluating the likelihood of change, at least for those cases where there is a prospect for safe contact between the fabricator and the child. The circumstances and qualities that might increase or decrease the risk of maltreatment should be identified. This will involve taking all domains of risk into consideration along with the proposed strategies for intervention and treatment. An estimate of the likelihood of successful intervention should be attempted at this early stage, recognizing the constraints on accurate prediction. It is useful to outline a proposed process of change for the different individuals and the family, together with what treatment provision and interventions are envisaged. The criteria for evaluation of whether change has occurred and interventions have been successful (or otherwise) should be articulated as part of this phase of assessment. Assessment of the relative likelihood of change is a crucial part of risk management. The expectation is that assessment of risk will then be modified in the light of new data and findings deriving from the intervention process itself. Thus, risk assessment is not a single 'once and for all' entity, but can be revised in the light of treatment response.

A time-scale for change, sensitive to the age and needs of the individual child, is important and should be set out at the beginning of the intervention, in order to obviate drift in case planning and to keep the child's welfare in centre stage (Jones, 1997 and 1998; Adcock, 1998).

By this point some families will have been identified as too dangerous for significant contact between child and parent to occur. Plans will need to be made for substitute care for these children, while also evaluating the risk of harm to any existing or future siblings. For others, intervention can be considered, using the approach to risk outlined above, and a series of stages set up to evaluate progress.

Management of severe cases

The remainder of this chapter will now concentrate on those children and families where the possibility of reunification remains. The process of change will be described in terms of three phases: an initial acknowledgement phase; a second phase comprising improvement in parental sensitivity and effectual parenting; and finally a resolution phase, moving in the direction of either alternative care or care within the family (Jones, 1997). This sequence is proposed as a means of analysing the process of change in a way that is manageable for the practitioner and provides a framework for children and families involved in the task of change.

By no means all serious cases of MSBP abuse can be responded to in this way, as already discussed above. Sometimes, the risk of harm to the child is simply too great, parental denial too entrenched or the likelihood of timely psychological treatment too slim. For the children of these parents, it will be essential that protective action is taken at an early stage and a clear assessment of the reasons for this action is given. Not only does this afford maximum protection for the index child but it also ensures that appropriate consideration can be given to the welfare of siblings or future children born to the family.

In serious cases, but where intervention may be feasible, the present author thinks it is essential that a period of in-patient stay be part of the treatment plan. This enables the family to be assessed and treated across the whole range of daily activities, with the accompanying accumulation of stress this involves. Opportunities for intervention occur across the whole day, and a timely intervention in an informal setting when the issue is very much alive for the mother and child can have great therapeutic potential. For some parents a mealtime may be the most stressful time of the day, particularly with mothers who have their own eating disorders. For others, bedtime with a child who does not settle can be the most stressful period and, therefore, the most vulnerable time for the child. Out-patient appointments cannot achieve the breadth and depth of assessment that is essential in cases where the risk posed is very high. In addition to this, high risk cases that have involved serious physical harm to the child require twenty-four hour observation initially, while the effectiveness of intervention is being assessed.

The detail of the process outlined above will now be described, for those considered amenable to it.

Acknowledgement

Parents' denial of the fact of maltreatment is often the first therapeutic hurdle to overcome in the process of establishing a focus of agreement on which to base a treatment programme. As an essential prerequisite for later work, the parents must be encouraged not only to acknowledge that harm has been done and take appropriate responsibility for it, but also to develop a genuine appreciation of the child's experience of abuse and their accompanying parenting problems. This abusive experience includes not only the immediate effects of direct suffering and unnecessary medical investigation and/or treatment, but also the indirect consequences of parent–child disruption, substitute care and related distress.

Can families be worked with where denial is intact and parents united in the view that 'the doctors have got it wrong'? The initial task is to find a way of engaging with the parents and developing trust over a period of time in an out-patient setting, with the aim of moving towards a more realistic acceptance of the problem. A significant proportion of referred parents are considered to be too firmly entrenched in denial to anticipate sufficient progress within a time-scale appropriate to the child's needs. This fact alone is often enough to prevent the psychiatrist embarking on an attempted treatment plan. An example of such a situation is described below.

A mother persisted in her conviction that her child had suffered epileptic seizures, despite thorough medical investigations, which produced no evidence of organic abnormalities. Despite never having witnessed any seizure activity, her husband, a somewhat distant father who was content to delegate most of the parenting role to his wife, did not question her story and colluded with her anger that she was being accused when in reality her child was suffering some as yet undiagnosed serious medical condition. The couple united in anger against the medics and child welfare agency, and could not allow themselves to consider the severity of parenting failure which was placing their child at risk.

In the field of serious abuse, persisting denial of responsibility is a bar to progress. In MSBP abuse, involving induction or tampering, persisting denial would spell the end of any efforts in the direction of family reunification. In MSBP abuse involving fabrications of symptoms only, much depends on the extent of harm to the child. This includes the degree to which his/her health and welfare have been sacrificed by the fabricator in the pursuit of satisfying personal needs (by proxy), together with any other accompanying maltreatment or parenting difficulties. The decision to pursue family reunification when denial persists is hazardous in MSBP abuse because of the likelihood of recurrence (Davis *et al.*, 1998), poor outcome among untreated cases (Bools, Neale and Meadow, 1993), and the degree and extent of personality disorder (Bools, Neale and Meadow, 1994). In selected cases, following assessment of all domains of risk, reunification can be embarked upon where harm to the child has been limited. However, it can only occasionally be justified to be in the child's best interests, and only then with a very clear risk management policy, agreed by the multi-disciplinary team of professionals who will be providing follow-up.

Findings of fact made by a judge within the family justice system may enable progress to be made, weakening denial which has hitherto been unmovable, or where paediatric opinion is divided. Establishing a focus for, and engagement with, psychological treatment is a key task in this phase, in addition to overcoming the parents' denial of problems.

During this initial phase a comprehensive review of all the case material, including access to past medical and psychiatric records relating to all family members, is undertaken if it has not already been done. This can be time consuming, but has proved invaluable in gaining a full understanding of the family history and especially any tendency towards somatization behaviour or other personal and interpersonal difficulties in the fabricator's life. The process does not merely yield information, however, but is part of the therapy in itself. Involving parents in understanding their life history, and how somatization, fabrication and other personality difficulties have developed, leading finally to the current picture of MSBP abuse, is a central component of the therapeutic work.

All medical records, both general practice and hospital, including obstetric, should be obtained and scrutinized by a doctor with both child health and adult mental health experience. Nursing notes can help to reveal the fabricator's style of presentation. School records are also useful, if available, and any records of criminal activity. Written release from the fabricator is obtained prior to seeking records, in order to emphasize the partnership approach and joint commitment to understand the route to MSBP abuse.

Our task is to understand the abuse and its wider background as clearly as possible, in order to minimize the possibility of collusion between ourselves and the family. Maltreatment perpetrated in this way relies on the abuser's plausibility and potential to deceive, and we must guard against being used by families to disprove the paediatric diagnosis and basis for concern (Schreier and Libow, 1994).

In addition to these initial efforts to engage the family, it is necessary to establish the boundaries of our work in relation to the wider professional system. An early meeting of professionals is essential to the foundation of joint understanding and planning, as well as setting the scene for working together. With respect to the author's own professional 'setting', the in-patient treatment programme at the Park Hospital is intensive and short term, and necessitates the use of professional links to establish effective plans for follow-up psychological work and monitoring of the child's welfare at discharge. All mental health teams need to work out their relative roles and responsibilities in relation to other agencies. Not only does this prevent the isolation of any one agency, but it also permits early identification of untenable perspectives, and identifies areas of agreement and disagreement. Regular subsequent meetings obviate problems of inter-disciplinary feuding, and provide opportunities for the professionals to understand that such tensions often reflect collective anxieties in managing serious child abuse, or mirror conflicts and disharmony within the family itself.

This initial process of multi agency working also enables different groups to voice their concerns and formulate an agreed set of aims and objectives for treatment. In this way, the agencies collectively establish those aspects of risk which have to change in order for a consensus to emerge concerning criteria for family reunification.

Acknowledgement, in psychological terms, is not a one-off confession by an abuser but rather a process by which a person faces the reality of their situation, takes responsibility for causing harm and makes a commitment to understanding the impact of their actions on their child. Initially, this is less about the search for a full admission of all the facts, and more about a willingness to work with mental health professionals towards a trusting relationship focused on a safe outcome for their child. Will it be possible to agree a set of criteria for change with this family, taking as the joint focus the child's long term welfare? Co-operation with the process of assessment is only the first step towards a positive engagement within which to predict appropriate change within the child's time-scale. Not only are the facts of the situation considered, but a detailed assessment of the personality of the abuser and non-abusing partner (if present) is also made, looking as much for strengths on which to build as for deficits to help understand the maltreatment.

In the Park Hospital programme, once a basis for work is established, the family are admitted to the Family Unit for an intensive period of treatment. In many cases the child comes to this admission from a foster care placement and is reunited with his parents in a highly supervised setting. It must be recognized that not only has the child been vulnerable to actual harm but, usually, he or she has also been victim to generalized deficiencies of parenting, including emotional unavailability and neglect of appropriate care (Erikson and Egeland, 1996). It is this total picture that the psychiatrist strives to understand with parents. It is not enough to understand the actual mechanism of abuse; an acknowledgement of overall parenting problems or failure must also be established. Parents are asked to address both the incidents leading to actual abuse, the abuse itself and its consequences for the child and themselves. In addition, they are gradually helped to face the personal difficulties that made it possible for abuse to occur. There may be deep-rooted psychological difficulties that this particular child has aroused, leading to early attachment disruption between mother and child and subsequent catastrophic events. Such a situation is described in the following vignette.

A mother who was eventually charged with the attempted murder of her child through poisoning was helped to acknowledge her personal sense of failure as a mother. Her third planned, but difficult to conceive pregnancy, coincided with a period during which her husband was frequently absent from the home due to increased work pressure. The pregnancy was characterized by threatened miscarriage and a feeling within the mother that the baby was fragile and that she had to hold on to him for his survival. As the pregnancy continued, he became increasingly depersonalized and a constant reminder to her of her own inadequacies. After birth, the mother and child relationship deteriorated into a vicious circle of failure to thrive and severe feeding difficulties, and an extended period of therapy was needed to enable the mother to acknowledge and face her feelings of guilt and remorse.

It is only when this picture is built up that one can move with any optimism towards further phases of treatment and the prospect of eventual family reunification.

In addition to this focus on intensive acknowledgement work with the fabricator, progress with the non-abusing carer is also required if family reunification is to be achieved. Is it possible for this person to recognize both the deeds of their partner and also their own deficiencies in terms of parenting responsibilities, resulting in a failure to see what was happening? And could they protect the child from future harm? If the couple decide to remain together, will the partner (usually the man) be able to put the child's future safety above the adult relationship and ally himself with the professional system sufficiently enough to be relied on to 'blow the whistle' if repeat harm is suspected? Confidence in this respect is invaluable to the process of managing risk, but there is inevitably much painful work to be done in acknowledging guilt and anger, and translating these into understanding and a positive way forward. It is, however, the author's contention that a full and extensive acknowledgement of the entire range of parenting difficulties is essential to effective treatment. This approach applies to the whole family, its different internal alliances, and individual members (Bentovim, 1998).

Improving parental sensitivity and competence

This phase is grounded in a comprehensive evaluation of parent–child relationships, especially the quality of parent–child attachment. However, broader family dynamics also need to be considered, including the overall pattern of relationships, the marital partnership, the parental partnership and sibling relationships, in addition to the parent–child relationships (Bentovim, 1998; Jones, 1997). This phase also involves substantial work with the parents, individually.

It follows from what was said earlier in this chapter that a child who has become a victim of MSBP abuse will almost inevitably be suffering some degree of emotional neglect and/or abuse. One of the most important factors in the prevention of any child abuse, or re-abuse, is a parent–child relationship that is characterized by an appreciation of the individuality of the child as a person in his own right, and a warm sensitivity to the child's communication of his needs (DeWolff and Van Izendoorm, 1997). Sensitivity is emphasized, along with a mother's awareness of her infant's signals and her accurate interpretation and appropriate and prompt response to them. Any assessment of parenting must identify where the problems lie in the parent–child relationship in order for attempts at intervention to have the potential for success.

It is not difficult to spot grossly insensitive responses to a child's needs. The child's distress and despair, which can go unnoticed by the parent, can be a clear and loud indicator that the relationship is in difficulty. Identifying subtle problems is more difficult, and a number of complementary approaches are necessary. For instance, a mother's ability to accurately interpret her infant's signals relies firstly on her awareness and accessibility to the infant, secondly on her capacity to acknowledge her own moods and feelings (which threaten to distort perceptions) and thirdly on her capacity for empathy, i.e. her capacity to see things from his point of view (a child's eye view). In addition, inappropriate responses may ensue if a mother is unable to temper the intensity and length of her responses to the infant's communications about how much he needs and can deal with. An example would be of a mother able to judge the length of any contact required to comfort a child if that child is to be satisfied. Ignorance and lack of understanding contribute to insensitive responses. In working with parents, one often witnesses those whose expectations of their child are age-inappropriate.

At the Park Hospital a number of approaches are employed which complement each other and, overall, contribute both to accurate assessment of the parent–child relationship and to the treatment of the same. Individual therapy with the parent (sometimes with the child in the room) is undertaken, often twice weekly. Observation and treatment in formal and informal settings organized around key periods of interaction in the parent–child relationship, such as mealtimes, bedtimes, playtimes, separations and reunions, are integral components of this phase of treatment. Direct work with the older child can lead to a better understanding of the impact upon the child of his experiences. This work may be therapeutic for the child, but will also inform feedback to the parent in attempting to educate them as to their child's needs and to facilitate a better understanding of the tasks facing the child in integrating these experiences into his perception of himself and the world around him.

As outlined above, acknowledgement involves a full appreciation of the impact of the abuse and neglect upon the child and this is explored fully in the parent's individual therapy/sessions. Fraiberg, Adelson and Shapiro (1975) pioneered therapy with the parent and child and commented on how it can be excruciatingly painful for the observer when, for instance, witnessing a mother appear oblivious to her infant's cries of distress and the infant's ensuing despair. However, the reasons for this failure to hear her own child's cry may be quite complex. Fraiberg, Adelson and Shapiro described a case in which the therapists involved posed themselves the question: 'Why doesn't this mother hear her baby's cries?'. The answer lay in the mother's history, in that her own cries had gone unheard and now, in the face of her baby's distress which threatened to put her in touch with her own grief and pain, she defended against this by distancing herself from her baby's pain. As the mother was facilitated in the expression of her own feelings of anguish and grief, her capacity to hear and tolerate her baby's distress underwent a corresponding development.

In the therapy the parent has opportunities to explore what meaning the child holds for them and how this has influenced their perception of the child's communications. One mother spoke of her conviction that her baby son would grow up to abuse her and other women in the way his father abused her within the marriage and her uncle abused her as a child. Separating out her projections from the actual reality of the child and identifying that his bids for contact were not abusive, proved essential in achieving a reasonable degree of sensitivity to his needs.

MSBP abuse involves sacrificing the child's needs for the sake of the parents', and now the parent has the choice to place the child's needs above their own. For this to occur, the child has to be perceived as a person in his own right, and parents are therefore encouraged to interpret accurately their child's communications about states of mind and feelings, along with wishes and needs. This often leads to an understanding that their previous perception of their child's state and nature was distorted by overwhelming personal needs and problems. A situation illustrating this is described below.

A mother of two boys could not bear to touch the eldest boy through loathing and fear of a wish to re-enact her own sexual abuse when a child. She rebuffed his bids for physical contact and was reluctant to let go of the youngest boy, but clutched him to her chest. Neither child was being perceived and responded to in terms of their own personalities and needs, but each was used as a receptacle for different projections of the mother's. One was in receipt of very negative communications including the mother's identification with her abuser, while the other was in receipt of her lonely, frightened baby self. To an outside observer the second child seemed less at risk, as the mother's responses could be seen as appropriate to the child's needs. However, both children's attachments were insecure: the first disorganized, and the second child anxious in type.

Formal observations and interventions by the occupational therapy team take place alongside daily informal observation and assessment. Parent–child therapists are with the family throughout the day, present to observe and offer intervention during nursery and play sessions, mealtimes, bathtimes, bedtimes and so on. Their daily observations are recorded in a standardized way. Video-recorded sessions are analysed and fed back to the parent to facilitate the development of more sensitive parenting, building on positive interchanges and sensitive care-taking. Both occupational therapists and parent–child therapists also act as role models to parents, offering suggestions as to how they might interpret a child's behaviour (for instance by magnifying the child's response: 'Oh look how he holds his arms up to you, he really wants mummy to pick him up') and how to respond to their child's communications. Inviting the parent to look at the child's experience at any given point of the day can be an important intervention, helping the parent to identify more clearly an expression of a need or to reinforce the correct response to that need. Examples of such 'prompts' might be: 'I wonder what your baby was feeling when you left the room just now?' and 'How do you think he felt just now when you cuddled him?'

During this phase it is essential that all agencies involved in the future care and supervision of the family are in discussion. There needs to be agreement about the levels of risk, and a shared understanding of the factors that contribute to increased and decreased risk. This allows future supervision and intervention in the community setting to continue to facilitate the developing sensitivity and competent parenting initiated in the hospital setting. Often, agencies will have to struggle to change their perceptions of the parents in the same way and at the same time that the parents undergo changes in their perceptions of their babies. In some cases it has proved more difficult to 'release' a mother from the projections of the agencies involved (witch mother) than it has been to release the child from the mother's projections (devil's child).

Resolution

The child's future safety is the primary focus that guides recommendations about long term placement, either back with his/her parents, within the extended family, or in substitute care. A successful outcome for treatment is therefore defined in terms of securing a permanent, safe upbringing for the child, not merely reunification. Whether recommendations involve a cautious family reunification or permanent separation of the child from his/her parents, there will still be much long term planning and follow-up to be done. If the child returns to the care of previously abusing parents, how will the maintenance of healthy relationships be ensured and how can the parents guard against reversion to old styles of interaction and help-seeking? How will the mother be able to seek appropriate medical attention when she has previously deceived a range of health professionals with factitious or fabricated symptoms? Perhaps most crucially, whatever the treatment outcome, what should the child be told about early abuse and what might he/she remember of it?

The overall task, if the option of family reunification is pursued, is to do everything possible to maintain the lowered risk into the long term future. For these cases, this will mean an active approach towards relapse prevention, particularly in view of the outcome studies of maltreatment generally, emphasizing the recurrence of ineffectual and problematic parenting difficulties even if the index abuse does not recur (Jones, 1998). Where substitute care for the child appears the only safe option, there are still significant treatment and management implications for the fabricator, as well as for the index child. The issue of the risk to future children argues the need for therapeutic work if it will be accepted, with an eye to lowering the risk of future maltreatment. Equally, for some children, while substitute care renders them safer, significant emotional and behavioural difficulties may well persist, particularly in those cases where diagnosis of MSBP abuse has been delayed (Bools, Neale and Meadow, 1993; Maguire and Feldman, 1989; Meadow, 1982).

Whatever the placement outcome for the abused child, an understanding of his past and the decisions that were taken on his behalf is likely to be important to his future psychological health. A significant number of the parents with whom the author has worked with towards reunification, have realized, as treatment has progressed, that their child may, realistically, have some memory of past trauma and that it will be their task to respond to questions in the future. These very severe cases of abuse may often attract media and community attention at the early investigative stages, and subsequently, if criminal proceedings result. Despite attempts at anonymity during proceedings, it may well be that the local community has pieced together the story and, of course, the child protection process will have alerted the professional system to the potential risks. Parents, in facing the enormity of the abuse, will also have to consider how best to talk to their child in the knowledge that what they do not remember for themselves may well be told to them as they return to the home community, now or in the future. Many of the parents the author has worked with have talked about this dilemma as they begin to plan for discharge, and have often shown their commitment to addressing this excruciating reality despite the obvious pain it causes them. Some children have recalled their abuse and asked their parents about it. It has been impressive how parents have responded to this issue.

> A boy whose mother fabricated epileptic fits and induced physical symptoms said to be the result of a fall while fitting, remembered an incident which occurred when he was only eighteen months old. At the age of five years he asked his mother why she had hurt him. She was able to acknowledge that the incident had occurred, that it was wrong and that she alone was responsible for it. She also apologised to her son and explained that she was unwell when the incident had occurred, but had now had help to get better.

For those children who do not return to their parents' care it is equally important that they have an understanding of their past in order to comprehend and assimilate their feelings about being in substitute care. It is known, from long-standing experience in the field of adoption generally, that a knowledge and understanding of the past is essential for children to settle into a long term alternative, and it may be that parents who cannot be considered as safe carers could play some part in providing this explanation. If not, a professional will need to impart the information to the child.

In working with this issue, a number of guiding principles have been developed. The first is based on the child's need to have accurate and adequate information about what has happened to them. Closely linked to this is their right to have an explanation. Both the information and its explanation will need to be developmentally sensitive so that it is within the child's understanding. Naturally this will change over time and the whole issue will need to be revisited at different stages in the child's life. These principles apply not only to the index child but also to siblings. However, the information needs to steer a course between honesty and accuracy on the one hand, and avoiding disturbing the child's security on the other. To some extent this will always involve a compromise, which will need to be carefully and explicitly worked out with the child's parents. The movement towards honest explanations and accurate information must not be merely to satiate a parental need for alleviating guilt through ventilation of memories, or from a desire for self punishment. Sometimes these are the primary motivating forces rather than a concern for the child. Above all, however, the information and explanations need to be considered from a family perspective, for they will involve index children, fabricators, siblings and other family members. It will be particularly important to involve those family members who are part of the process of maintaining future safety, who must know what the child knows.

There are further issues for those families moving towards reunification, particularly concerning ways of helping parents to maintain the changes they have made and, with risk management in mind, finding ways to prevent 'slippage' in the direction of old problems as the family return to their home environment.

Not only must re-abuse (of the same kind) be prevented but also the possibility of more general parenting dysfunction. It will always be necessary for the health and development of these children to be closely monitored, and for the professional system to be aware of possible future risk in the widest sense and to have an agreed response plan if difficulties arise.

The role of the primary health care team is crucial to this stage of the process. The GP and health visitor are in the dual position of encouraging a previously abusive and deceiving mother to seek appropriate medical care for her child, as well as being in the front line of detecting future patterns of inappropriate illness presentations. Having perhaps been duped in the past, they will inevitably wish to be cautious and thorough as the patient returns to their community care. A meeting between the specialist mental health treatment providers and the primary health care team, as well as the paediatrician who will follow up the children, is a helpful way of reviewing the management of the fabricator's future health seeking behaviours. It also enables risks of future maltreatment, both MSBP abuse and other forms, to be evaluated. Re-abuse may be via an alternative method of fabrication (Jones and Bools, 1999), which raises significant issues for health surveillance.

A clear and informed inter-agency system needs to be established not only to help the parents deal with the problems of being ordinarily ill but also to support its own professional members as these families are brought back together. It will be necessary for professionals to retain a realistic perspective on current risk throughout this process. There is a tendency to move precipitously from the stance that the family are untreatable to one of unsubstantiated optimism following intensive psychological treatment.

In the authors' experience with a small group of families who have been reunited, there is a need for ongoing, less intensive, out-patient treatment and the best way to provide this will have to be decided in each case. The original team can provide this for local cases, while for others close links with locally based child psychiatric teams can enable continuing work to occur. Whatever arrangements are agreed, direct but infrequent involvement with the family has to be maintained, often combined with a consultative role for professional colleagues. This can encompass both discussion relating to longer term treatment and a continuing role in the risk management task.

Outcome

All psychological and social work inputs need to be seen as part of an integrated intervention, rather than in hierarchical terms, if these potentially high risk situations are to be managed effectively. Continuing social casework and family support services are of equal importance to the intervention's success, as is in-depth psychological work. It is contended that the whole treatment approach is necessary. The research does not allow us to assert that one particular component makes a crucial difference. In fact, given the developmental and ecological perspective on child abuse, it is unlikely that one particular intervention, focused on one element of the multifaceted problem of MSBP abuse, would be the agent of change. Hence, in keeping with the model selected, we emphasize the range of psychological and social contributions, working with parents and extended family, involved in achieving the overall aim of a safe outcome for the child.

There have been single case reports of family reunification following identification of MSBP abuse (Jones and Bools, 1999). These reports have usually concentrated on apparently successful cases, because in general authors do not write up, nor journals publish, case reports of unsuccessful interventions. Reports have involved cases where the parent has been able to take responsibility for her actions and has been assessed as amenable to psychological treatments. These have mostly been psychoanalytically orientated psychotherapies.

The Great Ormond Street group has described the outcome of their management strategy within the paediatric unit and the subsequent arrangements for child protection in a case series involving forty-one children (Gray and Bentovim, 1996). Although they were not principally focused on family reunification, the authors note that, in cases with a successful outcome, there was a balanced combination of child protection work and therapeutic input for the mother and wider family.

Berg and Jones (1999) have described a follow-up of seventeen consecutive children where child and family psychiatric intervention occurred. Four of these seventeen were assessments, but thirteen involved treatment directed towards family reunification. Of these thirteen, ten children were reunited with their biological parents; three were considered to be too risky for reunification and substitute care was recommended. These recommendations were followed in all cases. The children were assessed at an average of twenty-seven months following discharge from the unit. Overall, the children had done well in terms of their development, growth and psychological adjustment. One child had been re-abused by her mother, fortunately leading to only mild physical harm which was rapidly detected and led to the immediate separation of the child from the fabricator (her mother), to be solely cared for by her father thereafter. From the child's perspective, there was continuous care by her father, but of course the mother left the household. An important finding from this work was that, in a minority of cases, the fabricators continued to have mental health difficulties, particularly depression and persistent anxiety symptoms, and tended to exaggerate symptoms of their personal ill health and were frequent doctor attendees. However, the only evidence of continuing factitious ill-health by proxy was the one incident mentioned above. Berg and Jones cautiously conclude that family reunification is feasible for a selected subgroup of cases of MSBP abuse, but only where there can be long term follow-up involving continuing health monitoring, social casework, and psychological treatment. In order to prevent the possibility of poor parenting practices recurring (Bools, Neale and Meadow, 1993; Davis *et al.*, 1998), long term follow-up is necessary to detect future deterioration in maternal mental health and health care seeking behaviour, as well as to monitor the child's health and development. For those who have made successful changes in both their personal life and family functioning subsequent to the identification of MSBP abuse, the outcomes for the children have been positive, and surely better than the results associated with untreated cases. While awaiting the outcome from long term follow-up of successfully treated cases, it may still be concluded that the goal of family reunification is feasible for a selected minority of cases, provided a long term approach to risk management can be mustered by the professionals and the family itself.

References

Adcock, M. (1998) Significant harm: implications for local authorities. In *Significant Harm: Its Management and Outcome*, 2nd Edn (Adcock, M. and White, R., eds), pp. 33–56. Significant Publications.

Bentovim, A. (1998) Significant harm in context. In *Significant Harm: Its Management and Outcome*, 2nd Edn (Adcock, M. and White, R., eds), pp. 57–89, Significant Publications.

Belsky, J. (1993) Etiology of child maltreatment: a developmental/ecological analysis. *Psychological Bulletin*, **114**, 413–434.

Berg, B. and Jones, D.P.H. (1999) Outcome of psychiatric intervention in factitious illness by proxy (Munchausen's syndrome by proxy). *Archives of Disease in Childhood* (in press).

Bools, C.N., Neale, B.A. and Meadow, S.R. (1993) Follow-up of victims of fabricated illness (MSBP). *Archives of Disease in Childhood*, **69**, 625–630.

Bools, C.N., Neale, B. and Meadow, R. (1994) Munchausen syndrome by proxy: a study of psychopathology. *Child Abuse and Neglect*, **18**, 773–788.

Cicchetti, D. (1989). How research on child maltreatment has informed the study of child development: perspectives from developmental psychopathology. In *Child Maltreatment: Theory and Research on the Causes and Consequences of Child Abuse and Neglect* (Cicchetti, D. and Carlson, V., eds), pp. 377–431. Cambridge University Press.

Davis, P., McClure, R.J., Rolfe, K. *et al.* (1998) Procedures, placement and risks of further abuse following Munchausen syndrome by proxy, non-accidental poisoning, and non-accidental suffocation. *Archives of Disease in Childhood*, **78**, 217–221.

De Wolff, M.S. and Van Ijzendoorn, M.H. (1997) Sensitivity and attachment: a meta-analysis on parental antecedents of infant attachment. *Child Development*, **68**, 571–591.

Erickson, M. and Egeland, B. (1996) Child neglect. In *The APSAC Handbook on Child Maltreatment* (Briere, J., Berliner, L., Bulkley, J., Jenny, C. and Reid, T., eds), pp. 4–20. Sage.

Fraiberg, S., Adelson, E. and Shapiro, E. (1975) Ghosts in the nursery: a psychoanalytic approach to the impairment of infant–mother relationships. *Journal of the American Academy of Child Psychiatry*, **14**, 387–421.

Gray, J. and Bentovim, A. (1996) Illness induction syndrome: Paper 1. A series of 41 children from 37 families identified at the Great Ormond Street Hospital for Children NHS Trust. *Child Abuse and Neglect*, **20**, 655–673.

Jones, D.P.H. (1997) Treatment of the child and the family where child abuse or neglect has occurred. In *The Battered Child*, 5th Edn (Helfer, R., Kempe, R. and Krugman, R., eds), pp. 521–542. University of Chicago Press.

Jones, D.P.H. (1998) The effectiveness of intervention. In *Significant Harm: Its Management and Outcome*, 2nd Edn (Adcock, M. and White, R., eds). pp. 91–119. Significant Publications.

Jones, D.P.H. and Bools, C.N. (1999) Facititious illness by proxy. In *Recent Advances in Paediatrics* (David, T., ed.), pp. 57–71. Churchill Livingstone.

Jones, D.P.H. and Ramchandani, P. (1999) *Child Sexual Abuse: Informing Practice from Research*, pp. 1–4. Radcliffe Medical Press.

McGuire, T.L. and Feldman, K.W. (1989) Psychological morbidity of children subjected to Munchausen syndrome by proxy. *Pediatrics*, **83**, 289–292.

Meadow, S.R. (1985) Management of Munchausen syndrome by proxy. *Archives of Disease in Childhood*, **60**, 385–393.

Meadow, S.R. (1982) Munchausen's syndrome by proxy. *Archives of Disease in Childhood*, **57**, 92–98.

National Research Council (1993) Aetiology of child maltreatment. In *Understanding Child Abuse and Neglect* (Panel on Research on Child Abuse and Neglect, National Research Council, eds), Chapter 4. National Academy Press.

Parnell, T.F. and Day, D.O. (1998) *Munchausen by Proxy Syndrome: Misunderstood Child Abuse*, pp. 105–112. Sage.

Schreier, H. and Libow, J. (1994) Munchausen syndrome by proxy: a clinical fable of our times. *Journal of the American Academy of Child and Adolescent Psychiatry*, **33**, 904–905.

14

Picking up the pieces

Hilary Lloyd and Anne MacDonald

Introduction

The title of this chapter clearly implies that something is broken or parts have been separated. Our subject covers the effects on health care staff of their involvement in cases of Munchausen syndrome by proxy abuse and how these effects might be minimized and best managed.

On the whole, the research literature pays little reference to such issues, although many articles comment upon staff reactions. Considerably more has been written in the nursing than in the medical literature, although most of this is descriptive rather systematic research, and is based on single or, at best, a few cases.

Such articles as there are, plus the authors' own direct experience of cases and experience of talking to nursing staff about their own encounters, suggest that this is an important area. Moreover, there appear to be a number of common effects on staff and the working of clinical teams, and a consideration of these suggests ways in which the negative effects may be proactively reduced or at least partially redressed. The area of concern includes the effects on individuals and on staff teams, both in hospitals and in community settings. This chapter focuses on nursing staff because they are so often the health professionals with the most direct contact with the families, and are therefore the group most likely to be affected. However, the same issues are relevant to doctors and other health care staff.

Perhaps what is most obviously vulnerable to breakage in cases of MSBP abuse is trust. Three main areas are seen to be at risk: the paediatric health care professional's trust in the parent (or other perpetrator), trust in the judgement and support of others in the clinical team (in one's own discipline or another) and trust in one's own judgement and ability to spot deception. Ultimately, from the professional standpoint, the potential consequences may be serious. Excessive suspiciousness of parents may compromise the professional's relationships with other parents. Loss of confidence in others may lead to splitting within and between professional groups. Loss of confidence in one's own judgement may compromise professional working in many respects. In addition, there is potential for substantial personal distress in individual team members.

Extracts from the transcripts of interviews with hospital nursing staff and health visitors undertaken specifically in preparation for this chapter are used to illustrate points throughout the text.

Tables 14.1 and 14.2 suggest proactive and reactive measures that can be taken to facilitate team functioning when dealing with MSBP abuse.

Issues for individuals

Blix and Brack (1988) conducted one of the few systematic enquiries into this area in the USA. Twenty nurses on one paediatric unit completed a questionnaire

Table 14.1 Proactive measures to assist staff with the emotional burden of involvement in cases of MSBP abuse

---

Training
- MSBP abuse should be covered in nurse and medical training.
- Such training should cover common effects on staff (so that reactions can be expected, understood and recognized in self and others), and advice given about methods of dealing with such issues.
- Continuing education/continuing professional development for children's health care personnel should cover MSBP abuse.

Up to date information on MSBP abuse
- Should be to hand on wards, and included in child protection policies and procedures.
- Should be included in formal orientation and induction programmes.

Communication
- Psychosocial or other ward meetings to act as a regular multi-disciplinary forum in which issues can be raised and discussed at an early stage, and a culture developed which encourages staff to reflect on the emotional demands of cases and promotes the recognition and labelling of the emotions evoked.
- Careful liaison between departments, between hospital and community teams, and between agencies.

Paired working
- In complex cases and where index of suspicion is high, to provide opportunity for 'checking out' experiences and impressions.

Clinical supervision systems
- To enable nurses and other staff to voice suspicions in a safe environment and examine evidence at an early stage.
- Adequate resourcing of such systems is essential.

Audit
- All of the above should be effected in individual case review format and in the context of wider audit.

All of the above measures aim to increase awareness, encourage questioning and reflection and reduce isolation.

Table 14.2 Reactive measures to assist staff with the emotional burden of involvement in cases of MSBP abuse

Communication
- May be enhanced by the involvement of fewer, rather than more staff.
- Once suspicions are voiced, multi-disciplinary (MD) meetings of involved staff to discuss formulation and management plans, to afford the opportunity to question and to acknowledge some of the conflicts and anxieties experienced by the staff.
- After events, meetings for staff to continue and tie up relevant issues. If MD meetings did not occur whilst the case was 'active', then a meeting or series of meetings may still be useful at this stage.

Clarity
- Of management plan, including how to deal with parents while suspicions remain covert.
- Of lines of responsibility.

Paired working
- To reduce isolation of staff and to afford opportunities for 'checking out' impressions and experiences.

Clinical supervision systems
- When effective, can provide added support and containment to staff.
- Supervisors should monitor the reactions of their supervisees.

External support
- After particularly traumatic cases, the opportunity to speak to someone outside the clinical team may be valuable, either individually or as a group.

Audit
- Post facto audit of all cases of MSBP abuse to promote 'learning from experience'.

after a particular case of MSBP abuse had unfolded on the ward. The commonly reported reactions from involvement with the case were shock, disbelief and anger. The anger was identified as being towards the parent (usually), themselves (for having been deceived) and the doctors. This anger towards the doctors was for having given less support than the nurses felt they should, for having left the nurses at the 'sharp end' and, sometimes, for having been slow in taking the nurses' concerns seriously.

Whelan-Williams and Baker (1997) emphasize that staff may feel anger, betrayal, hurt and denial. They warn that, without an understanding of family dynamic issues, knowledge about MSBP abuse and 'resolution of the often intense personal emotions these cases can stimulate', staff will encounter problems. They may not only have difficulties in adequately protecting a child-victim whose parent still has contact, but they might also be reluctant to acknowledge fabrication of illness in future cases, or, conversely, they might become over-zealous in their suspicions.

Herzog, in a case discussion (Sugar *et al.*, 1991), notes that some of the paediatricians and nurses will feel guilty about their helplessness, their decision to separate mother and child, and their anger at the mother.

The nursing staff approached in preparation for writing this chapter, described having experienced the same sorts of emotional reactions to cases of MSBP abuse as those found by Blix and Brack and written about by Whelan-Williams and Baker and Sugar *et al*. These feelings were conveyed very strongly by the nurses in their interviews. Even several years after the cases, staff made comments that conveyed a sense of the power of the impact made on them, such as 'I can remember it as if it were yesterday'.

Parent–professional relationship

The paramount importance of patients and parents being able to have trust in their clinical staff is generally acknowledged. The reciprocity of trust in these relationships, perhaps understandably, is less often discussed. Verbal enquiry of the parent is an essential and major means of informing the diagnostic process and case management at almost every level in child health. The ability of health care professionals to be of assistance to patients, indeed their ability to do their jobs, would suffer a major compromise if they were unable to rely on history taking. A particularly potent example of this is epilepsy, which remains a clinical diagnosis based largely on history. There are many others.

Skill in medical history taking rests on a style of enquiry that becomes increasingly specific as it attempts to define facts more precisely. Whilst the process is aimed at clarifying and defining, and allows for patients' and parents' subjectivity, it can easily be allowed to rest on the assumption that patients and parents tell the truth or their perception of the truth. If health care staff start from this premise, then it is hardly surprising that they are shocked when they find that they have been duped.

There is, however, a different angle that is at once more dispassionate and less judgemental of parents: that parents tell health care staff what they want them to believe. This may be how things appeared to them, or what they believe, or for some, purely what they want staff to believe. After all, most human communication involves one person informing another of what they think or believe, or of trying to persuade the other round to their own point of view, or of persuading the other person to do as they wish.

There seems to be little reason to doubt that the vast majority of parents want to, and do, assist health care professionals in doing their job of diagnosing and treating the child's ailments. However, any but the least experienced of clinical staff will have encountered occasions of apparent substantial subjectivity or even bias put on histories because of the parent's anxiety, or depression, or desperation to receive state benefit. These cases are, for the most part, readily understandable to us, and so do not shock. Meadow (1985) has described exaggeration and mild deception by parents as being 'part of everyday behaviour'. Conversely, the deliberate, covert induction of symptoms in a child by a parent to serve the parent's own needs, such as occurs in MSBP abuse, can be shocking unless one is aware of such capability (see the vignette below and that on p. 312). The greater the risk posed to the child's life by the perpetrator's activities and the later the suspicions of a fabrication are aroused, the greater the shock is likely to be.

> The health visitor had not suspected that Carol's symptoms might be facti-
> tious until she was contacted by the hospital staff who raised the possibility
> that the father was inducing the illness. Her first reaction was to think that
> there must have been a mistake. She could not contemplate a parent doing
> such a thing, and she sought alternative explanations in her mind, hoping
> that the salt in the feed might have been an accident.

However, difficulty in believing is unlikely to be simply a basic problem of believing that a parent could harm their child in such a manner, or of ignorance. Rather, it could be that the ways in which the parents appear so credible, so dependent on ward staff, so solicitous of their child and, perhaps, so personable, are factors that may make staff particularly reluctant to suspect abuse. The same factors will also increase their shock when evidence is before them (see the next two vignettes). Blake (1990) describes the disbelief experienced by nurses in a case in which the family of the victim had made 'a good relationship' on the ward. The present authors have come across cases in which ward staff have continued to disbelieve despite clear, objective evidence. Such denial may be manifest in continued searching for an alternative explanation, such as that the laboratory must have made a series of mistakes, or that the administration of unprescribed medication was accidental. Alternatively, an individual's disbelief may put them at odds with the majority of the team, and friction may be explicit. It is important that this is recognized and sensitively addressed, not only for the sake of the individuals and the functioning of the team, but also for the effective management of the case.

> Lois's mother was in a wheelchair and was said to have rheumatoid arthritis.
> She appeared sociable and settled whilst in hospital. She got on to first name
> terms with the nurses, and was 'in and out of the kitchen'. One of the nurses
> described her as 'oozing contentment and fulfilment'. She 'talked non-stop
> about Lois and her life and of how only she could care for her'.
>
> After incontrovertible evidence of the mother suffocating Lois was
> recorded during covert video surveillance, the nurses were shocked and
> could not believe it. They had felt sorry for Lois's mother because of her inva-
> lidity. However, these nurses did not recall feeling guilty that it had taken so
> long for their suspicions to be aroused (her child had been admitted about
> five times over six to eight months). They saw this as having been due to the
> mother's plausibility and deception.

> Initially Anne's mother came across to nursing staff as 'an attractive, socia-
> ble person who got on well with the staff'. She was thought to be typical of
> the mother of a handicapped child, in that she appeared knowledgeable
> about Anne's needs and anticipated aspects of treatment. Anne's mother
> became very friendly with staff and even joined them on their Christmas night
> out (by this time she had spent several weeks on the ward). Eventually, the
> nurses noticed that she began to dress like them, wearing similar trousers
> and a hospital sweatshirt. At times she seemed somewhat demanding but,
> on the whole, the staff thought they had a good relationship with her, and she
> was well liked.

Szajnberg *et al.* (1996) describe a reaction in clinicians interviewing known perpetrators of MSBP abuse characterized by 'an uncanny, ego-dystonic and cognitively dissonant sense that the parent could not be the perpetrator, despite all clinical/forensic evidence'. The authors relate this to character pathology in the parent. That is to say, they suggest that the abusing parent may have developed a style of interaction with health professionals that may be particularly seductive and persuasive, and evokes empathy. Such characteristics, which are a function of the abuser's personality, will make it particularly difficult for the professional to accept that the person before him or her has, in fact, abused the child, even in the face of the most powerful objective evidence.

When discussing how to improve health professionals' ability to recognize MSBP abuse presentations, Horwath and Lawson (1995) suggest looking for a 'credibility gap', that is, any incongruity between what we are told and what we observe (see also the discussion in Chapters 2 and 3). This appears to be a useful concept. It may also be useful in minimizing the shock experienced by professionals when MSBP abuse is eventually recognized.

Nursing staff to whom the authors talked described having felt uneasy and sometimes even guilty when they first came to realize that they were developing suspicions that the parent might be inducing the child's illness (see the following two vignettes).

> Several of the nurses individually came to realize that they each had some
> doubts about Anne's mother, caused, for example, by how she had become
> so 'hospitalized' and the way in which she kept saying she would be back
> each time Anne was discharged home. Their suspicions at this stage made
> them feel uneasy, because they had always seen her as a caring person.
>
> One of the nurses said that, at first, it was 'very confusing, and very frus-
> trating' and caused 'some personal conflict'. The evidence appeared to be
> conflicting, and this nurse still felt that the mother was in need (even if she
> turned out to be a perpetrator of abuse).

One nurse had come to be suspicious of Carol's father because of his apparent familiarity with medical expressions and she felt that he exaggerated his care of Carol.

The nurses interviewed described having felt relieved when the abuse had been confirmed and Carol's safety secured. They had felt some guilt early on, when they had begun to feel a mistrust and dislike of her father because, at that stage, they wondered if they were misjudging him.

Effects on the care of other children

It might be thought that the breach of trust in parents that has been discussed above in cases of fabrication may lead staff to become overly suspicious. Whelan-Williams and Baker (1997) note this as a possibility when staff are ignorant of MSBP abuse, have little understanding of family dynamic issues or are left with intense, unresolved emotions that have been aroused by a case. Errors could be serious in either direction. On the one hand, failure to recognize MSBP abuse allows continued abuse or even the death of the child. On the other hand, wrongful suspicion might have its dangers if acted upon prematurely. Certainly the parents' trust in clinical staff may be damaged, but unnecessary separation of a child and parent should be unlikely without there being sufficient evidence to convince the social services department that there is a reasonable and serious child protection case. The essential need for sufficient evidence in these cases is covered elsewhere in this book.

In fact, nursing staff interviewed about their involvement with cases of MSBP abuse have not identified difficulties in trusting other parents as actually becoming an enduring problem. Transient 'over-suspiciousness' was identified by one nurse after reading The Allitt Inquiry. However, there have been situations in which changes of policy and procedures were implemented after individual cases. For example, after a case in which a parent had put salt in the child's feeds, it was made ward policy that parents would not be allowed to make up infant feeds. This apparent attempt to avoid a repetition of the exact circumstances of the case appears understandable, but it is difficult to see how it would realistically prevent further cases of MSBP abuse, help earlier detection or protect children. If the parent in that case had not been making up the feeds in hospital, then one would expect that the child would still have been abused. An alternative means would have been found.

Emotional reactions

Far more notable than concerns that their ability to form appropriately trusting working relationships with parents might have been compromised, was the fact that nursing staff often described experiencing intense shock and anger at having been deceived (see the vignette on p. 312 and that below), and guilt for having been taken in by the deceiving parent (see the next but one vignette).

'It's incomprehensible that a parent could do such a thing as poison their child.'
'No-one wants to bite the bullet – it's so horrendous.'
'You don't want to think negative thoughts – it's as though we need permission to express fears or thoughts.'
'Despite twenty years as a health visitor, I was hoodwinked.'
When recollecting her shock at having realised a parent had induced symptoms in a child, one health visitor suggested that it might be particularly hard for nurses to suspect parents might do this because it is a prerequisite of the work 'to be able to see the good in people' so that one does not give up on parents who are difficult to engage.

The nurse described having felt both guilt and anger when she realized that this was a case of induced illness. She described other ward staff as having felt similar emotions. She felt the shock had been heightened because they had viewed Sammy's mother particularly sympathetically as a bereaved parent (an older child had died some eighteen months previously). The guilt was attributed to a belief that they had missed the diagnosis and had been taken in by the deception. Staff came to wonder if the older child had also been a victim.

In community settings, shock can be great because contact with the abusing parent may have endured over very long periods before the abuse was recognized. Health visitors may have seen the parents to be competent in other respects and with other children.

One of the prime roles of health visitors is the early detection of deviations from normal development. Hence, health visitors, having been deceived by parents who have induced illness in their child, may see that they themselves were unwilling but instrumental agents in putting the child forward for medical investigations and into the hospital arena. Health visitors may feel that they are under a heavy burden of responsibility for surveillance in cases where suspicions have been raised but remain unresolved (see below).

Susan was a few months old when she started to present with respiratory difficulties. A previous baby had suffered a presumed 'cot death'. The health visitor had not had suspicions of anything untoward in relation to the first baby, but with this one, 'things just didn't add up'. Susan seemed to become ill unusually quickly. On one occasion, a junior doctor thought there was evidence of petechial bruising around Susan's neck, but the consultant did not think there was sufficient evidence to warrant action and Susan was sent home. The health visitor felt extremely concerned for Susan's safety from this point on. It was a time of immense anxiety for the health visitor who felt she was being given responsibility for supervising the baby without adequate support.

Few of the nurses spoken to had had such intense emotional reactions to involvement in a case that they needed time off work. The emotions evoked were often intense and memorable to them, but there is no evidence to suggest that their professional functioning was impaired in serious ways. The price was personal distress and, sometimes, less than optimal team working. One senior nurse, for instance, still felt that she had 'let the team down' because of feeling confused by the case. Normally being very sure of herself, she had come to feel 'inadequate' and 'a loss of control'. Another described having felt 'in a turmoil'. One nurse did have several weeks off work following her involvement in a case. She recollected having had a series of viral infections but, in retrospect, came to wonder if the stress of the case had been a contributory factor.

Nurses mentioned instances of responses from senior staff and management that they perceived as having been supportive (see the next vignette). However, there were also comments such as 'management hasn't the same time to listen' (i.e. compared with colleagues).

Despite not having met such circumstances in the interviews undertaken here, it is recognized that, for psychologically vulnerable staff who are unsupported, there is the potential for more severe psychological consequences (the precipitation of intense adjustment reactions or depressive episodes, for example).

The chief nurse of the hospital saw the staff and offered them the opportunity for any counselling and support they felt they needed, and impressed upon them that expressing such a need was not to be regarded as a sign of weakness. In fact, none of the staff did seek external support, but they valued its having been available, and perceived the senior nurse's response to have been very supportive in itself.

Concerns about the legal position

Staff may also worry about the legal position in the interim between the acknowledgement of suspicions by the team and the confirmation of fabrication by the parent. Likely concerns include responsibility if further harm is done to the child whilst he or she remains on the ward (see the vignette below and that on p. 306), and having to deceive parents whilst investigation remains covert. These issues are discussed further in Chapters 4 and 5.

Eventually it was decided to refer Lois to another hospital for covert video surveillance. During the period of waiting for this transfer, Lois was 'specialled' (1:1 nurse:patient ratio). It was explained to the mother that a very careful eye had to be kept on Lois. The nurses described the period of 'specialling' as having been quite stressful. They were still feeling shock at the suspicions, and could not quite believe that the apnoeic attacks were being induced by the mother. 'Specialling' Lois had been very different from 'specialling' a physically sick child, as there was nothing for the nurses to do except observe, and, because the mother was always there, they felt awkward. The nurses felt that the 'specialling' 'added an extra pressure and tension on the ward'. One of them described a 'sense of fear for the child'. They recalled considerable anxiety about whether they would be criticized or even held responsible if Lois were endangered during this period (i.e. despite their observation).

Another source of tension they identified was the importance of care about what they said and about what they wrote in the bedside care plans. It was difficult to appear natural with the mother whilst they were suspicious of her.

Problems of concealment

Several nurses described their discomfort at being less than frank with parents (see the vignette above and the two following). They talked about the evidence gathering in such cases as challenging the principle of working in partnership with parents – a principle that is so emphasized in contemporary nurse training. Facey (1993) describes ward staff feeling anxious about having to deceive parents for just these reasons. It is the nursing staff, and to a lesser extent perhaps, junior doctors, who are most likely to be affected by this, again because of their continual contact with the parents.

One nurse recalled having felt unhappy that things were intentionally being kept back from Anne's mother. Having to continue to relate to her despite the doubts and whilst being privy to the fact that the team was continuing to collect evidence was stressful for the ward staff. During the period of covert observation, the nurses continued to feel uncomfortable. They only left Anne's mother unsupervised when the father was present. This appeared to be particularly hard for the younger qualified nurses who wanted to believe the mother. The nurses kept separate notes in the office and this enhanced their feeling that they were being 'underhand'. One nurse described how awkward it had felt when, during the period of covert observation, the nursing staff had had to take over simple tasks that had previously been left to the mother.

Other ethical issues

Interestingly, all of the children's nurses spoken to said that they saw a place for covert video surveillance in some cases, although it had been employed in only two of the cases here, and in only one was it implemented in the same hospital.

All the nurses clearly placed concerns for the child's safety above all else (see the next vignette).

There is an ongoing debate within the nursing profession concerning the ethics of covert video surveillance. It appears here that those who are actually involved in the nursing of child victims of MSBP abuse or have working involvement of child protection are rarely, if ever, among its outspoken critics. Issues pertaining to covert video surveillance are dealt with elsewhere in this book (see Chapter 4).

> The nursing staff knew that they had to continue to treat the mother professionally even after their suspicions had been aroused, but this was stressful especially in the interim before the covert video surveillance began. The nurses described having felt 'in a turmoil whilst struggling not to show it'. Covert video surveillance was then instituted. Jenny was taken for a scan whilst it was set up. This was particularly difficult for the nurses because of the frank deception they were having to act out.
>
> Nevertheless, the nurses welcomed the use of CVS, because it was expected to be a means of ending the abuse and, ultimately, of protecting the child. The time between the suspicions being realized and the CVS being implemented was remembered as an extremely anxious period for the staff, when there was real concern that Jenny might be injured, or even killed, on the ward.

Contact after the confrontation

After the invocation of child protection procedures, but whilst the child remains on the ward, another period of potential disquiet for nursing staff may ensue. Circumstances here vary very much from case to case, but parents may, for example, be arrested on the ward, or return to the ward unexpectedly and vent some of their emotions on unprepared staff (see the next vignette).

> Seeing Jenny's mother handcuffed upset the staff. They felt that she needed help, but was being treated like a criminal. Later, they learned about the difficulty in treating perpetrators of MSBP abuse.
>
> After being charged by the police, Sammy's mother returned to the ward and was abusive to the nurse. The nurse remembered feeling sorry for the mother at this time.
>
> After the introduction of the foster parents, the nurses had to teach them how to look after Anne (who had cerebral palsy). Anne's mother still had supervised contact with Anne, and she appeared to 'hate' the foster mother. This created another tension for the nursing staff, because they had to develop a relationship with the foster mother whilst maintaining relations with the natural mother. Anne had a birthday during this period. One of the nurses described this as 'an extremely traumatic day'. None of the nurses could bear to watch as the sister accompanied the tearful mother into the cubicle to see her child.

For health visitors, these issues may be particularly difficult. Health visitors may have to continue working with the family in the aftermath of child care proceedings. When the abused child has been removed, the siblings who remain with the parents may continue on the health visitor's case load (see the following vignette).

> The health visitor had supported Susan's mother at the time of the first child's death, and had seen her as a bereaved parent in tragic circumstances. As suspicions about Susan's welfare developed, the health visitor came to suspect that the first child may have been killed by the mother. The health visitor came to feel guilt about this child's death, although she could be reassured by her colleagues that she had not been responsible. The health visitor had to give Susan's MMR immunization in the mother's presence after care proceedings had been instituted, but the mother would not speak to her.

The most powerful emotion evoked by the case for this health visitor appeared to be anger – both towards the doctors for, in her eyes, not having acted decisively early on, and at the hospital staff for not having shared information with her.

Clinical supervision

An important means of assisting staff in dealing with the emotional issues is good clinical supervision and/or mentoring. Clearly the supervisor or mentor needs to be sensitive to and aware of the likely issues. He or she should be able to tell when an individual's reaction is extreme (and impairs functioning), and should be able to point the person being mentored in the direction of more specialist help if necessary. Clinical supervision has been on the nursing agenda since 1993, but has attracted much greater attention since publication of The Allitt Inquiry (1994). Faugier and Butterworth (1994), in a position paper about clinical supervision in nursing (commissioned by the Department of Health), describe three functions of clinical supervision: formative, restorative and normative. The formative function is defined as the development of the skills, understanding and abilities of the supervisee. The normative function is the assurance of the highest professional standards. The restorative function is specifically defined as the support needed by nurses because of the stressful environment in which they work.

At the time of writing, clinical supervision is not implemented to anything like the degree that Butterworth and Faugier envisage, and it seems that this is a national problem. Good intentions are insufficient in this matter. There are serious resource issues to be addressed. Good supervision entails time and the training and commitment of supervisors.

These issues are just as relevant to medical staff. The requirements for the establishment of the Specialist Registrar grade emphasize the training needs of junior doctors. Mentoring systems are being more widely introduced, and there is an expectation that junior doctors will be given names and contact points for 'those who will be responsible for providing guidance and counselling...' (Department of Health, 1998). Whilst these are welcome developments, it appears to remain variable as to whether consultant trainers can, and do, provide their juniors with opportunities to discuss aspects of difficult consultations or complex cases other than the strictly technical or intellectual. These are surely important issues for good clinical supervision, and are of particular concern in cases of factitious illness, both to assist the juniors in recognizing and dealing with their own reactions, and to facilitate learning about case and team management.

In health visiting systems, peer group support appears to be particularly and systematically utilized. In such systems there is often a regular forum in which health visitors can voice their suspicions at an early stage for discussion with their colleagues. The authors are aware of one community child health nursing service that appears to be rather in advance of some hospitals in both its implementation of clinical supervision generally and in child protection in particular. In this service, a senior nurse appointed to work in child protection routinely arranges 'debriefing' sessions for community nurses in the aftermath of all child protection cases, including MSBP abuse.

On the other hand, health visitors are usually lone operators in their actual direct contact with families. Although there may be useful peer support, colleagues will not usually be having direct contact with the same child or parents contemporaneously. Hence there is no opportunity for checking out one's reactions and experiences of the family by direct comparison with those of a colleague. On wards, although one nurse may have greater contact with a family, several others will also have direct contact for comparison. It is therefore suggested that, in difficult, complex cases such as those where factitious illness may be an issue, the principle of joint or paired working by health visitors may be useful.

Issues for teams

The effects on teams cannot be wholly separated from the effects on their individual members. However, some important issues warrant consideration under this heading.

Splitting

One issue frequently described here has been the splitting of clinical teams (see the vignettes on pp. 309–11). In the lead up to confirmation of fabrication of illness, this was sometimes irrespective of discipline, resulting in two camps: those who thought the suspicions ill-founded and those who thought they were correct. Such splits may be emotionally charged, with staff either championing or condemning the parent. Splits may also occur between nurses and doctors (see the vignette on p. 311), usually when the nurses, with so much greater opportunity for contact with the parent and for observation (and therefore for detecting a 'credibility gap'), voice suspicions that are initially dismissed by the doctors (see the next vignette).

> In the earlier admissions, the nursing staff had had no qualms about the genuineness of the situation. At the third admission, however, one of the nurses felt 'uneasy': 'Things just didn't seem right'. Carol's father stayed on the ward as the mother stayed at home to look after their other three children. The father began to tell the nurse about his own health problems in a way that she felt was inappropriate and hypochondriacal. She recalled expressing her concerns to the consultant who was, at first, frankly dismissive, saying, 'Oh, you nurses!'.

Personal distress and strains on teamwork may also arise during the period after suspicions are acknowledged but before sufficient evidence has been collected. As mentioned above, nursing staff may rightly feel that the burden of the deceit is put on them. Here it would appear that good communication between staff is of paramount importance, it being necessary to have clear management plans and discussion of how parents are to be approached, and how and by whom parents' queries are to be answered. For example, it may be prudent to agree that certain types of questions posed by the parents will be deferred to one or two key staff. These cases, perhaps more than any others, cry out for a multi-disciplinary care plan approach, i.e. a single, clear management plan subscribed to by all the disciplines. The opportunity for discussion of the reasoning behind such management plans is also important. Particular support for staff may be warranted in dealing with the conflicts aroused when acting in the best interests of the child means that parents have to be deceived.

However, there are occasions in the management of such cases on wards when, according to level of suspicion and severity of risk, it is important that only members of a small core team, and not all staff, are privy to all the information. That is to say that effective communication and case management may be enhanced by the involvement of fewer staff rather than more. Such issues must be addressed in the management plan, and the senior staff need to impress upon the core team the importance of the containment of the information. The core team should be afforded opportunities to discuss the difficulties of having to be less than frank with one's junior colleagues who are outside of the core (see the next vignette). In such circumstances, where junior staff have been purposefully excluded from the core team, it may be particularly important that there is a multi-disciplinary meeting for all staff in the wake of the case.

Although, as mentioned above, the nursing staff are more likely than others to have contact with the abusing parent after the 'confrontation', the consultant is likely to be the one to bear the brunt of responsibility for and to take the lead in the 'confrontation'. He or she may be exposed to remonstrations and counter-accusations by the parents that intensify the already substantial difficulties of such an interview.

> One of the nurses described a period of 'low morale' on the ward when there was felt to be a lot of conflict between various individuals and groups. The nurses felt 'caught between the parents and the other professionals'. There seemed to be a lot of 'unpleasantness' between Anne's parents, the doctors and the other professionals. The senior nurses had to withhold certain information from junior staff, and this brought further tensions. One of the nurses still experienced some doubt as to the mother's guilt. Another said that she felt it was important to accept that it was normal to feel confused and unsure in such cases, and would encourage her junior staff 'not to fight such feelings' in future cases. These nurses recalled that another nurse had appeared particularly unhappy and had argued with the others, acting as an advocate of the mother.

It seems possible that, particularly in cases where suspicions are slowly raised over a protracted period, there is potential for splitting (see the next vignette) or for the development of ill-feeling between hospital and community staff (see the next but one vignette). Cases of MSBP abuse are not common in hospital paediatric settings, but staff in an average general practice are likely to encounter frank MSBP abuse even more rarely. It is suggested that, where health care staff in community settings have had any substantial involvement in a case where the evidence of abuse is found in hospital, then particular efforts should be made to ensure good communication. This would include appraising the community staff of the reasons for suspicion and the management rationale at an appropriate time. Time given to direct discussion between ward and community nursing staff, and between hospital paediatrician and the general practitioner is likely to be time well spent. Community staff may have highly relevant information that would aid the hospital team's management and vice versa. It is important to be aware, of course, that community teams may be the first to recognize evidence of MSBP abuse.

> On one occasion, Anne came in at the request of the district nurse. She was drowsy for no apparent reason, and urine was sent for toxicology. This showed evidence of an anticonvulsant that had not been prescribed for some time. A strategy meeting was called without the knowledge of the parents. Social services, police, community nurses and special school staff attended, and new information came to light. For example, it was disclosed that the mother had factitious illness. The family's GP declined to attend the case conference, and was reported to be in support of the parents and did not wish to be party to the proceedings.

> When Susan was admitted to another hospital with a further episode, suspicions of MSBP abuse were raised, and a professionals' meeting was called. The health visitor felt 'on trial' at this meeting. Staff from the first hospital revealed information about the illness and death of the first child, suggesting that there had been suspicions about that child's symptoms at the time. The health visitor felt very strongly that she should have been given this information previously. Being privy to only pieces of information and not the whole picture both increased anxiety and prevented effective action.

Community staff are also excellently placed to gather information over time in the less dramatic, less acute cases. Indeed, as described elsewhere in this book (see Chapters 7 and 9), cases in the 'hinterland' of MSBP abuse may not come to in-patient wards, and may be wholly managed in the community. Some health visitors keep a 'concern register' where issues and events about particular cases can be logged and systematically reviewed so that, over time, a composite view, that may tend to support or refute suspicions, is built. This system appears to assist the confidence of staff, whilst also serving the functions of communication and documentation.

There is also the potential for splits between agencies, as illustrated in the next vignette.

> The nurses described a major tension between themselves and the social workers (who were not hospital based). It seemed to the nurses that the social workers resented the good relationship that the nurses had with Anne's mother. The nurses were disappointed that the social workers did not share the responsibility for the surveillance.

The importance of communication

Communication is probably the most powerful means of minimizing the potential for, and the effects of, splitting. In the interviews here, staff frequently emphasized the value of communication within the clinical team. They mentioned how crucial they believe it is, both in terms of actual clinical management of cases of MSBP abuse and in helping staff reactions. Furthermore, they mentioned it irrespective of whether they felt that the communication within their own team at the time of their involvement with the cases had been adequate. Some hospital wards do not always appear to have opportunity for multi-disciplinary discussion (see the following vignette). Indeed, there are clinical teams in which discussion, or questioning, of the doctor's diagnosis is regarded as heresy or revolt rather than welcome professional stimulation, enhancement of patient care and informal audit. Some senior nurses also too readily feel challenged by questioning juniors.

> Initially the nurses were not told the differential diagnosis. They were told to treat John as a normal boy, and to offer a normal diet. There were no clear or specific instructions, and no defined care plan for the nurses to follow. On ward rounds, the junior doctors bypassed the cubicle. The senior doctors went in to talk with the mother about twice a week. The nurses were not invited to join in these consultations, and got little, if any, feedback about them. The nurses recalled that they were 'just told to carry on', and that they felt patronized by one doctor who told them that they were doing 'a good job'. There was a sense of anger at the doctors for what was felt to be markedly inadequate communication over the course of a very lengthy admission.

On the other hand, some children's wards have excellent models of ward rounds and regular meetings away from the bedside wherein these issues can be discussed. Such wards have a culture and ethos that encourage reflection by staff and have a high awareness of relevant issues. When MSBP abuse cases occur (usually on wards that deal with particularly chronic and complex medical conditions), regular psychosocial meetings can provide a useful forum for support, reflection and planning. On one ward, the nursing staff interviewed had a useful model which they found of assistance in a case of MSBP abuse. They met after the child had been discharged in the way that they would normally meet to talk about the death of a child.

> The nurses came to argue amongst themselves, and splits appeared in the team. There were two camps: those who felt so unsure about what was going on that there was no alternative other than that they be guided by the doctors; and those who felt so strongly that John was being avoidably harmed that they should tell the doctors that the nurses were no longer prepared to continue in this way.

If there is no regular forum already in place, once suspicions are acknowledged, it may be essential that one is created. The benefits and necessity of good communication in such cases extend far beyond the pastoral care of the staff group and the optimal functioning of the team in interpersonal terms. Child and adolescent psychiatrists experienced and skilled in paediatric liaison may be appropriately approached to be of assistance. Indeed, Herzog (Sugar *et al.*, 1991) describes a role for child psychiatrists in facilitating communication amongst the clinical team: 'The child and adolescent psychiatrist often provides the glue that keeps the medical/nursing team working together in such a case'. He suggests that the psychiatrist may have a role in assisting the team to manage feelings that can adversely affect care.

It is essential that suspicions are dealt with judiciously within teams. Suspicion is not assumption of guilt. The proper consequences of suspicion are the gathering and consideration of evidence that may tend either to refute or further the suspicion. Sustaining the team's collective objectivity and professionalism is essential, not only to ensure that actions taken are appropriate and necessary, but also to enhance team functioning when there is a danger of splitting. It is incumbent on senior staff, of whatever discipline, to be instrumental in shaping team attitudes and ethos. An objective, professional attitude towards the evaluation of evidence and management planning is by no means incompatible with a team ethos that allows discussion of conflicts and emotions.

Information, education and training

Chan *et al*. (1986) suggest that hospital staff should be helped to understand the dynamics of families where MSBP abuse has taken place, and be educated about the likely responses of parents once confronted. The rationale behind these suggestions is that such steps are expected to assist staff in dealing with the conflicts commonly aroused by such cases.

Meadow (1985) views giving ward staff reprints of articles about MSBP abuse as useful. The nurses interviewed here all stated that they considered that they had had too little training about MSBP abuse. Some had had none. They shared the view that not only case management, but also individual coping and team functioning would have been helped by their having had greater knowledge (see the following vignette).

It is, of course, a truism that ignorance of a possibility is likely to increase the risk of shock when that possibility is realized.

> None of the nurses had received any formal training about MSBP abuse. Some had been aware of such cases from articles and from other cases. The sister said that more knowledge would have helped her to assist junior staff in understanding such cases and their management.
>
> Whilst Anne remained on the ward, it was arranged that a child psychiatrist would speak with the nurses. They recalled this as having been very informative: 'It brought us up short when the psychiatrist said that some parents in such situations go on to kill their children'.

On one hospital ward, the nurses had taken their own actions in an attempt to ensure that staff would not again feel so handicapped by lack of knowledge (see following page).

In the wake of one case, information about the MSBP abuse had been included in ward manuals and in the child protection guidance. All new nursing staff were expected to read the information, but it was also ready at hand so that staff could refamiliarize themselves with the issues if new cases presented.

The high profile of the Allitt case and inquiry may have gone some way towards encouraging nursing and paediatric medical staff to educate themselves. MSBP abuse is now mentioned in nurse training within modules about child abuse, but it often seems to be included in rather wide-ranging lectures, rather than having at least a whole lecture or seminar dedicated to it. It remains the case that paediatric nurses could complete their training with scant specific and formal education about MSBP abuse. The present authors are firmly of the view that this should be redressed. Furthermore, in both medical and nursing staff education about MSBP abuse, the common psychological reactions of individuals and teams should be included. This would raise awareness of and encourage a pre-paredness in staff for the reactions that they are likely to experience themselves or see in others.

Summary

In summary, from the discussions with nursing staff who have experience of dealing with MSBP abuse, the following were identified as the sorts of provisions that they found were, or that they would expect to be, of assistance in dealing with the powerful emotional and team dynamic issues aroused by MSBP abuse:

- Support from senior staff (nursing and consultants).
- Information about MSBP abuse in training (student or continuing education) and on the ward.
- Clinical supervision (which should allow staff to discuss and reflect on emotional or interpersonal issues raised by cases).
- Clear management plans.
- Multi-disciplinary ward/team meetings.

These suggestions have been expanded and added to, and divided into proactive and reactive measures, and are set out earlier in the chapter in Tables 14.1 and 14.2, respectively.

References

Blake, P. (1990) Munchausen syndrome by proxy. *Paediatric Nursing*, **2** (2), 17–18.

Blix, S. and Brack, G. (1988) The effects of a suspected case of Munchausen's syndrome by proxy on a pediatric nursing staff. *General Hospital Psychiatry*, **10**, 402–409.

Chan, D.A., Salcedo, J.R., Atkins, D.M. and Ruley, E.J. (1986) Munchausen syndrome by proxy: a review and case study. *Journal of Pediatric Psychology*, **11** (1), 71–80.

Department of Health (1998) A Guide to Specialist Registrar Training. NHS Executive.

Facey, S. (1993) Munchausen syndrome by proxy. *Nursing Times*, **89**, 54–56.

Faugier, J. and Butterworth, T. (1994) Clinical supervision: a position paper. Manchester University School of Nursing Studies.

Horwath, J. and Lawson, B. (1995) Conclusion: affirming, challenging, linking and developing practice. In *Trust Betrayed? Munchausen Syndrome by Proxy, Inter-agency Child Protection and Partnership with Families* (Horwath, J. and Lawson, B., eds), pp. 210–218. National Children's Bureau.

Meadow, R. (1985) Management of Munchausen syndrome by proxy. *Archives of disease in Childhood*, **60**, 385–393.

Sugar, J., Belfer, M., Israel, E. and Herzog, D. (1991) A 3-year-old boy's chronic diarrhea and unexplained death. *Journal of the American Academy of Child and Adolescent Psychiatry*, **30** , 1015–1021.

Szajnberg, N.M., Moilanen, I., Kanerva, A. and Tolf, B. (1996) Munchausen by proxy syndrome: countertransference as a diagnostic tool. *Bulletin of the Menninger Clinic*, **60**, 229–237.

The Allitt Inquiry (1994) Independent inquiry relating to deaths and injuries on the children's ward at Grantham and Kesteven General Hospital during the period February to April 1991. HMSO.

Whelan-Williams, S. and Baker, T.D. (1997) A multidisciplinary hospital response protocol. In *Munchausen by Proxy Syndrome: Misunderstood Child Abuse* (Parnell, T.F. and Day, D.O., eds), pp. 253–264. Sage.

Index